Pediatric School Psychology

Series Editor:

Paul McCabe
Brooklyn College
School of Education
Brooklyn, NY, USA

The Pediatric School Psychology series presents evidence-based research and practices for prevention, intervention, and treatment of pediatric health issues in school settings. As school psychologists and other educational professionals apply their skills to promote the social and academic success of all students, the information presented in each book in the series facilitates their efforts to understand various health and mental health disorders and target educational delivery to maximize success. Each volume in the series provides analysis by leading experts, who evaluate, synthesize and summarize key research findings and school-related considerations on a specific pediatric disorder. Volume authors critically assess the quality and scholarly design of the extant literature and provide readers with a comprehensive, in depth review of the topic. The information presented in each volume helps scholars and practitioners make informed decisions about identification, evaluation, and treatment of the pediatric health or mental health issue. The overarching goal of the series is to inform and facilitate efforts to enhance the health, mental health, and educational development of students.

More information about this series at http://www.springer.com/series/13561

Steven R. Shaw • Anna M. Jankowska

Pediatric Intellectual Disabilities at School

Translating Research into Practice

Springer

Steven R. Shaw
McGill University
Montreal, QC, Canada

Anna M. Jankowska
University of Gdańsk
Gdańsk, Poland

ISSN 2524-8278 ISSN 2524-8286 (electronic)
Pediatric School Psychology
ISBN 978-3-030-02990-6 ISBN 978-3-030-02992-0 (eBook)
https://doi.org/10.1007/978-3-030-02992-0

Library of Congress Control Number: 2018961746

This Springer imprint is published by the registered company Springer Nature Switzerland AG
The registered company address is: Gewerbestrasse 11, 6330 Cham, Switzerland

Preface

Both authors of this volume have extensive clinical experience providing educational, social, and mental health services to a diverse population of children and their families. Even though our training and clinical experiences took place in different parts of the world with differing cultures, systems, beliefs, and languages (Poland and Spain for AMJ, the southern United States, French and English-speaking Canada for SRS), we saw similar challenges of meeting all the needs of children with intellectual developmental disabilities and how quickly professionals were to dismiss these children as having low potential for success. As we moved from careers as clinicians to researchers, we saw three major areas of challenges.

Professionals researching developmental disabilities focus much of their attention on autism spectrum disorder (ASD) and minimize research on intellectual developmental disabilities. The frequently heard arguments were that research on ASD is dynamic and exciting whereas research on intellectual development has stagnated and advanced little over the last 20 years.

Another frequent refrain is that research in intellectual developmental disabilities has advanced in fields of genetics and neuroscience, but there is no change in implementing these ideas or applying advanced research to classrooms or therapy.

The third concern is that much work on intellectual developmental disabilities has focused on advocacy, disability rights, and legal reform. As such, advances in scholarship may be specific to a nation, legal system, or culture. An international perspective in improving the details of educational and mental health service delivery to persons with intellectual developmental disabilities is lacking.

As we began collaborating and focusing on children with low general mental ability, it became clear that a volume was required that identified the wide breadth and depth of new research focusing on intellectual developmental disabilities. Far from being stagnant, the field is dynamic and has provided multiple advances in areas ranging from genetics and neuroscience to family and community supports. We also identified the need for a volume that focuses on how this information can be directly applied to ideas for implementing research for teachers, therapists, policymakers, parents, pediatricians, and other professionals and stakeholders in the lives and development of persons with intellectual developmental disabilities.

Finally, we wanted to integrate our international perspectives and review the best and most recent scholarship from around the world and summarize this information in a single volume.

This volume addresses several issues for school psychologists, educators, therapists, and researchers that require a new book-length treatment on the topic of providing rehabilitative and educational services to children with intellectual developmental disabilities. There are many children in school systems with idiopathic severe to profound intellectual disabilities or autism who are sometimes considered to be untestable, unteachable, and unknowable. This volume describes and addresses the following issues:

- There have been many advances in genetic and medical research with direct implications for children with intellectual disabilities. Yet, most of these findings appear in medical and genetic journals that are not immediately accessible to most school psychologists and educators. Moreover, the application of the findings to the provision of advanced educational and mental health services in a school setting is not clear. This book reviews the latest advances in the detection, understanding, and medical treatments for children with intellectual disabilities and transfers this knowledge to an audience of educators and school psychologists in a clear and applied manner.
- In addition to advances in genetics and medicine, there have also been major advances made in the psychology, education, and technology for assessment, education, therapies, implementation of innovation, evidence-based interventions, and medical management of children with low incidence developmental disabilities. These advances require translation of research to practice.
- The role of mental health for children with intellectual developmental disabilities has received more attention and research over the last 5 years than before. Rather than simply considered a behavior management issue, there is significantly new thinking about the understanding of assessment and treatment of emotional and behavioral therapies for people with intellectual disabilities.
- There are new classification systems from the American Psychiatric Association, World Health Organization, and the American Association on Intellectual and Developmental Disabilities. These classification systems require integration and application to school settings. Ramifications of these changes for assessment, education, service delivery, and funding are discussed and suggestions made.
- In a dynamic area of research, such as intellectual disabilities, there is a host of new research and clinical questions, unresolved research areas, and more unknowns than ever. As an analogy: as the balloon of what is known expands due to new research findings, an ever-greater surface area of the balloon encounters the unknown. New and future research questions and methods to address future questions are discussed.
- As in other areas of clinical practice, the answer to providing quality research-to-practice school psychological, educational, and mental health services is via a team approach. Methods of developing and using multidisciplinary, interdisciplinary, and transdisciplinary teams for providing improved services to children with intellectual developmental disabilities are discussed.

There is often a false dichotomy set up in books, professional training, education, and clinical practice. This false dichotomy is the "practical versus research" problem. This false dichotomy results in psychologists and educators chasing unfounded ideas because they are practical and intuitive. Likewise, research is more likely to be developed to test a theoretically relevant hypothesis and ignore potential applications. The move toward evidence-based practice has resulted in meretricious ideas and interventions that are bolstered by carefully cherry-picked supportive scientific studies of questionable quality, all the while ignoring studies not supporting the idea or intervention of the moment. The Lewin quote "There is nothing so practical as good theory" has never been more relevant than for children with intellectual developmental disabilities. The purpose of this book is to mobilize theory and research in the service of evidence-based practice for this population and combat questionable and even dangerous practices. Only when research and its application inform each other will the quality of education and service delivery advance.

The purpose of this book is to integrate the interdisciplinary advances in the frontiers of research on intellectual developmental disabilities into a coherent and easy-to-read volume. We have prioritized the most important new research in medical, sociological, pedagogical, psychological, administrative, legal, biological, and genetic arenas for critical review. The goal is not simply to engage in knowledge transfer. The goal is to identify and describe exactly how teachers and researchers can integrate the wide range of new research and implement these findings into classrooms, therapeutic settings, and policy development arenas. We would like to erase the common, but false dichotomy between research and practice. Therefore, our primary audiences are teachers, psychologists, therapists, physicians, and other providers of services to children with intellectual developmental disabilities. Researchers may also benefit simply because we are providing a review of advances in science and identifying fertile ground for new research and weaknesses in the current research literature. Yet, the primary goal is to assist educators and other professionals to develop the most innovative and evidence-based approaches to providing services to children with intellectual disabilities based on new thinking, basic science, and published action research available.

Montreal, QC, Canada
Gdańsk, Poland

Steven R. Shaw
Anna M. Jankowska

Acknowledgments

We would like to acknowledge several people in the development and completion of this project. The graduate students and members of the Connections Lab at McGill University have been invaluable in providing direct support to this project and picking up the slack on our other research projects as I was away completing this volume.

Finally, many thanks to my family for their unfailing patience and support. Special thanks to Isabel for keeping me disciplined and focused.

S.R.S.

No project can be successful without the strong support of an editorial staff. Paul McCabe, Judy Jones, and Garth Haller have provided invaluable feedback to improve the focus and nature of this volume. Their kindness, rigor, timeliness, and professionalism have made this project an enjoyable one.

A.M.J.

Acknowledgments

Contents

About the Authors

Steven R. Shaw is associate professor in the Department of Educational and Counselling Psychology at McGill University in Montreal. He earned a Ph.D. in School Psychology from the University of Florida in 1991. At McGill University, he is director of the Resilience, Pediatric Psychology, and Neurogenetics Connections Lab and co-director of the McGill Developmental Research Lab. Before entering academia, he had 17 years of experience as a school psychologist in school, hospital, medical school, and independent practice. From 1997 to 2004, he served as lead psychologist and associate professor of pediatrics at the Children's Hospital in Greenville, South Carolina (developmental pediatrics and pediatric oncology units), and the Medical University of South Carolina. Dr. Shaw is a Nationally Certified School Psychologist. His current research work focuses on improving methods of implementation of innovative ideas and evidence-based practices in education, improving instruction for children with borderline intellectual functioning and intellectual disabilities, and improving education for children with acute and chronic medical problems. He has over 220 scholarly publications and presentations and has published four books. He co-edited (with Paul McCabe) the Pediatric School Psychology book series for NASP/Corwin Press (2010). He is co-editor (with Andrea Cantor and Leslie Paige) of the book *Helping Children in Home and School*, 3rd edition (NASP 2010). He is on the editorial board of six international scholarly journals, editor of the *Canadian Journal of School Psychology*, and is the former editor of *School Psychology Forum*.

Anna M. Jankowska is assistant professor in the Institute of Psychology at the University of Gdańsk and adjunct assistant professor at City University of New York Brooklyn College. She earned her Ph.D. in Developmental Psychology from the University of Gdask. Her doctoral thesis investigated cognitive and psychosocial development of children with borderline intellectual functioning, for which she received multiple awards. Her research interests are in the field of developmental and educational psychology, and she holds interests in education and school adaptation of students with developmental delays with special emphasis on the development of self-regulation. In parallel to her academic career, she has 10 years of clinical work experience with children with developmental and neurodevelopmental disabilities while practicing in numerous settings. In addition, she is also dedicated to therapeutic work with foster care families and children who experienced trauma and abuse. Her professional and academic experience has been international. Dr. Jankowska participated in exchange programs, international internships, served as a visiting scholar in foreign research centers, and has lectured at various universities, including those in Spain (University of Santiago de Compostela, University de Complutense de Madrid), Canada (McGill University), and the USA (Brooklyn College). She is a member of European Association of Developmental Psychology, Polish Psychologists' Association, and National Association of School Psychologists and serves on the editorial board of several international scholarly journals.

Chapter 1
Introduction and Overview

Abstract This chapter explores what is meant by intellectual developmental disabilities, intellectual disabilities, mental retardation, and similar terms. The primary focus is less on the terminology than on the complexity, diversity, and humanity of people with intellectual disabilities. Common characteristics of persons with intellectual disabilities are described, and the range of function is considered. The evolution of the science of intellectual disabilities and the contribution of disability studies in the application of science provide a context for further research. Also, detailed understanding of the different available definitions for intellectual disabilities is required to understand the details of research and how to apply new findings. Ultimately, the details of this socially defined construct affect the direction of the science of intellectual developmental disabilities and how the science is applied to classroom and clinical practice.

Case Study

Amanda was the third child of Mr. and Mrs. Schmidt. The pregnancy was challenging because of frequent nausea and dehydration throughout the pregnancy. Amanda was born at 39 weeks of gestation and delivery was unremarkable. Immediately after Amanda was taken home, her parents noticed that she was different from her older siblings. Amanda had low muscle tone, made few sounds, cried little, and was lethargic. The pediatrician noticed slightly dysmorphic facial features such as smooth philtrum (the groove between the upper lip and base of the nose), deep set eyes, and large ears. The primary care pediatrician referred Amanda and her family to a developmental pediatrician. The developmental pediatrician included a neurodevelopmental genetics team to have multiple professionals involved in the diagnostic process. The team included a clinical geneticist, developmental pediatrician, pediatric neurologist, psychologist, speech and language therapist, social worker, and occupational therapist. Multiple genetic disorders were considered. Based on chromosome microarray analysis, the diagnosis of 22q13.3 deletion syndrome (i.e. Phelan-McDermid syndrome) was made. This genetic syndrome is characterized by intellectual disabilities, lack of speech, and multiple

S. R. Shaw, A. M. Jankowska, *Pediatric Intellectual Disabilities at School*,
Pediatric School Psychology, https://doi.org/10.1007/978-3-030-02992-0_1

medical issues. Amanda was 13 months old at the time of her diagnosis. At this point, the parents began preparing emotionally for a lifetime of providing care. Mr. and Mrs. Schmidt had many questions as they began planning.

- What is the most effective and evidence-based forms of educational, speech and language, medical, and motor therapies to improve the quality of life for Amanda?
- Many people with 22q13.3 deletion syndrome are diagnosed with autism spectrum disorder, and nearly all have intellectual disabilities. How can we diagnose whether Amanda has autism spectrum disorder or intellectual disabilities?
- Although understanding the genetic cause of Amanda's problems has many advantages, to receive therapies, supportive services, educational services, and social security supports, there are different definitions of intellectual disabilities. Which definition of intellectual disabilities is most helpful?
- People with 22q13.3 deletion syndrome have varying degrees of intellectual disabilities ranging from mild to profound. How is the severity of intellectual disability determined?

People with Intellectual Disabilities

People with intellectual disabilities represent approximately 2% of the general population. This population has functional impairments in cognitive abilities that begin in childhood, which are pervasive and are lifelong. This population also has a long history of discrimination, isolation, abuse, and being ignored by societal policymakers. Although clinicians, educators, parents, and many other stakeholders are aware, people with intellectual disabilities represent a heterogeneous group of individuals. Sometimes scientists focus too heavily on the specific type of genetic cause of the intellectual disability or the meaning of low scores on a standardized and norm-referenced test of intelligence. Not to underestimate the importance and functional challenges of cognitive abilities that dramatically affect the ability to function socially, economically, and educationally, but cognitive abilities do not define the complexity of this population. People with intellectual disabilities have their own wants, needs, joys, strengths, and flaws. Scholars advancing the science and the application of science to classroom and therapy settings do their best work when integrating overall scientific information with the needs of individuals.

Common Characteristics

Despite the heterogeneity of this population, there are common issues that allow us to have a common language, understanding, and approach to providing services to people with intellectual disabilities. For this population, nearly all aspects of cognition are affected and are significantly below average. Cognitive processes such as attention, memory, working memory, storage of information, and retrieval of information all have some degree of impairment. General rules for providing services and improving the functioning of people with intellectual disabilities are:

- The more abstract concepts are, the more difficult learning and application are.
- Inefficient storage of information is common and is a major reason why retrieval of information is so difficult.
- Although there are often impairments in attention, not knowing how or where to direct attention is a major reason for challenges in formal and informal methods of instruction.
- Generalization of learned activities is extremely challenging and should be planned and specifically taught.

These four basic rules seem to apply to most individuals with intellectual disabilities. However, the relative importance of each rule is in large part determined by the severity of the cognitive impairments, history of instruction and early experiences, individual personality and cognitive strengths and weaknesses, and the cause of the functional cognitive impairments. The primary challenges are integrating new science in these areas, understanding the individual and environmental needs of the person with disability, and converting all of this information into the implementation of an effective and comprehensive approach towards improving the functioning of the individual.

Evolving Science, Evolving Social Perspectives

Intellectual disabilities have long been considered with the lens of a biopsychosocial model in which some impairment that affects the central nervous system causes a deviation from typical development. The social model of disability focuses on systemic barriers, societal attitudes, and exclusion by society as the primary factors that create a disability. The academic field of disability studies has had a valuable effect on how research is considered and applied. The focus of disability studies is about cultural, social, political, linguistic, and economic factors that influence how a person who differs from typical is considered and treated by society (Baglieri, 2017, pp. 33–36). The focus is on destigmatizing what the medical model might refer to as disease, impairment, illness, or genetic anomaly. Disability studies has also served a powerful function by placing ideas and constructions of disability within the context of national and international histories, politics, culture, literature, and other depictions that provide insight into how deviations from the norm on any construct interact with society. The third positive impact of disability studies is a strong encouragement of participation and self-advocacy for persons with disabilities to access physical, academic, intellectual, and cultural resources of society.

Referring to disability studies as ignoring biological and medical-based research or minimizing the functional effects of intellectual disabilities is incorrect and something of a caricature. By strongly considering societal context of disability, the field of disability studies has helped to create a path by which research-based innovation can be implemented in classrooms, community, and other clinical settings (Goodley, 2016, pp. 13–16). In addition, the area of disability studies has brought significant attention to civil rights, humanity, acceptance, inclusion, opportunity, dignity, habilitation, self-advocacy, and education of people with intellectual disabilities. The social justice emphasis of disability studies is best thought of as a reminder to researchers and clinicians who tend to work in a biopsychosocial model: people with intellectual disabilities are a population whose rights require advocacy and protection. Even the most basic genetic or neuroscience research is at its most useful when there is respect and advocacy for the humanity of people with intellectual disabilities.

Although often garnering media attention, advances in the science of intellectual disabilities are not all about neuroscientific findings or complex genetic advances. The purpose of this book is to consider advances in a variety of areas ranging from assessment, education, team work, mental health, and family dynamics. The tools of science have advanced these areas as well. Such topics tend not to be reported in popular scientific press at the same volume as neuroscience and genetics, but are just as helpful in advancing the cause of people with intellectual disabilities. Describing and integrating new scientific information from multiple domains are necessary for advancing the education and mental health of people with intellectual disabilities. Classroom teachers, therapists, psychologists, administrators, policymakers, and other stakeholders in the provision of services to people with intellectual disabilities are aided by integrated approach to understanding advances across domains.

Defining Developmental Intellectual Disabilities

The role of evidence-based practices is critical in improving the quality of life for people with intellectual disabilities. However, one of the great challenges for all problem-solving activities is to accurately define the problems being solved. Although labelling or diagnosing persons with intellectual disabilities is not universally respected and can be problematic in some circumstances, accurate definitions of intellectual disabilities can be preliminary and provide shorthand methods for professionals to communicate and begin to define the problems to be addressed (Simeonsson, Granlund, & Bjorck-Akesson, 2003). Defining intellectual disabilities brings with it many challenges. Of course, one of the biggest problems is that intellectual disabilities is a heterogeneous set of problems that one label is insufficient to describe. In addition, there is a long history of stigma associated with a diagnosis of intellectual disabilities (Devlieger, 2003). That stigma still exists. Discussing the nature and varieties of definitions for intellectual disabilities is an activity that can bring professionals closer to defining and then solving problems using the rubric of evidence-based interventions.

Labelling/Euphemism Treadmill

Interpreting research in intellectual disabilities is challenging due to issues in labelling and definition. There are multiple definitions from multiple agencies that change over time. For example, the International Classification of Diseases (ICD-10/ICD-11) (WHO, 1993, 2018), *Diagnostic and Statistical Manual of Mental Disorders, Fifth Edition (DSM-5)* (American Psychiatric Association, 2013), and the American Association of Intellectual and Developmental Disabilities (AAIDD, 2011), Social Security Disability Insurance (Social Security Administration, 2016), and the Individuals with Disabilities Education Act (2004) each have their own definitions of intellectual disabilities, which have evolved over time. Any interpretation of research literature requires that consumers understand exactly which definition of intellectual disabilities were being used in the study. Many times, the operational definition defining intellectual disabilities is not stated in research. The most common diagnostic labels that are currently used are intellectual disabilities, intellectual developmental disabilities, and mental retardation. There is significant overlap among these terms. However, a lack of agreement in labelling and definition can hinder scientific progress. Although the concept of social constructivism (i.e. that knowledge is constructed by social interaction and shared experiences) is *en vogue* in the field of education, the socially accepted definition of intellectual disabilities has a profound effect on the scientific exploration and findings in the field.

In the area of labelling and terminology, intellectual disabilities have been more influenced by the concept of "euphemism treadmill" (Pinker, 2002) than maybe any other field. The terms imbecile, moron, and idiot were once emotion-free scientific labels used to describe the severity of intellectual disabilities. These terms became pejorative. The labelling changed to mental retardation. This term also became a pejorative and is rarely used. Yet, ICD-10, the most common diagnostic manual used in the field of medicine, still uses the term mental retardation. ICD-11 will change the label to disorders of intellectual development in 2018. AAIDD uses the term intellectual disabilities. And *DSM-5* uses the term intellectual developmental disabilities. It is yet to be determined whether these terms will eventually become pejorative, and labels will be changed again in the future. However, based on historical precedent, this seems likely. Given that labelling surrounding persons with intellectual disabilities has become a part of the euphemism treadmill, there is some indication that society deems persons with intellectual disabilities as lesser or lacking in some important characteristic. The label of intellectual disabilities is considered by the general population be unfortunate and to be avoided. There is no question that the socially constructed popular beliefs have affected the definition and therefore the science behind intellectual disabilities.

There are two examples of how social constructivism has influenced the science of intellectual disabilities: the use and influence of intelligence testing in the diagnosis and the rise of the diagnosis of autism. Intelligence testing has long been one of the most reliable and stable measures in all of psychology (Ritchie, 2015).

Even when compared to measures used commonly in biology and medicine such as white blood cell count, total blood cholesterol, and body weight, intelligence testing compares favourably in terms of reliability and stability (Ritchie, 2015). However, this measure has been marginalized by social narrative. There are the philosophical narratives that are especially influential in the United States: the American dream that all children regardless of background can grow up to be whatever and whoever they wish and the Marxist narrative that all people are created equal and are born with equal opportunities to have success (Carlson, 2009, pp. 105–108). Intelligence testing of individual differences challenges both narratives. As in many cases of social constructivism, it is easier to demonize and marginalize threats to the narrative rather than change the narrative itself. As such, common beliefs about intelligence tests are that they are biased in such a manner to disadvantage ethnic minorities and persons of lower socioeconomic class, are a tool to keep non-white and lower socioeconomic status persons from social mobility, are used as a tool to segregate schools, and create a fixed mindset that acts as a barrier to cognitive growth of children. There is little to no evidence supporting any of these claims, yet it is the prevailing social narrative (Ritchie, 2015). The result of this narrative is that for diagnosing intellectual disabilities, the role of intelligence testing has been dramatically reduced. Although most definitions currently use intelligence testing, the role of adaptive behaviour, teacher and parent checklists of functioning, functional behaviour analysis, work samples, developmental and language history, and response to academic interventions all play significant roles in diagnosis of intellectual disabilities. The primary consequence of the reduction of the influence of intelligence testing in diagnosing intellectual disabilities is that less reliable measures with less predictive power are used to make diagnoses, thereby reducing the reliability, stability, and accuracy of diagnosis (Sattler, 2008).

The dramatic rise in the incidence and prevalence of autism also has an influence on the incidence and prevalence of intellectual disabilities. In 1981, the incidence of autism was calculated at 1 per 2000 individuals (Rutter, 2005). In 2014, the incidence of autism was calculated at 1 in 68 (Centers for Disease Control, 2014). There have been a variety of hypotheses proposed to explain this exponential rise in the number of children diagnosed with autism. Environmental causes such as air pollution, food additives, vaccinations, maternal stress, increases in psychotropic drug use by parents, and a host of other factors have been implicated. However, most scholars in the field believe that simple redefinition of autism is responsible for the changes in incidence (e.g. Wazana, Bresnahan, & Kline, 2007). Moreover, other factors include the use of a single instrument that is considered the "gold standard" in diagnosing of autism (i.e. Autism Diagnostic Observation Schedule; Lord, Rutter, DeLavore, & Risi, 2008) and Autism Diagnostic Interview-Revised (Rutter, LeCouteur, & Lord, 2008), massive public awareness and publicity on the importance of early intervention for autism, and dramatic increase in the number of professionals who specialize in autism. The social construct of autism is critical in understanding issues surrounding intellectual disabilities. This is because the increase in the numbers of autism is mirrored exactly by a decrease in the number of children being identified as having intellectual disabilities (Centers for Disease Control, 2014).

Sociological Influences

Reconciling the social constructivist nature of nosological algorithms for diagnosis with scientific research is sometimes difficult. This is especially true when attempting to differentiate autism from intellectual disabilities. In the opening case study, Andrea was definitively diagnosed with a rare micro-genetic deletion disorder (22q13 deletion disorder or Phelan-McDermid syndrome), she had adaptive behaviour and general intellectual ability scores of more than three standard deviations below the mean, and she also presented with concurrent medical issues such as polycystic kidneys and gastro-oesophageal reflux disease. As a long-time researcher and clinician working with persons with Phelan-McDermid syndrome, one of the authors (SS) has seen Andrea for several years. When she saw SS at an annual parent support group meeting, she smiled widely and initiated a hug. However, she was diagnosed with autism spectrum disorder for purposes of schooling and for her formal medical diagnosis. Nearly every 9-year-old child with moderate-to-severe intellectual disabilities is likely to meet a diagnostic interpretation of the definition for autism spectrum disorder. Andrea has no oral communication, signing, communication board, or formalized gestural communication skills, which are common characteristics for children with Phelan-McDermid syndrome. Her social skills are also significantly impaired compared to other 9-year-old children. There are also some occasions where Andrea will repetitively tap her foot, experience dislike of certain food textures, and be extremely sensitive to loud or unusual sounds. As such, Andrea was given a diagnosis of autism spectrum disorder. Intellectual disabilities were considered to be a comorbid condition rather than her primary diagnosis. Arguing about whether intellectual disabilities or autism spectrum disorders are primary versus secondary for purposes of diagnosis is likely not a worthwhile discussion. However, there are very real reasons why so many children previously diagnosed with intellectual disabilities are now being diagnosed as having autism spectrum disorder.

When in clinical practice, one of the authors (SS) experienced significant parental pressures to make a diagnosis of autism spectrum disorder and not a diagnosis of intellectual disabilities. There are multiple reasons for these pressures. First, several parents expressed the belief that children with autism spectrum disorder have a fully formed typical personality, intact cognitive skills, and are otherwise typical children that are trapped by forces crudely labelled as autism. Their belief was that a child diagnosed with intellectual disabilities is extremely impaired with no hope of uncovering their true selves. Therefore, autism spectrum disorder was viewed as a hopeful diagnosis where there was a potential to uncover their true child. Second, due to effective lobbying and legislative efforts by parenting and autism advocacy groups, the diagnosis of autism spectrum disorder resulted in the provision of far more types of therapy paid for by the government (Stuart et al., 2017). For example, children diagnosed with autism spectrum disorder were eligible to receive government funding for applied behaviour analysis therapies, occupational and sensory integration therapies, and speech and language therapy. However, in this community the same children with a diagnosis of intellectual disabilities would be eligible for none of the services. Third, due to strong and effective public awareness efforts, parents would see the psychologist or pediatrician and immediately request a diagnosis of autism. Autism spectrum disorder is a phrase that they had heard many times on television, on the Internet, at daycare, and through the word of mouth of other parents. The phrase intellectual disabilities or mental retardation has a much lower profile. In addition, there is a stigma to intellectual disabilities and mental retardation that is different for the diagnosis of autism spectrum disorder.

Another likely reason for children with intellectual disabilities being labelled as having autism spectrum disorder is that there are many professionals who specialize in autism. Professionals who are experts in autism frequently do not have expertise in other easily conflated diagnoses such as intellectual disabilities, speech and language disorder, movement and tic disorder, childhood schizophrenia, severe and early onset of attention deficit hyperactivity disorder, and other related disorders of childhood. With so many experts in autism available, the phrase, "When all you have is a hammer everything looks like a nail," seems appropriate (Evans, 2017).

This social trend in increased social advocacy and awareness of autism spectrum disorder has also affected research. Well-funded foundations supporting autism research have been a major driver of an increase of professional scientific journals related to autism and the number of research studies focusing on autism spectrum disorder (Chiang, 2017; Evans, 2017). This makes the review of research on intellectual disabilities especially difficult in that many samples of research studies may have intellectual disabilities but are labelled as children with autism spectrum disorder. Much like in clinical practice, there is a tendency to define children with developmental disabilities that affect cognition, language, and social skills as having autism spectrum disorder rather than intellectual disabilities.

Discussion of whether autism spectrum disorder is now overdiagnosed and intellectual disabilities underdiagnosed is unlikely to shed any light on the discussion as diagnosis is a socially constructed concept that is subject to social and pragmatic pressures that change rapidly over time (Wazana et al., 2007). However, this book will address issues related to all children with intellectual disabilities, those also diagnosed with autism spectrum disorder, and those who only have the diagnosis of intellectual disabilities. Although there have been significant changes in the diagnostic criteria for intellectual disabilities, in general the lowest 2% of the general population in cognitive ability, adaptive behaviour, and general functioning within society are considered to have intellectual disabilities. The value of a social constructivist definition that focuses on the functionality of individuals is a positive development for service delivery, advocacy, self-advocacy, and societal integration. However, when it comes to science and research, such fluid definitions are much like aiming at a constantly moving target.

The comorbidity of autism spectrum disorder and intellectual disabilities is another factor that has changed with the redefinition of autism. In the mid-1980s, over 80% of persons diagnosed with autism also had intellectual disabilities (Centers for Disease Control, 2014; Rutter, 2005). However, in 2014 estimates are that less than 50% of those diagnosed with autism also had intellectual disabilities (Centers for Disease Control, 2014). The diagnosis of autism spectrum disorder also has as one of the qualifying descriptions "with intellectual disabilities or without intellectual disabilities."

Definitions in Current Use

There are several major organizing nosological symptoms for intellectual disabilities. This chapter will review the *Diagnostic and Statistical Manual of Mental Disorders, Fifth Edition*; the International Classification of Diseases, 11th edition; the American Association on Intellectual and Developmental Disabilities, 11th edition; Social Security Disability Insurance definition; and the federal law defining special education in the United States, the Individuals with Disabilities Education Act. These definitions are primarily for administrative eligibility for earmarked programs and services and funding for individuals with disabilities (Richards, Brady, & Taylor, 2014). Yet, there are subtle variations in the definitions that can influence exactly what combinations of behaviours professionals are discussing when using the phrase "intellectual disabilities" (MacMillan & Siperstein, 2003).

Diagnostic and Statistical Manual of Mental Disorders, Fifth Edition

The *DSM-5* was developed by the American Psychiatric Association (2013) to catalogue and describe mental health issues addressed by psychiatrists and other mental health professionals. Diagnostic criteria for each disorder are organized and developed by working groups of experienced psychiatric professionals. The purpose of *DSM-5* is to define and classify mental disorders to improve diagnoses, treatment, and research.

Under *DSM-5* the diagnosis of intellectual disability (i.e. intellectual developmental disorder) requires that three criteria be met: (1) deficits in intellectual functions confirmed by both clinical assessment and individualized, standardized testing (functions such as reasoning, problem-solving, abstract thinking, academic learning, learning from experienced); (2) marked deficits in adaptive functioning that lead to inability to meet developmental and sociocultural standards for personal independence and social responsibility (e.g. communication, social participation, independent living); and (3) onset of intellectual and adaptive deficits during the developmental period (childhood and adolescence; many consider 18 years of age the cut-off point, although not specified in the *DSM-5*).

Cases of intellectual disability are classified based on the severity of intellectual impairment, but this classification is no longer dependent upon an intelligence test score in *DSM-5*. Mild intellectual disability, which accounts for 85% of all intellectual disability cases, may not become apparent until a child is of school age and has difficulty meeting educational demands. Moderate intellectual disability occurs in approximately 10% of individuals with intellectual disability. These individuals usually develop communication skills during early childhood, slightly later than those with mild intellectual disability, who generally acquire both communication and social skills during the preschool years. Individuals with moderate intellectual disability can be trained to perform unskilled work under close supervision. Individuals with severe intellectual disability constitute 3–4% of the intellectually disabled population. In severe intellectual disability, communicative speech usually does not develop during early childhood, although it may be acquired during the school-age years. Individuals with severe intellectual disability can learn basic self-care but need additional supervision. Profound intellectual disability occurs in approximately 1–2% of people with intellectual disability. Communication skills and sensorimotor functioning are significantly impaired. These individuals need nearly constant supervision and generally benefit from a one-to-one relationship with a caregiver. Intellectual disability involves impairments of general mental abilities that influence adaptive functioning in three domains: conceptual, social, and practical. These domains determine how individuals cope with everyday tasks.

The conceptual domain includes skills in language, reading, writing, math, reasoning, knowledge, and memory. The social domain refers to empathy, social judgement, interpersonal communication skills, the ability to make and retain friendships, and similar capacities. The practical domain centres on self-management in areas such as personal care, job responsibilities, money management, recreation, and organizing school and work tasks. Although intellectual disability does not have a specific age requirement, an individual's symptoms must begin during the developmental period and are diagnosed based on the severity of deficits in adaptive functioning. The disorder is considered chronic and often co-occurs with other mental conditions like depression, attention deficit/hyperactivity disorder, and autism spectrum disorder.

Co-occurring diagnoses to consider are major depressive disorder, which may occur throughout the range of severity of ID, attention deficit hyperactivity disorder, bipolar disorders (with and without aggression), anxiety disorders, autism spectrum disorder, impulse control disorders, major neurocognitive disorder, and stereotypic movement disorder (with or without self-injurious behaviour). Self-injurious behaviour requires prompt diagnostic attention and may warrant a separate diagnosis of stereotypic movement disorder. Individuals with severe intellectual disabilities are more likely to demonstrate self-injury, aggression, and disruptive behaviours. Finally, individuals with a diagnosis of intellectual disabilities with co-occurring mental disorders are at risk for suicide attempts.

An important aspect of any diagnosis is to differentiate between similar and related diagnoses. This is clearly the case when it comes to autism spectrum disorder and intellectual disabilities. In addition, social (pragmatic) communication disorder shares characteristics of both autism spectrum disorder and intellectual disabilities. However, social (pragmatic) communication disorder stands apart from autism spectrum disorder and intellectual disabilities. In many cases, this form of communication disorder can be mistaken for both autism and intellectual disabilities, but is not appropriate in cases where limitations of communication can best be asked blamed by autism spectrum disorder or intellectual disabilities. By reviewing the criteria for these two related disorders, it is easy to see how there can be confusion in diagnostic accuracy among these three disorders.

Social (Pragmatic) Communication Disorder 315.39 (F80.89) is a form of communication disorder that includes persistent difficulties in the social use of verbal and nonverbal communication as manifested by all the following:

- Deficits in using communication for social purposes, such as greeting and sharing information, in a manner that is appropriate for the social context.
- Impairment of the ability to change communication to match context or the needs of the listener, such as speaking differently in a classroom than on the playground, talking differently to a child than to an adult, and avoiding use of overly formal language.
- Difficulties following rules for conversation and storytelling, such as taking turns in conversation, rephrasing when misunderstood, and knowing how to use verbal and nonverbal signals to regulate interaction.
- Difficulties understanding what is not explicitly stated (e.g. making inferences) and nonliteral or ambiguous meanings of language (e.g. idioms, humour, metaphors, multiple meanings that depend on the context for interpretation).

The deficits result in functional limitations in effective communication, social participation, social relationships, academic achievement, or occupational performance, individually or in combination. The onset of the symptoms is in the early developmental period (but deficits may not become fully manifest until social communication demands exceed limited capacities).

The symptoms are not attributable to another medical or neurological condition or to low abilities in the domains or word structure and grammar and are not better explained by autism spectrum disorder, intellectual disability (intellectual developmental disorder), global developmental delay, or another mental disorder.

Autism Spectrum Disorder 299.00 (F84.0) as described in the *DSM-5* represents a change from previous editions of the DSM. The current edition also considers the severity of the impairment. Diagnostic criteria for this disorder include two components: (a) social communication and social interaction and (b) restricted, repetitive patterns of behaviour, interests, or activities.

Persistent deficits in social communication and social interaction across multiple contexts, as manifested by the following, currently or by history:

- Deficits in social-emotional reciprocity, ranging, for example, from abnormal social approach and failure of normal back-and-forth conversation to reduced sharing of interests, emotions, or affect and to failure to initiate or respond to social interactions.
- Deficits in nonverbal communicative behaviours used for social interaction, ranging, for example, from poorly integrated verbal and nonverbal communication to abnormalities in eye contact and body language or deficits in

understanding and use of gestures to a total lack of facial expressions and nonverbal communication.

- Deficits in developing, maintaining, and understanding relationships, ranging, for example, from difficulties adjusting behaviour to suit various social contexts to difficulties in sharing imaginative play or in making friends to absence of interest in peers. Restricted, repetitive patterns of behaviour, interests, or activities, as manifested by at least two of the following, currently or by history.
- Stereotyped or repetitive motor movements, use of objects, or speech (e.g. simple motor stereotypes, lining up toys or flipping objects, echolalia, idiosyncratic phrases).
- Insistence on sameness, inflexible adherence to routines, or ritualized patterns of verbal or nonverbal behaviour (e.g. extreme distress at small changes, difficulties with transitions, rigid thinking patterns, greeting rituals, the need to take the same route or eat the same food every day).
- Highly restricted, fixated interests that are abnormal in intensity or focus (e.g. strong attachment to or preoccupation with unusual objects, excessively circumscribed or perseverative interests).
- Hyper- or hyporeactivity to sensory input or unusual interest in sensory aspects of the environment (e.g. apparent indifference to pain/temperature, adverse response to specific sounds or textures, excessive smelling or touching of objects, visual fascination with lights or movement).

Additional diagnostic criteria and differential diagnosis information include:

- Symptoms must be present in the early developmental period (but may not become fully manifest until social demands exceed limited capacities or may be masked by learned strategies in later life).
- Symptoms cause clinically significant impairment in social, occupational, or other important areas of current functioning.
- These disturbances are not better explained by intellectual disability (intellectual developmental disorder) or global developmental delay. Intellectual disability and autism spectrum disorder frequently co-occur; to make comorbid diagnoses of autism spectrum disorder and intellectual disability, social communication should be below that expected for general developmental level.

Note: Individuals with a well-established *DSM-4* diagnosis of autistic disorder, Asperger's disorder or pervasive developmental disorder not otherwise specified should be given the diagnosis of autism spectrum disorder. Individuals who have marked deficits in social communication, but whose symptoms do not otherwise meet criteria for autism spectrum disorder, should be evaluated for social (pragmatic) communication disorder. The final criterion can be somewhat confusing and difficult to assess. If the language difficulties and repetitive and restrictive behaviours, interests, or activities are due solely to intellectual disabilities, then the diagnosis of autism spectrum disorder is not appropriate. However, making this determination is difficult to operationalize. The result is that most clinicians make a diagnosis of autism spectrum disorder with a specifier of accompanying intellectual impairment.

The *DSM-5* recognizes that autism spectrum disorder is a heterogeneous collection of behaviours. Therefore, a list of specifiers and degree of severity of the disorder are well described. This detailed description of specifiers and severity are new to this edition of the *DSM*. Specifiers include:

- With or without accompanying intellectual impairment.
- With or without accompanying language impairment.
- Associated with a known medical or genetic condition or environmental factor.
- (Coding note: Use additional code to identify the associated medical or genetic condition.)
- Associated with another neurodevelopmental, mental, or behavioural disorder.
- (Coding note: Use additional code[s] to identify the associated neurodevelopmental, mental, or behavioural disorder[s].)
- With catatonia (refer to the criteria for catatonia associated with another mental disorder, pp. 119–120, for definition) (Coding note: Use additional code 293.89 [F06.1] catatonia associated with autism spectrum disorder to indicate the presence of the comorbid catatonia.)

- Severity is based on social communication impairments and restricted repetitive patterns of behaviour.

Levels of support are somewhat like the criteria and framework developed by the American Association on Intellectual and Developmental Disabilities framework involving the functional effects of the disorder. Including levels of support in the diagnostic criteria creates an acknowledgement that additional environmental supports can assist persons with autism spectrum disorder function more effectively in a variety of environments.

- Level 1—Requiring support—Without supports in place, deficits in social communication cause noticeable impairments. Has difficulty initiating social interactions and demonstrates clear examples of atypical or unsuccessful responses to social overtures of others. May appear to have decreased interest in social interactions. Rituals and repetitive behaviours (RRBs) cause significant interference with functioning in one or more contexts. Resists attempts by others to interrupt RRBs or to be redirected from fixated interest.
- Level 2—Requiring substantial support—Marked deficits in verbal and nonverbal social communication skills; social impairments apparent even with supports in place; limited initiation of social interactions and reduced or abnormal response to social overtures from others. RRBs and/or preoccupations or fixated interests appear frequently enough to be obvious to the casual observer and interfere with functioning in a variety of contexts. Distress or frustration is apparent when RRBs are interrupted, difficult to redirect from fixated interest.
- Level 3—Requiring very substantial support—Severe deficits in verbal and nonverbal social communication skills cause severe impairments in functioning, very limited initiation of social interactions and minimal response to social overtures from others. Preoccupations, fixated rituals, and/or repetitive behaviours markedly interfere with functioning in all spheres. Marked distress when rituals or routines are interrupted, very difficult to redirect from fixated interest or returns to it quickly.

International Classification of Diseases, 11th Edition

The International Classification of Diseases 11th edition has recently been updated 2018 (WHO, 1993, 2017, 2018). Intellectual developmental disabilities (IDD) are characterized by a marked impairment of core cognitive functions necessary for the development of knowledge, reasoning, and symbolic representation of the level expected of one's age peers and cultural and community environment. Nevertheless, different patterns of cognitive impairments appear for subtypes and causes of IDD. In general, persons with IDD have difficulties with verbal comprehension, perceptual reasoning, working memory and processing speed (Hodapp & Burack, 2006). The cognitive impairment in persons with IDD is associated with difficulties in different domains of learning, including academic and practical knowledge. Persons with IDD typically manifest difficulties in adaptive behaviour, that is, meeting the demands of daily life expected for one's age peers and cultural and community environment. These difficulties include limitations in relevant conceptual, social, and practical skills. Persons with IDD often have difficulties managing their behaviour, emotions, and interpersonal relationships and maintaining motivation in the learning process. IDD is a lifespan condition requiring consideration of developmental stages and life transitions.

Within this approach, cognitive skills are assessed through tests, semi-structured observations, and direct clinical examination. The tests should combine the measurement of general mental ability with that of several aspects of executive functioning, perceptual reasoning, processing speed, verbal comprehension, as well as the assessment of attention, perception, and working memory. The evaluation should aim to identify the cognitive dysfunctions that have the greatest negative impact in terms of behaviour, adjustment, autonomy, and above all quality of life, across the lifespan. The instruments to assess specific cognitive functions should have a low cost, to allow rapid assimilation by professionals practicing in low-income countries. The definition of intellectual developmental disability is a group of developmental conditions characterized by significant impairment of cognitive functions, which are associated with limitations of learning, adaptive behaviour, and skills.

A mild disorder of intellectual development is characterized by significantly below-average intellectual functioning and adaptive behaviour that are approximately two to three standard deviations below the mean (approximately 0.1–2.3 percentile), based on appropriately normed, individually administered standardized tests or by comparable behavioural indicators when standardized testing is unavailable. Affected persons often exhibit difficulties in the acquisition and comprehension of complex language concepts and academic skills. Most master basic self-care, domestic, and practical activities. Persons affected by a mild disorder of intellectual development can generally achieve relatively independent living and employment as adults but may require appropriate support.

A moderate disorder of intellectual development is a condition characterized by significantly below-average intellectual functioning and adaptive behaviour that are approximately three to four standard deviations below the mean (approximately 0.003–0.1 percentile), based on appropriately normed, individually administered standardized tests or by comparable behavioural indicators when standardized testing is unavailable. Language and capacity for acquisition of academic skills of persons affected by a moderate disorder of intellectual development vary but are generally limited to basic skills. Some may master basic self-care, domestic, and practical activities. Most affected persons require considerable and consistent support to achieve independent living and employment as adults.

A severe disorder of intellectual development is a condition characterized by significantly below-average intellectual functioning and adaptive behaviour that are approximately four of more standard deviations below the mean (less than approximately the 0.003rd percentile), individually administered standardized tests or by comparable behavioural indicators when standardized testing is unavailable. Affected persons exhibit very limited language and capacity for acquisition of academic skills. They may also have motor impairments and typically require daily support in a supervised environment for adequate care but may acquire basic self-care skills with intensive training. Severe and profound disorders of intellectual development are differentiated exclusively based on adaptive behaviour differences because existing standardized tests of intelligence cannot reliably or validly distinguish among individuals with intellectual functioning below the 0.003rd percentile.

A profound disorder of intellectual development is a condition characterized by significantly below-average intellectual functioning and adaptive behaviour that are approximately four of more standard deviations below the mean (approximately less than the 0.003rd percentile), based on individually administered standardized tests or by comparable behavioural indicators when standardized testing is unavailable. Affected persons possess very limited communication abilities, and capacity for acquisition of academic skills is restricted to basic concrete skills. They may also have co-occurring motor and sensory impairments and typically require daily support in a supervised environment for adequate care. Severe and profound disorders of intellectual development are differentiated exclusively based on adaptive behaviour differences because existing standardized tests of intelligence cannot reliably or validly distinguish among individuals with intellectual functioning below the 0.003rd percentile.

Disorder of intellectual development, provisional is diagnosed when there is evidence of a disorder of intellectual development but the individual is an infant or child under the age of 4, or it is not possible to conduct a valid assessment of intellectual functioning and adaptive behaviour because of sensory or physical impairments (e.g. blindness, prelingual deafness), locomotor disability, severe problem behaviours, or co-occurring mental and behavioural disorders.

American Association on Intellectual and Developmental Disabilities

Intellectual disability is a disability characterized by significant limitations in both intellectual functioning and in adaptive behaviour, which covers many everyday social and practical skills. Only based on multidimensional assessment can professionals determine whether an individual has intellectual disability and tailor individualized support plans. Based on a disability perspective, the American Association on Intellectual and Developmental Disabilities has assembled a comprehensive definition, classification, and system of supports that focus mainly on functioning, adaptive behaviour, and support needs (2011). This disability originates before the age of 18. Important components of the definition are:

- Intellectual functioning—Also called intelligence—Refers to general mental capacity, such as learning, reasoning, problem-solving, and so on.
- One way to measure intellectual functioning is an intelligence test. Generally, an intelligence test score of around 70 or as high as 75 indicates a limitation in intellectual functioning.
- Adaptive behaviour is the collection of conceptional, social, and practical skills that are learned and performed by people in their everyday lives.
  - Conceptual skills—language and literacy; money, time, and number concepts; and self-direction.
  - Social skills—interpersonal skills, social responsibility, self-esteem, gullibility, naïveté (i.e. wariness), social problem-solving, and the ability to follow rules/obey laws and to avoid being victimized.
  - Practical skills—activities of daily living (personal care), occupational skills, healthcare, travel/transportation, schedules/routines, safety, use of money, the use of the telephone.
- Additional considerations in defining and assessing intellectual disability, the AAIDD stresses that additional factors must be considered, such as the community environment typical of the individual's peers and culture. Professionals should also consider linguistic diversity and cultural differences in the way people communicate, move, and behave.
- Finally, assessments must also assume that limitations in individuals often coexist with strengths and that a person's level of life functioning will improve if appropriate personalized supports are provided over a sustained period.

A major focus of the AAIDD approach to intellectual disabilities is the focus on supports required for individuals to be functional in certain environments (Schalock et al., 2012). Rather than a static diagnostic condition, the definition focuses on interactions between the skills of the individual and the skill requirements of their environment. As such, a complete report and diagnosis of a person with intellectual disabilities requires information concerning (1) exceptional medical support needs, (2) exceptional behaviour support needs, (3) the number and complexity of the settings in which a person participates, and (4) the number and complexity of the life activities in which a person participates. Although traditional measures of adaptive behaviour and general intelligence are useful, this definition allows for understanding of individual variation and strengths and weaknesses for certain functional tasks. Inferring a person's pattern and intensity of support needs from traditional measures of personal competence is unlikely to result in specific and practically useful conclusions because intelligence test scores and adaptive behaviour measures do not provide a complete measure of personal competence, nor do they account for the other four influences on support needs (Greenspan, 1997; Schalock et al., 2010).

Individuals with Disabilities Education Act

The Individuals with Disabilities Education Act (2004) is a US federal law that provides funding to local educational agencies (i.e. school boards/districts) to offset the extra funds needed to educate students with disabilities to provide them with a free and appropriate education. This law recognizes 13 disabilities (i.e. specific learning disabilities, intellectual disabilities, autism spectrum disorder, emotional disturbance, speech or language impairment, visual impairment, blindness, hearing impairment, deafness, other health impairment, orthopaedic or motor impairment, traumatic brain injury, multiple disabilities). The federal law provides a basic description that is to be implemented by each state's Department of Education and further operationalized by each local educational agency.

Although the major definitions of intellectual disabilities are social constructs, school-based definitions are not only driven by expert opinion but also by funding considerations with a long history of case law in the United States. A reasonable way to think about the definition of intellectual disabilities in a school setting is less of a diagnostic category and more of a determination of eligibility to receive additional federal funding for that student. Despite being operationally defined by the diagnostic criteria of *DSM-5*, ICD-11, and AAIDD, it is quite possible to receive a diagnosis of intellectual disabilities under one of these sets of diagnostic criteria via assessment by medical or psychological professional in private practice, but not be eligible for a school-based categorization under IDEA criteria for intellectual disabilities due to the differences in the criteria. Many children must be reassessed using school-based criteria even after receiving the diagnosis from a psychologist or physician.

For purposes of the specific description in the federal law, intellectual disabilities mean significantly subaverage general intellectual functioning, existing concurrently with deficits in adaptive behaviour and manifested during the developmental period, that adversely affects a child's educational performance. This definition varies across states and across local educational agencies. Most states use the definition provided by *DSM-5*. However, some states (e.g. Iowa) use a noncategorical special education system that is based on the level of support required to be functional in a classroom. This form of determination of support is referred to as response to intervention. This model is most consistent with the American Association on Intellectual and Developmental Disabilities definition. For purposes of research and understanding, the definitions of intellectual disabilities may vary dramatically across nations and regions.

Social Security Disability Insurance

A common reason for assessment for a possible diagnosis of intellectual disabilities is to determine eligibility for Social Security Administration Disability Insurance (2016). This program is designed to provide financial support to meet the needs of individuals with intellectual disabilities. As a federal program, similar to IDEA, there is a specific definition and specific criteria designed to determine eligibility.

Intellectual disability refers to a measured, below-average intelligence, to the extent that the individual lacks the skills necessary to perform basic daily functions. Intellectual disability is usually diagnosed during childhood and will persist throughout a person's entire lifetime. As with many conditions, the spectrum of intellectual disability can range from mild to profound.

Intellectual disability can be caused by many things, but genetics and problems related to pregnancy and birth are the most common causes.

Those with intellectual disabilities have a very low intelligence test scores, usually scoring less than 70 (i.e. two standard deviations below the mean). A diagnosis usually occurs after a medical professional has documented delays in learning, problem-solving, memory, and speaking. In all but the most severe cases, these individuals can still learn these skills but require much more time and practice to do so.

Because intellectual disability itself is not a disease, it is not treated as though it is an illness. Instead, children and adults with intellectual disabilities may need occupational or physical therapies, supervision, and specially tailored educational environments to help them succeed. The Social Security Administration evaluates intellectual disabilities in the Blue Book under Section 12.05—intellectual disability—within the mental disorder category. The listing requires that one of the following be met to receive benefits:

- Mental incapacity, as shown by a dependence on others for basic personal needs and inability to follow directions, such that the use of standardized measures of intellectual functioning is precluded.
- A valid verbal, performance, or Full Scale IQ of 59 or less.
- A valid verbal, performance, or Full Scale IQ of 60 through 70 and a physical or other mental impairments that imposes an additional and significant work-related functional limitation.
- A valid verbal, performance, or full-scale IQ of 60 through 70, resulting in at least two of the following:

- Marked restriction of activities of daily living.
- Marked difficulties in maintaining social functioning.
- Marked difficulties in maintaining concentration, persistence, or pace.
- Repeated episodes of decompensation, each of extended duration.

If an individual with an intellectual disability does not meet this listing, he or she may be eligible to qualify under a medical vocational allowance. This often occurs to disabled individuals who may not meet a Blue Book listing but have a condition that reduces their functional capabilities to the point that they are unable to perform work. An individual who is unable to work and function independently due to an intellectual disability could be a candidate for Social Security Disability Benefits, provided their case can be clearly and objectively presented to the Social Security Administration.

Conclusions

The first step in a scientific approach to improving the understanding, assessment, and treatment of persons with intellectual disabilities is to have an agreed-upon definition of exactly what intellectual disabilities are. The definition can be conceptual, empirical, or operational (preferably all three). However, the current definitions are marked by a strong social constructivist movement in which definitions are developed by medical, psychiatric, advocacy groups, and educational institutions, each with their own goals and perceptions of this population. Although this is not unreasonable, creating generalizable scientific findings is extremely challenging. All evidence used must be interpreted considering the different definitions used to define the population and samples used in research. Moreover, considering whether the sample used in the research has co-occurring, autism spectrum disorder diagnosis will also need to be considered. Throughout this book research will be interpreted based on the definition for each study. For effective evidence-based practices to take place, not only must research be sound in terms of research methods and internal validity, the sample in the research must to some degree reflect the target population of any intervention. This relevance of research is a key variable on whether the concept of evidence-based practices will result in a positive set of outcomes for children with intellectual disabilities.

References

American Association on Intellectual & Developmental Disabilities. (2011). *Intellectual disability: Definition, classification, and systems of supports* (11th ed.). Washington, DC: Author.

American Psychiatric Association. (2013). *Diagnostic and statistical manual of mental disorders* (5th ed., pp. 74–85). Arlington, VA: American Psychiatric Publishing. ISBN 978-0-89042-555-8.

Baglieri, S. (2017). *Disability studies and the inclusive classroom: Critical practices for embracing diversity in education* (pp. 33–36). London, England: Taylor & Francis.
Carlson, L. (2009). *The faces of intellectual disability: Philosophical reflections* (pp. 105–108). Bloomington, IN: Indiana University Press.
Centers for Disease Control. (2014). *Prevalence of autism spectrum disorder among children aged 8 years autism and developmental disabilities monitoring network, 11 sites, United States, 2010.* (2014, April 25). Retrieved May 18, 2017, from https://web.archive.org/web/20140425185152/http://www.cdc.gov/mmwr/preview/mmwrhtml/ss6302a1.htm?s_cid=ss6302a1_w
Chiang, H.-M. (2017). Current trends and future directions. In *Curricula for teaching students with autism spectrum disorder* (pp. 291–295). Cham, Switzerland: Springer. https://doi.org/10.1007/978-3-319-69983-7_13
Devlieger, J. P. (2003). From "idiot" to "person with mental retardation": Defining differences in an effort to dissolve it. In J. P. Devlieger, F. Rusch, & D. Pfeiffer (Eds.), *Rethinking disability: The emergence of new definitions, concepts, and communities* (pp. 169–188). Antwerp, Belgium: Garant Publishers.
Evans, B. (2017). *The metamorphosis of autism*. Manchester, England: Manchester University Press. https://doi.org/10.26530/OAPEN_625488
Goodley, D. (2016). *Disability studies: An interdisciplinary introduction* (pp. 13–16). London, England: SAGE.
Greenspan, S. (1997). Dead man walking? Why the 1992 AAMR definition needs redoing. *Education and Training in Mental Retardation and Developmental Disabilities, 32*, 179–190.
Hodapp, R. M., & Burack, J. A. (2006). Developmental approaches to children with mental retardation: A second generation? In D. Cicchetti & D. J. Cohen (Eds.), *Developmental psychopathology, Vol. 3: Risk, disorder, and adaptation* (2nd ed., pp. 235–267). Hoboken, NJ: Wiley.
IDEA. (2004). *Regulations: Subpart E – Procedural safeguards*. Retrieved May 17, 2017, from http://www.wrightslaw.com/idea/law/idea.regs.subparte.pdf, Individuals with Disabilities Education Act, 20 U.S.C. § 1400 (2004).
Lord, C., Rutter, M., DeLavore, P. C., & Risi, S. (2008). *Autism diagnostic observation schedule*. Los Angeles, CA: Western Psychological Services.
MacMillan, D. L., & Siperstein, G. N. (2003). Children with mental retardation. In H. N. Switzky & S. Greenspan (Eds.), *What is mental retardation?* (pp. 242–261). Washington, DC: American Association on Mental Retardation.
Pinker, S. (2002). *The blank slate*. New York, NY: Viking.
Richards, S. B., Brady, M. P., & Taylor, R. L. (2014). *Cognitive and intellectual disabilities: Historical perspectives, current practices, and future directions*. London, England: Routledge.
Ritchie, S. (2015). *Intelligence: All that matters*. London, England: Hodder & Stoughton.
Rutter, M. (2005). Incidence of autism spectrum disorders: Changes over time and their meaning. *Acta Paediatrica, 94*(1), 2–15. https://doi.org/10.1111/j.1651-2227.2005.tb01779.x
Rutter, M., LeCouteur, A., & Lord, C. (2008). *Autism diagnostic interview – Revised.* Los Angeles, CA: Western Psychological Services.
Sattler, J. M. (2008). *Assessment of children: Cognitive foundations* (5th ed.). San Diego, CA: Sattler.
Schalock, R. L., Borthwick-Duffy, S., Bradley, V. J., Buntinx, W. H. E., Coulter, D. L., Craig, E. M., … Yeag, e. M. H. (2010). *Intellectual disability: Definition, classification, and systems of supports* (11th ed.). Washington, DC: American Association on Intellectual and Developmental Disabilities.
Schalock, R. L., Luckasson, R., Bradley, V., Buntinx, W., Lachapelle, Y., Shogren, K., … Wehmeyer, M. L. (2012). *User's guide to accompany the 11th edition of Intellectual Disability: Definition, Classification, and Systems of Supports: Applications for clinicians, educators, organizations providing supports, policy makers, family members members and advocates, and health care professionals*. Washington, DC: American Association on Intellectual and Developmental Disabilities.

Simeonsson, R. J., Granlund, M., & Bjorck-Akesson, E. (2003). Classifying mental retardation: Impairment, disability, handicap limitations, or restriction? In H. N. Switzky & S. Greenspan (Eds.), *What is mental retardation?* (pp. 309–329). Washington, DC: American Association on Mental Retardation.

Social Security Administration. (2016). Revised medical criteria for evaluating mental disorders; final rule. *Federal Register, 81*(186), 66138–66178.

Stuart, E. A., McGinty, E. E., Kalb, L., Huskamp, H. A., Busch, S. H., Gibson, T. B., ... Barry, C. L. (2017). Increased service use among children with autism spectrum disorder associated with mental health parity law. *Health Affairs, 36*(2), 337–345. https://doi.org/10.1377/hlthaff.2016.0824

Wazana, A., Bresnahan, M., & Kline, J. (2007). The autism epidemic: Fact or artifact? *Journal of the American Academy Child Adolescent Psychiatry, 46*(6), 721–730. https://doi.org/10.1097/chi.0b013e31804a7f3b

World Health Organization. (2017). *ICD-11 Beta draft - Mortality and morbidity statistics.* Retrieved May 17, 2017, from http://apps.who.int/classifications/icd11/browse/l-m/en#/http%3a%2f%2fid.who.int%2ficd%2fentity%2f605267007

World Health Organization (WHO). (1993). *International statistical classification of diseases and related health problems* (10th ed.). Geneva, Switzerland: Author.

World Health Organization (WHO). (2018). *International statistical classification of diseases and related health problems* (11th ed.). Geneva, Switzerland: Author.

Chapter 2
Causes and Symptoms

Abstract This chapter explores the causes and symptoms of intellectual disabilities. The discussion addresses the complex and multifaceted interaction of genetic, biological, neurological, and environmental factors that lead to intellectual disabilities. This chapter also discusses advances in how the causes of intellectual disabilities are determined, typical symptoms, and course. The language of the chapter assumes a medical model of intellectual disabilities. That is, the primary cause of disability is physiological and functional deficits due to a disordered or pathological state. The entire research model in this chapter focuses on neurological and genetic underpinnings of functional cognitive deficits. Due to new research tools and models, the focus on neuroscience and genetics has led to exponential change in the understanding of the causes of intellectual disabilities. The understanding of causes and symptoms has also led to diversity of training and backgrounds in multidisciplinary teams that provide comprehensive services to individuals with intellectual disabilities and their families.

Case Study

Jonah is a 17-month-old male who has concerned his parents from the first day that they brought him home from the hospital. His parents were worried about his "rigidness". He was late to sit, crawl, orient to sound, and babble. At 17 months, he stands with assistance, but does not take more than one or two steps before losing balance and falling. Sometimes his muscles appeared to be trembling for no apparent reason. He has shown no evidence of speaking, and his babbling is unsophisticated in that it consists mostly of crying and making vowel sounds. Jonah's parents have not heard any more sophisticated babbling such as "bababa" or "mamama". Jonah's parents called him a happy child who smiles frequently.

Jonah's pediatrician referred him to the neurodevelopmental assessment team at a regional teaching hospital. The neurodevelopmental assessment team is an interdisciplinary approach to assessment of young children with complex developmental disorders that have proved challenging for primary care pediatricians. The team consists of a developmental pediatrician, clinical geneticist, pediatric

S. R. Shaw, A. M. Jankowska, *Pediatric Intellectual Disabilities at School*, Pediatric School Psychology, https://doi.org/10.1007/978-3-030-02992-0_2

neurologist, speech and language therapist, occupational therapist, and psychologist. In addition, psychiatry, genetic counselling, social work, counselling, physical therapy, and other professions are frequently invited to work with the team as needed. The purpose of the team is to make as early identification of developmental disorders as possible and begin to implement interventions. After each member of the team invested between 20 and 60 min assessing Jonah directly or interviewing the parents, the team met to discuss possible diagnoses. In most cases for this team, diagnoses are complex and require discussion, consensus building, and further study. The case of Jonah was a relatively simple diagnosis. All members of the team agreed that the likely diagnosis was Angelman syndrome. The clinical geneticist would have the appropriate diagnostic testing conducted to confirm the diagnosis. In this case, the purpose of the diagnostic test is to investigate evidence of a deletion or lack of visible inactivity on chromosome 15 by array comparative genomic hybridization (aCGH).

Although there is no known cure for Angelman syndrome, a treatment plan was put in place. Among the aspects of the treatment plan are genetic counselling for Jonah's parents, family counselling to help with adjustment, physical and occupational therapy to assist with motor movement for Jonah, consultation with neurology because epilepsy and other forms of seizure disorder are common, speech and language therapy to assist in the development of communication skills, and additional consultation with a developmental pediatrician to support likely sleep problems and provide general developmental consultation to parents.

The advances in research on Angelman syndrome have created an understanding of a cluster of behavioural and developmental symptom presentation to assist in the identification of the specific disorder. In addition, advances in genetics have helped to create a definitive genetic test for the disorder. Also, research in development provides a description of common behavioural characteristics (i.e. behavioural phenotype) that are not currently issues for Jonah's parents but may be in the future and allow for monitoring and rapid intervention (e.g. seizure disorders, sleep problems, overactivity). Although prevention or a cure may be a long-term goal for many, causes of intellectual disabilities, advanced research into the causes, symptoms, and diagnosis of specific forms of intellectual disability have led to improved management of symptoms and quality of life for the affected children and their families.

Introduction

Over the last 15 years, advancements in understanding neuroscientific substrates of behaviour, genetics, and environmental factors have led to dramatic changes in the identification of the causes, symptoms, and diagnosis of intellectual disabilities. Investigation into the causes of intellectual disabilities may be the area that has most changed over the last 10 years and is most likely to have the greatest impact in research and clinical practice during the next 10 years (The Deciphering

Developmental Disorders Study, 2015). Extraordinary advances in genetics and neuroscience have created answers to many questions that were common in the field and have allowed new questions to be asked.

At one time, over 80% of individuals diagnosed with intellectual disabilities had no known cause (Atwal et al., 2014). Currently, that percentage has been reduced to approximately 40% of persons with intellectual disabilities having no known cause (Black, 2015). Although understanding the cause does not necessarily lead directly to an appropriate clinical treatment as is assumed in a medical model of neurodevelopmental disabilities, it may improve understanding of development and allow anticipatory and prophylactic treatment of clusters of behaviour (Glover, Bernard, Branford, Holland, & Strydom, 2014). A simple example is the case of persons identified with Prader-Willi syndrome. This rare disorder is caused by partial deletion on the 15th chromosome (q11–13) location (Burnett et al., 2017). Prader-Willi is characterized by short stature, intellectual disabilities, low muscle tone, and an obsession with eating food (Clark, Boer, & Webb, 1995). Thus, persons with Prader-Willi frequently become obese, and subsequent related health problems arise. Knowing that these behaviours are extremely common, early diagnosis can lead to preventative methods of controlling diet and access to food at an extremely young age (Burnett et al., 2017). Other causal mechanisms have a distinct developmental pattern so that planning of services can more easily take place. For example, in the case of 22q11 deletion syndrome, there is a high probability of learning disabilities and mental health issues (e.g. bipolar disorder, anxiety disorder, attention deficit hyperactivity disorder; Zarchi et al., 2014). The learning issues manifest themselves in the early school years, and mental health issues most typically manifest themselves post puberty (Snijders Blok et al., 2014). Such knowledge can help arrange treatment by anticipating the high probability of these behavioural manifestations. Even in most cases in which knowledge of the cause of the intellectual disabilities does not lead to prophylactic clinical treatments or understanding of development and progression, knowledge of the causal mechanisms is productive in genetic counselling and family peace of mind (Van den Veyver, 2016).

Frequently, advocacy groups and parent support groups have interpreted the advances in genetics and neuroscience as evidence that a cure for the disorder is imminent. Development of a cure for some causes of intellectual disabilities is ambitious and far ahead of most research. Overcoming structural and neuroanatomical anomalies at the gross anatomical, microscopic anatomical, or physiological level presents extreme challenges (Wallace, 2016). For nearly all causes of intellectual disabilities, a cure may not be possible. Far more likely, early identification (i.e. less than 12-week gestation) may lead to in utero treatment and prevention of the presentation of intellectual disabilities. Prevention via genetic counselling and early identification of de novo (i.e. due to mutation rather than hereditary transmission) presentation of genetic disorders is one avenue of prevention. Identification of environmental interventions that can be used to minimize the effects of genetic disorders has proved valuable. For example, specialized diet for infants identified with phenylketonuria (PKU) results in a dramatic improvement of cognitive function and prevents intellectual disabilities (O'Brien, 2006). In addition, some causes of intellectual disabilities have a primary environmental cause and are well addressed via public health campaigns such as abstention from alcohol during pregnancy and reduction of exposure to lead, which have prevented large numbers of cases of intellectual disabilities (O'Leary et al., 2013). The desire to create a cure for intellectual disabilities is laudable but for nearly all cases far ahead of the research in this area. Yet, efforts to apply knowledge of the causes, symptoms, and diagnoses of intellectual disabilities to developing a cure are far from realization and reflect more wishful thinking than any near-term reality (Willemsen & Kleefstra, 2014). Nonetheless, a long-term goal of curing intellectual disabilities is worth pursuing, no matter how far the goal is from present-day reality.

Advances in research in intellectual disabilities involve multiple fields of study (Rizzo, 2014). However, commonly research does not translate across professions. Genetics, neuroscience, medicine, psychology, and education all tend to work in silos making the translation and utility of research in any one field difficult to interpret (Riggs et al., 2014). For determining and understanding the cause of intellectual disabilities, the major advances have been in genetics. Although there is overlap, there are six broad categories of genetic causes of intellectual disabilities: autosomal dominant, autosomal recessive, X-linked dominant and recessive, mitochondrial disorders, micro-deletion syndromes, and multifactor and polygenetic disorders. The advances may be less dramatic, yet understanding of the environmental causes of intellectual disabilities has also advanced significantly over the last 10 years (Lebel, 2014). Organization of environmental causes is often organized as prenatal, perinatal, or postnatal (Srour & Shevell, 2014).

Genetics

For purposes of organization, it is easiest to subdivide genetically caused intellectual disabilities into syndromic and non-syndromic cases. Syndromic intellectual disabilities involve symptoms and characteristics that are consistently present in nearly all cases (Kaasinen et al., 2014). Examples of syndromic intellectual disability include Down syndrome, Klinefelter syndrome, and fragile X syndrome among many others. Non-syndromic intellectual disabilities represent no consistent pattern of symptoms and characteristics that have been described in the research literature (Kaufman, Ayub, & Vincent, 2010). Non-syndromic intellectual disabilities are extraordinarily challenging to study and represent major research and clinical problems. Nearly all the major advances in identifying causes of intellectual disabilities have taken place around syndromic intellectual disabilities. This is clearly a moving target as advances in genetics, neuroscience, and psychology frequently mean that characteristics once thought of non-syndromic intellectual disabilities become syndromic as patterns are uncovered (Kaufman et al., 2010).

Autosomal Dominant

An autosomal disorder refers to any chromosomal disorder, other than sex chromosomes. There are over 1400 autosomal causes of intellectual disabilities (Tan et al., 2015). Autosomal dominant conditions are caused by the inheritance of a disease, condition, or trait that is transmitted through only one parent. Because people affected with autosomal dominant intellectual disabilities are unlikely to procreate, the causes of the genetic abnormalities are most frequently de novo (i.e. spontaneously arising and due to mutation) in nature. Autosomal dominant conditions are syndromal and relatively common and have been well understood for some time. However, there have been significant advances in some of our understanding of the long-term development for persons with autosomal dominant conditions. Some examples are provided in Table 2.1.

Autosomal Recessive

Autosomal recessive conditions are caused by the inheritance of a disease, condition, or trait transmitted through both parents. Autosomal recessive causes of intellectual disabilities are more common in cases of consanguinity and restricted gene pools (Harripaul et al., 2017). Most autosomal recessive causes of intellectual disabilities are non-syndromic (Harripaul et al., 2017). Quite likely, a large percentage of persons with idiopathic causes of intellectual disabilities have some form of autosomal recessive condition (Lee et al., 2014). A well-mapped example of an autosomal recessive condition is Carpenter syndrome (Jenkins et al., 2007). Research and clinical practice is improving dramatically in this area with at least 94 candidate genes to date being identified as potential loci of autosomal recessive conditions that can result in intellectual disabilities (Harripaul et al., 2017).

Table 2.1 Examples of Autosomal Dominant Conditions

Name	Sample citation	Mechanism	Primary signs	Prevalence
Tuberous sclerosis	Ridler et al. (2007)	9q34 16p13.3	Benign tumours in the central nervous system and vital organs	1 in 12,500
Neurofibromatosis	North et al. (1997)	17q11.2	Benign tumours in the central nervous system, café au lait spots	1 in 3500
Myotonic dystrophy	Meola and Cardani (2015)	19q13.32 3q21.3	Muscular disorders, motor issues	1 in 8000
Rubinstein-Taybi syndrome	Wójcik et al. (2010)	16p13.3	Short stature, distinctive facial features, broad thumbs and toes	1 in 125,000

Table 2.2 Examples of Trisomies and Sex Chromosomal Causes

Name	Sample citation	Mechanism	Primary signs	Prevalence
Down syndrome	Patterson (2009)	Trisomy 21	Growth delays, hypotonia, characteristic facial features	1 in 700
Edwards syndrome	Papp et al. (2007)	Trisomy 18	Heart defects, microcephaly, overlapping fingers	1 in 5000
Patau syndrome	Janvier, Farlow, and Wilfond (2012)	Trisomy 13	Microcephaly, holoprosencephaly (failure of the forebrain to divide properly)	1 in 20,000
Turner syndrome	Donaldson, Gault, Tan, and Dunger (2006)	45, X	Webbed neck, short stature, heart defects	1 in 2500 females
Klinefelter syndrome	Visootsak, Aylstock, and Graham (2001)	XXY	Symptoms usually noticed initially at puberty: Sterility, low muscle tone	1 in 800 males

Others

To some degree, differentiating between dominant and recessive autosomal causes is an artificial categorization. The terms dominant and recessive are reserved for traits that can be transmitted from parents to child (i.e. Mendelian inheritance; Redin et al., 2014). In many cases, there is mutation that damages chromosomal structures and that mutation cannot be found in the DNA of either parent (Vissers, Gilissen, & Veltman, 2016). In common cases, there is not a specific set of genes that is involved but an abnormal number of chromosomes (i.e. aneuploidy). These abnormalities may be in the autosomal or in the sex chromosomes (Vissers et al., 2016). Some examples are reported in Table 2.2.

X-Linked Inheritance

X-linked inheritance is similar in some respects to autosomal recessive conditions. Because the gene in question is located on the X chromosome, anomalies on the X chromosome are manifest in males because they have only one copy of the X chromosome (Ge, Kwok, & Shieh, 2015; Lubs, Stevenson, & Schwartz, 2012). Females are typically considered to be carriers and only manifest the results of the genetic anomaly when there are two affected X chromosomes (exactly as in an autosomal recessive characteristic). There are dozens of X-linked inheritance causes of intellectual disabilities (Møller et al., 2013). Some examples are provided in Table 2.3.

Mitochondrial Disorders

Mitochondrial disorders are chronic, genetic disorders that occur when the mitochondria of the cell fail to produce enough energy for cell or organ function (Valenti, de Bari, De Filippis, Henrion-Caude, & Vacca, 2014). Mitochondrial diseases can develop because of mitochondrial (mtDNA) or nuclear DNA (nDNA) mutations;

Table 2.3 Examples of X-linked Disorders

Name	Sample citation	Mechanism	Primary signs	Prevalence
Fragile X syndrome	Bassell and Warren (2008)	Xq27.3	Delayed speech, long and narrow face, large ears	1 in 4000 males 1 in 8000 females
Aarskog-Scott syndrome	Pilozzi-Edmonds et al. (2011)	Xp11.21	Short stature, facial abnormalities	1 in 1,000,000
Coffin-Lowry syndrome	Rojnueangnit, Jones, Basehore, and Robin (2014)	Xp22.2	Microcephaly, small jaw, cardiac abnormalities	1 in 40,000
MAO-A deficiency behaviour	Vishnivetskaya, Skrinskaya, Seif, and Popova (2007)	Xp11.3	Extreme aggression, often does not cause intellectual disabilities	Wide variety depending on alleles affected
Glycerol kinase deficiency	Rahib, MacLennan, Horvath, Liao, and Dipple (2007)	Xp22.3	Strabismus, seizures, general abnormalities	1 in 1700
Rett syndrome	Hardwick et al. (2007)	Xq28	Short stature, hypotonia, language delay, motor delay	1 in 10,000 females

however, in many cases, no mutations are found (Wortmann, Koolen, Smeitink, van den Heuvel, & Rodenburg, 2015). These mutations are uncommon in the general population and have an estimated prevalence of around one in 8500 (Wortmann et al., 2015). Persons with intellectual disabilities and a mitochondrial disease generally present several symptoms that are rarely observed in idiopathic intellectual disabilities, which can include tremor, ataxia, pancreatic or liver dysfunction, cardiac or haematological alterations, growth retardation, and/or ophthalmological or auditory signs. Mitochondrial disorders typically lead to overall metabolic disorders that affect multiple organ systems in addition to the brain (Wortmann et al., 2015). In some cases, other identified genetic disorders such as Down syndrome and fragile X syndrome have affected mitochondrial functioning. However, other idiopathic causes of intellectual disabilities may have their primary roots in disorders of mitochondria (Valenti et al., 2014). Children with intellectual disabilities or autism with tremors, hypertonia, and other muscular and motor issues may benefit from assessment for mitochondrial disorder (e.g. muscle biopsy; He et al., 2014). Overall development, medical status, and multiple organ systems are affected in addition to the central nervous system.

Metabolic Syndromes

The two most common metabolic syndromes are Tay-Sachs syndrome and PKU (Antoni et al., 2014). Both causes result in metabolic conditions involving the processing of amino acids. The failure to process these amino acids effective leads to accumulation of toxic substances that leads to impairment of function of the central nervous system (Wortmann et al., 2015).

Micro-Deletion Syndromes

Micro-deletion syndromes are caused by chromosomal deletions less than five million base pairs (5 Mb) and are typically too small to be detected by high-resolution karyotyping or conventional cytogenetic methods of detection (Rump et al., 2016). However, most micro-deletion syndromes are also autosomal dominant in nature (Gilissen et al., 2014). They are distinguished from the above-described autosomal dominant syndromes by the methods used to detect them. There are an extraordinarily large number of micro-deletion syndromes, many of which may have only a few known cases. Uncovering of micro-deletion syndromes has been a major factor in determining causes of intellectual disabilities that were previously considered idiopathic or without known cause (de Ligt et al., 2012). Micro-deletion syndromes are also either autosomal dominant or autosomal recessive (Coe et al., 2014). However, for terms of classification, they are considered a different category than the autosomal causes of intellectual disabilities listed above.

There are well over 900 micro-deletion syndromes that have been identified (Boycott, Vanstone, Bulman, & MacKenzie, 2013). As the quality of clinical and laboratory assessment continues to improve, it is quite likely that the number of identified micro-deletion syndromes will increase dramatically. Some syndromes are quite common, and other syndromes may have had only two or three confirmed clinical cases reported (Carvalho et al., 2014). Table 2.4 catalogues the 12 most common micro-deletion syndromes.

Multifactorial and Polygenetic Causes

Multifactorial and polygenic disorders are the most common causes of mild intellectual disabilities (Lelieveld et al., 2016). Rather than being caused by a single genetic mutation or other anomaly, low general intelligence tends to run in families with multiple generations being affected by low levels of functional and adaptive behaviour (Magnin et al., 2014). Quite likely, multiple genes are involved in this process (Larson, 2007). In addition, persons with low general mental ability are frequently of low socioeconomic status with low levels of intellectual stimulation creating a situation where there are multiple contributing factors in the functional outcome of intellectual disability (Palmer et al., 2014).

Environmental Causes

Although genetics and neuroscience are areas most associated with research advances in intellectual disabilities, environmental causes remain important considerations for research and practice (Emerson, 2007).

The prenatal period begins at conception and extends through at least 22 weeks of gestation (Heuvelman et al., 2017). This period is generally divided into three stages: the germinal stage, the embryonic stage, and the fetal stage. Most prenatal

Table 2.4 Examples of Microdeletion Disorders

Name	Sample citation	Location	Primary signs	Prevalence
Velocardiofacial syndrome (DiGeorge syndrome)	Kobrynski and Sullivan (2007)	22q11	Cardiac defects, cleft palate	1 in 4000
Williams syndrome	Morris (2010)	7q11.23	Characteristic facial features, cardiac abnormalities, overly friendly	1 in 12,000
Prader-Willi syndrome	Clark et al. (1995)	15q11.23 (paternal)	Hypotonia, obesity	1 in 20,000
Angelman syndrome	Williams et al. (2006)	15q11.23 (maternal)	Lack of speech, stiff smiling, small head	1 in 20,000
Wolf Hirschhorn syndrome	Dufke et al. (2000)	4p16.3	Microcephaly, hypotonia, seizures	1 in 95,896
Smith-Magenis syndrome	Girirajan et al. (2006)	17p11.2	Deep set eyes, sleep disturbance, aggression	1 in 25,000
17q21.31 micro-deletion syndrome	Koolen et al. (2006)	17q21.31	Low birth weight, low muscle tone, poor feeding	1 in 16,000
Phelan-McDermid syndrome	Wilson et al. (2003)	22q13.3	Microcephaly, esophageal reflux	2% of people diagnosed with autism spectrum disorder and intellectual disabilities
Cri du chat syndrome	Sheth et al. (2012)	5p15.2	Characteristic crying, feeding problems, low birth weight	1 in 50,000
1p36 syndrome	Battaglia et al. (2008)	1p36	Hypotonia, seizures, limited speech	1 in 5000

causes of intellectual disabilities during the prenatal period are genetic in nature that typically influence the germinal and embryonic stages (Huang, Zhu, Qu, & Mu, 2016). However, there are environmental prenatal causes as well. The most common problems are fetal alcohol effects. Prenatal ingestion of alcohol is the leading preventable cause of intellectual disabilities (Strandberg-Larsen, Andersen, & Kesmodel, 2017). Malnutrition, maternal cigarette smoking, environmental toxins (especially heavy metal exposure), and maternal illness (such as toxoplasmosis, rubella, syphilis) are other environmental causes that occur during the prenatal period (Mann et al., 2009; Shah, 1991). Most environmental causes of intellectual disabilities that occur during the prenatal period can be prevented via improved maternal nutrition, early screening and treatment of maternal illness, and cessation of smoking, alcohol, and drug intake (O'Leary et al., 2013).

Perinatal causes of intellectual disabilities have decreased dramatically with improvements in obstetrics and education of expectant mothers (Landrigan,

Lambertini, & Birnbaum, 2012). The perinatal period is defined as the period immediately before and after the birth process. Although there are multiple definitions of the perinatal period, the World Health Organization defines the beginning of the perinatal period at approximately 22 weeks of gestation and ending approximately 1 week after birth (Shah, 1991). Problems that lead to intellectual disabilities that are associated with the perinatal period include low birth weight, birth asphyxia, a variety of birthing-related injuries, low birth weight, placenta previa, respiratory distress, infectious illness (especially pneumonia), fetal blood loss, neonatal jaundice, anemia hypothermia, and feeding problems (Adams et al., 1993; Baird & Sadovnick, 1985). Perinatal period excludes chromosomal abnormalities, nutritional issues, metabolic diseases, and external injuries (Kerr-Wilson, Mackay, Smith, & Pell, 2012). Effective prenatal nutrition, prenatal wellness visits, cessation of smoking, and improved obstetric care have all led to a decrease in the percentage of children diagnosed with intellectual disabilities that are directly attributable to perinatal causes. Current estimates are that approximately 9.5% of children with intellectual disabilities have the primary cause in perinatal events (Huang et al., 2016).

Postnatal causes of intellectual disabilities are also declining as a percentage (Huang et al., 2016). Common postnatal causes of intellectual disabilities include poisoning, accidents, injuries, infection and high fever, and malnutrition (van Bokhoven, 2011). Due to the proliferation of vaccines, childhood diseases such as measles, chickenpox, and mumps are far less common than they were 40 years ago (Decoufle & Boyle, 1995). Effective vaccines and treatments for hepatitis, meningitis, and encephalitis also reduce the number of children affected by high fevers (McLaren & Bryson, 1992). Fevers due to these childhood diseases were common causes of intellectual disabilities. These postnatal causes are now quite rare (Langridge et al., 2013). Parent education concerning storage of poisonous materials and prescription drugs is helpful in reducing postnatal causes. Brain injuries due to physical abuse are among the most common postnatal causes of intellectual disabilities. Shaken baby syndrome (SBS) remains a relatively common causal factor (Ludvigsson, 2017). The reported incidence of SBS ranges from 14 in100,000 to 40 in 100,000 children younger than 1 year old (Peterson et al., 2014). Postnatal causes of intellectual disabilities are estimated to range from 3% to 15% (Huang et al., 2016).

Advances in Practice

In practice, most parents want an answer to the question "Why?" It is extraordinarily frustrating when there is no answer for these parents. There is often guilt, family disruption, financial hardship, and intense fear related to a severe developmental problem with no known or communicated cause (Yang et al., 2013). For all the dramatic advances in the science of determining the genetic causes of intellectual disabilities, there is always a fundamental trade-off: Do the tests, many of which can be extremely expensive, result in improved outcomes for the child and the child's family? This is a complex question. Functionally, knowing the cause of intellectual disabilities does not always influence educational, psychological, or psychiatric treatment (Black, 2015). Sometimes tests can cost thousands of dollars and may or may not be covered by private or government insurance (Tzschach et al., 2015). As mentioned earlier, some cases may influence treatment or understanding of long-term development, yet many do not result in diagnosis-specific treatment (The Deciphering Developmental Disorders Study, 2015). The major question for many cases is determining how much "peace of mind" is worth to families. Moreover, genetic testing is often critical for genetic counselling (Bergen, 2008). There are also times where parents may feel guilty for contributing a genetic deletion or mutation to their child's outcome and wish to have firm answers at any cost. There are also practical issues for families. For example, knowledge that the cause of intellectual disabilities is something that can be transmitted reliably from parents (as opposed to a de novo mutation that is nearly random in transmission) may result in information concerning whether the family chooses to have additional children. Knowing exactly "why" a child has presented with intellectual disabilities often has limited utility. However there have been important influences in the areas of clinical genetics, genetic counselling, and psychology and education.

Advances in Technology, Screening, and Description of Behaviours

For educators and those providing interventions to children with intellectual disabilities and their families, the advances in genetics and neuroscience can be overwhelming. The relevance is often unclear. Moreover, there is often a great deal of hype and misleading overselling of scientific findings (Van den Veyver et al., 2009). Sometimes it can be discouraging to read that a new medication or new gene can be influenced and might provide a potential cure for intellectual disabilities or autism, only to find later that the study fails to be replicated or the ideas have only been attempted on mouse or computer models. Making things more challenging is that the technology of vocabulary of genetics and neuroscience studies is daunting.

Behavioural Phenotypes

Behavioural phenotypes are the expression of genotypes, in other words, exactly how all the different variations in genotype result in reliable and consistent patterns of behaviour (e.g. Tao et al., 2016). The course and presentation of behavioural phenotypes changes with development. Determining a characteristic pattern of medical, social, language, motor, and cognitive observations consistent with discrete genotypes is a valuable activity on many fronts (Scheepers et al., 2005). Most often, a constellation of behaviours and characteristics are observed, and then clinical geneticists work to identify the underlying genotype. However, with advances in screening and genetic testing, the reverse often occurs. That is, a specific genotype is identified from which predictable characteristics and behaviours can be predicted. In this fashion, educational, medical, and behavioural interventions can be developed to address problematic areas as early as possible. There is also the real possibility that interventions can be developed that may serve a prophylactic function and reduce the presence or severity of common behaviours before they occur. For example, for tuberous sclerosis, seizures become more common for some persons as they develop into later childhood (Ridler et al., 2007). Identification and control of seizures before they become problematic or lead to a progressive degeneration of cognitive skills can prevent some of the more severe cognitive outcomes. Likewise, in the case of children with Prader-Willi syndrome, interventions involving dietary management and anxiety-related issues can take place as early as infancy so that preventative forms of interventions can take place (Clark et al., 1995). There is much research to do in this area, and there are a wide variety of behavioural phenotypes for discrete genotypes, making generalization and treatment direction challenging. However, for teachers, therapists, and others providing interventions for children, behavioural phenotypes represent a mechanism by which complex research plays a fundamental role in the treatment and intervention development (e.g. Zarchi et al., 2014).

Genetic Testing

The majority of scientific and clinical advances is in genetic testing (Yang et al., 2013). The major diagnostic challenge is that presentation and behavioural phenotypes vary to such a large degree that clinical diagnosis is often impossible (Musante & Ropers, 2014). Due to advances in genetic testing, there are far fewer children with intellectual disabilities without an identified etiology than in the past. In a qualitative study of the reasons why families desire to have an etiological diagnosis made, the most common reasons were validation of the established problem as intellectual disability; information to help guide expectation and management, to acquire educational and habilitative services, and to develop emotional companionship with families experiencing similar problems with similar diagnoses; a strong "need to know"; and prenatal testing to be aware of future risks for current and future children (Makela, Birch, Friedman, & Marra, 2009). A secondary, but still important issue, is that advances in science have led to the reduction in costs of genetic testing due to increased efficiency (Vissers et al., 2016). However, there are still some geographic regions with limited access to laboratories that can conduct some genetic tests.

Based on guidelines developed by Moeschler, Shevell, and the AAP Committee on Genetics (2014), the most common approach to genetic testing is as follows:

Chromosome microarray (CMA) is now the first-line clinical diagnostic test for children presenting with intellectual disabilities (Palmer et al., 2014). This test supersedes standard karyotyping and fluorescent in situ hybridization sub-telomere tests, which were long the first line of genetic testing and still have significant supplementary value. This test can be done prenatally or postnatally. CMA represents significant advantages over standard karyotyping in that small deletions and duplications can often be detected with CMA that were nearly impossible to identify with standard karyotyping. Because CMA provides opportunities to consider multiple loci in one genome, interpretation of results can be difficult. Most typically a clinical geneticist works with the general pediatrician to interpret results. Interpretations of the copy number variants (CNV; i.e. deletions, duplications, or amplification at any specific locus) typically come back as either pathogenic, variants of unknown significance, or likely benign. Moreover, likely pathogenic reports from the CMA do not speak to the presenting severity of intellectual disability (Yang et al., 2013).

The second area is to screen for inborn errors of metabolism. As many as 1–5% of persons with intellectual disabilities have an identifiable metabolic disorder (Willemsen & Kleefstra, 2014). Although a low percentage, identifying metabolic disorders as early as possible can be critically important because many of these can be treated and have a resulting improved outcome. As such urinary screen for amino acids, organic acids, oligosaccharides, acid mucopolysaccharides, and uric acid and a serum test to screen for congenital disorders of glycosylation (Rahib et al., 2007) are often recommended. These are relatively simple and inexpensive laboratory tests that can be done in local hospital laboratories. Given the possibility that such disorders of metabolism can lead to an improved outcome, such assessment is widely recommended.

Genetic Screening and Testing

Prenatal screening for Down syndrome has been used for approximately 30 years (Tan et al., 2015). Analysis of specific analytes and maternal serum and ultrasound findings in the first or second trimester provide a risk estimate for Down syndrome and Edwards syndrome (trisomy 18). In addition, universal parental carrier screening for autosomal recessive disorder such as cystic fibrosis and ethnicity-based carrier screening such as for Tay-Sachs has been the most formal type of prenatal screening (Valenti et al., 2014). Technological advances in screening such as CMA and next-generation sequencing allow for screening and diagnosis of genetic abnormalities in the fetus (Atwal et al., 2014; Boycott et al., 2013). Hundreds of disorders such as fetal chromosomal aneuploidy (i.e. extra or missing chromosomes), some microdeletion syndromes, and some single-gene disorders can be identified routinely through genetic screening. Samples taken from amniocentesis and analysed via chromosome microarray analysis can be highly sensitive to minute chromosomal abnormalities that were not possible a few years ago with routine karyotyping (i.e.

chromosome analysis and mapping; Coe et al., 2014). Fluorescent in situ hybridization can also be employed to look for locus-specific chromosomal abnormalities. The challenge with this method is that the suspected location of the chromosomal abnormality must be identified in advance so the analysis knows exactly where to look.

Finding a Cure or Cause

Advances in understanding the causes of intellectual disabilities are unlikely to create a situation where there will be a cure for intellectual disabilities (Kaufman et al., 2010). Parents often place pressure on professionals to find a magic bullet or cure. There have been advances that have led valuable treatments that have reduced symptoms related to genetic causes of intellectual disabilities such as in the case of PKU (Kahn et al., 2016). Yet, in most cases, the advancement in understanding the causes will contribute to improving the quality of life for persons with intellectual disabilities and their families (Kahn et al., 2016). Providing support and comfort and reducing the severity of symptoms have all improved dramatically due to improved understanding of the cause and development of specific issues related to intellectual disabilities.

There is an oversimplification of genetic causes of intellectual disabilities and the relationship to a cure. A common belief is that if we completely understand the damage involved in a translocation, deletion, inversion, or duplication within a chromosome, future advances in genetics will be able to edit or otherwise fix that chromosome resulting in reduction of symptoms and a possible cure. To some degree, efforts to find a cure to intellectual disabilities are something like attempting to find cures for cancer. There is not a single type of intellectual disability with a single cause; there are hundreds, if not thousands, of causes and subtypes of intellectual disabilities. The probability is that dramatic advances in science, especially genetics, will be able to cure, prevent, or ameliorate each cause, albeit one at a time.

Even within a single micro-deletion disorder, there are magnitudes of complexity (Harripaul et al., 2017). Chromosomes may deviate from typical through heredity or mutation. Those deviations may be in the form of duplication, deletions of varying sizes, translocation (i.e. exchange of chromosomal material from one location to another), inversion (i.e. chromosomal material exist in reverse sequence), mosaic (i.e. some cells contain the atypical chromosome and some cells do not), and from which parent the disorder is inherited. These forms of a single gene disorder results in a variety of proteins that may be missing, disordered, or otherwise deviating from normal. Multiple proteins may interact, creating a new set of problems. The proteins created have a profound effect on energy metabolism (Au, Argiropoulos, Parboosingh, & Micheil Innes, 2014). These effects of energy metabolism can affect any organ structures and varied components of the central nervous system. Finally, changes in metabolism affect phenotypic expression of the genes. In each segment from chromosomal integrity to protein creation to metabolism to phenotypes, the variation grows increasingly diverse and complex. This level of complexity is within a single-gene defect. Given that there are at least hundreds of different genetic causes of intellectual disabilities, search for a cure is daunting.

For example, in the case of 22q13.3 deletion syndrome, the size of the deletion on the tip of the chromosome varies dramatically among individuals with this diagnosis. The size of the deletion ranges from 130 kb to over 9 Mb (Phelan et al., 2001). Therefore, the number of genes involved in this broad genetic diagnosis varies significantly as the breakpoint for the deletion is different for each person. The 22nd chromosome is completely mapped, and so the exact genes and locations, the proteins created by each gene, metabolism addressed by each gene, and the phenotypic response are often well-known. In this case, the gene entitled SHANK3 is on the very tip (i.e. telomere) of the chromosome, and all people diagnosed with this condition have only a single functional copy that does not produce effective proteins. This is known as haploinsufficiency, which is defined as when an organism has a single functional copy of a gene and that single copy does not produce enough product (i.e. protein) to display the phenotypic characteristics. SHANK3 is expressed as a structural and metabolism protein that involves the postsynaptic bouton (Wilson et al., 2003). The problem is that when the deletion creates haploinsufficiency of SHANK3, the ability of neural circuitry to accept neurotransmitters, specifically glutamate, is significantly impaired. Much of that impairment is concentrated in the hippocampus, an important neural structure in the formation and recall of memory (Wilson et al., 2003). The functional result is that the ability to learn is dramatically impaired for all persons with 22q13.3 deletion. However, there is some diversity of phenotype.

The effects of the size of the deletion depend upon which genes are affected. Some people with 22q13.3 deletion also have affected genes that have been associated with autism spectrum disorder, bipolar disorder, schizophrenia, learning disabilities, and a host of physical conditions as well (Wilson et al., 2003). Moreover, there are also a variety of alleles (i.e. alternate forms of each gene). Although 22q13.3 deletion syndrome is one of the simple micro-deletion syndromes, quickly it becomes clear that how many genes are impaired, which alleles are expressed, how deletions interact, how some of the basic genes deleted affect metabolism and protein creation, and how these deletions interact with environmental features and the variation in behaviours among people with 22q13 deletion syndrome are extraordinary. There have been successful efforts to create a mouse model with 22q13 deletion (Peça et al., 2011). The hope is that a mouse model could create a treatment or cure for intellectual disabilities. The effectiveness and value of a mouse model for such a low incidence genetic disorder are not entirely clear but is likely a valuable step forward. Development of a cure for persons affected by 22q13 deletion is far away, if it is possible at all. Nonetheless, there is a far higher likelihood that symptoms can be ameliorated and quality of life improved than an absolute cure be developed (Wilson et al., 2003).

Translating Basic Science to Classroom and Therapy

The basic science that has made such large gains in understanding the causes of intellectual disabilities can be overwhelming. Hundreds of papers every year make startling advances with important implications for screening, prevention, assessment, and treatment. The challenges in translating knowledge from basic or "blue sky" science to real-world interventions that can positively affect the lives of persons with intellectual disabilities, their families, and their communities are complex. Rather than being completely overwhelmed by the information, the vast amount of new information that no one person could effectively integrate necessarily means that multiple professionals must be involved in all treatment planning and execution. The massive influx of complex findings in the areas of genetics, epidemiology, and neuroscience requires an increasingly diverse group of professionals addressing functional impairments of persons with intellectual disabilities.

Once a professional knows why new research around causes and symptoms needs to be read and interpreted and understands exactly what those new findings are, the next difficult question is to understand how this is relevant to the practice of providing educational and psychological services to persons with intellectual disabilities (O'Brien, 2006).

No matter the causes of the intellectual disabilities, for the information to translate to the classroom, functional outcomes are the primary areas of interest (e.g. Maurin, Zongaro, & Bardoni, 2014). Yet, knowing the probability of specific functional issues, behavioural phenotype, and developmental course can assist in planning and allocation of resources for treatment. Typically, there are six major domains that describe functional outcomes for persons with intellectual disabilities:

1. *Severity of intellectual disabilities*. The significance of the impairment is also an important factor for determining the levels of support required for functioning effectively in schools and in daily living.
2. *Behavioural issues*. The frequency, severity, and duration of maladaptive behaviours are critical factors in any type of treatment plan. Due to limited social and language issues, any form of treatment requires some method of targeting prosocial skills. Some specific genetic disorders have high probabilities of mental health issues such as anxiety, depression, and thought disorders with identifiable genetic origins. However, persons with impaired language skills, reasoning skills, and social skills are also at extraordinarily high risk for maladaptive behaviours.
3. *Sensory disabilities*. Vision and hearing impairment are common across a variety of genetic disorders yet are extraordinarily difficult to assess in children with moderate to severe intellectual disabilities. Effective assessment of sensory issues is always a critical factor in planning any form of intervention.
4. *Motor impairment*. A host of motor issues including hypotonia, apraxia, motor spasticity, and other issues affects ambulation, orientation, speech, and manual manipulation of the environment. Most treatment plans will involve active

involvement or consultation with physical therapists, physiologists, and occupational therapists.

5. *Medical fragility*. Genetic and environmental issues that cause central nervous system damage to the point that there is intellectual impairment necessarily have negative outcomes for overall health. The more severe the impairment in intellectual functioning, the more likely there is to be structural neurological issues that can lead to seizure disorders and epileptiform seizures that are challenging to control. Many genetic disorders have midline impairments that affect heart, lungs, and digestive system. For purposes of educational treatment planning, limitations and accommodations to address medical fragility are worthy of placing in a formal treatment plan.
6. *Autistic features*. Due to sociological and diagnostic issues, more persons with intellectual disabilities receive a diagnosis of autism in addition to or instead of a diagnosis of intellectual disabilities. For purposes of treatment planning, social interaction, language skills, and stereotyped and restricted interests are common targets of intervention that are worthy of being addressed whether the diagnosis of autism is present or not.

Team Membership

The complexity of available information requires a team of experts to develop an effective educational and therapeutic program. Teamwork is always complex (see Chaps. 5 and 6), yet most people with intellectual disabilities have issues involving multiple domains. Improved understanding of the causes of intellectual disabilities can support the development of an effective multidisciplinary or interdisciplinary team (see Chap. 6).

Medical

The increase in genetics and neuroscience findings has implicated a variety of medical professionals that are important in the assessment and treatment of persons with intellectual disabilities. However, identifying exactly which subspecialties are relevant can be challenging.

Psychiatrists are physicians with specialization in medical management of mental health and psychiatric disorders. Persons with intellectual disabilities often have comorbid psychiatric issues as well, yet diagnosis of psychiatric issues in persons with significant cognitive impairments presents a variety of challenges. Rarely do psychiatrists have significant expertise for persons with intellectual disabilities, but such professionals can be extraordinarily useful in developing complex medical interventions.

Developmental pediatricians have expertise in developmental disorders affecting children. Developmental pediatricians have strong skills in medical management of behavioural and health issues for persons with disabilities. They frequently prescribe medications related to behaviour management like psychiatrists. In most cases, developmental pediatricians are ideal professionals to address the medical and behavioural issues of children with intellectual disabilities.

Pediatric neurologists have specialized training in developmental issues related to central nervous system disorders. Most often this subspecialty is valuable in assessing and treating seizure disorders, which are common for many types of intellectual disabilities. They also provide expertise in related issues such as stroke/infarct, corpus callosum agenesis, other atypical anatomical development, and infections related to the central nervous system. Pediatric neurologist may work closely with neurosurgeons and psychiatrists to provide comprehensive treatment to anatomical and physiological disorders in the central nervous system.

Clinical Genetics

Clinical geneticists are a subspecialty of physicians with expertise in identifying specific genetic disorders. They often work closely with genetic counsellors, pediatricians, neurologists, occupational therapist, speech and language pathologist, psychologists, and other diagnostic professionals. Clinical geneticists have an extreme challenge of staying current with the massive amounts of research that are currently being produced, especially around micro-deletion syndromes and the ability of cytology and genetics laboratories to test for newly developed syndromes (Van den Veyver, 2016). For purposes of treatment planning, clinical geneticists are extremely helpful in communicating developmental trajectories and behavioural phenotypes for specific disorders. This role has not been a traditional part of the clinical geneticists roll because of the dearth of information on developmental trajectories and behavioural phenotypes. However, because of the recent advancements in these fields, the ability of clinical geneticists to contribute to treatment planning has grown.

Other medical professionals may be involved as several genetic disorders are known to affect kidneys, liver, heart, digestive tract, musculature, and skeletal systems. An often forgotten professional in delivering medical services is dentistry. Plastic and oral surgeons are also helpful in addressing corrective issues related to cleft palate, which are common in disorders affecting midline such as 22q11 deletion disorder (i.e. velocardial facial disorder) (Kobrynski & Sullivan, 2007). Children with intellectual disabilities frequently lack the ability to communicate location of dental pain, which leads to distress and self-injurious behaviours. Dentists with specialties in addressing the needs of persons with intellectual disabilities are valuable members of medical teams.

Genetic Counselling

The advances in the science of detection of genetic disorders have profound influence on the field of genetic counselling. Genetic counselling involves families consulting with professionals with specialized education to make personalized decisions concerning genetic health. The extraordinary advances in genetic causes of intellectual disabilities provide a great deal of information to genetic counsellors. Among the many outstanding services are to discuss options concerning future pregnancies, may advise families on genetic testing to better understand familial origin of intellectual disabilities, may provide information on the likely developmental issues to be anticipated for children with intellectual disabilities, and have expertise in communicating complex genetic information to families. In many cases, genetic counsellors can provide important information to other therapists, psychologists, and educators. Genetic counselling remains a relatively small field with approximately 5000 practitioners (Stern, 2012). Historically, genetic counsellors provided valuable information around cancer risks and other medical issues with high risk of genetic transmission. Given the advances in knowledge concerning intellectual disabilities, genetic counsellors are now an essential opponent of the care and treatment team providing information and services to children, families, schools, and communities.

Psychology

Psychologists serve several functions on care and treatment teams for persons with intellectual disabilities. Among the most common roles for psychologists in treatment planning are the assessment of cognitive and behavioural functioning and the use of applied behaviour analysis to assist in the development of interventions for specific behaviours (Poncela-Casasnovas et al., 2016). However, roles can cover diverse domains such as parent education, sibling adjustment, daily living skills such as toilet training, neuropsychological assessment, individual or group counselling therapies, and many other domains (see Chap. 6). Psychologists frequently serve as liaison between medical and educational professionals. Many psychologists have developed the skills to effectively communicate medical findings to educational professionals.

Education

Children spend more time in schools than any other environment, except the home. Teachers have more opportunities to influence treatment programming than any other professional. As school-based treatment programs involve the development of an individualized educational plan, the teacher is often responsible for coordinating and carrying out the aspects of the plan. Treatment planning is most effective when those carrying out the plan have input in ownership into the details of treatment. The details of new research in genetics are typically beyond the training of most teachers. Yet, research in developmental trajectories and behavioural phenotypes provide important information for teachers to address the day-to-day needs of children with intellectual disabilities and to create the most effective possible treatment plans from a school setting.

Research

Investigations continue and are growing into understanding the causes, symptoms, and diagnoses of intellectual disabilities (Heuvelman et al., 2017). There are many avenues of research being pursued at high rates with potential to greatly influence the lives of persons with intellectual disabilities (Moeschler et al., 2014). Although all are potentially useful, the most immediately applicable involves early diagnosis to develop and apply the most effective early interventions with the purpose of ameliorating symptoms. Some examples include universal screening for phenylketonuria (PKU) (Kahn et al., 2016). Positive screen for PKU will result in administering a diet low in phenylalanine (an amino acid necessary for normal growth and development and found in high protein foods such as meat, dairy, and nuts). With strong adherence to diet, the major effects of PKU, which include brain damage, seizures, and intellectual disabilities, can be minimized to a great degree (Murgia & Adamski, 2017). With advanced research, perhaps other causes of intellectual disabilities can be identified that can be effectively treated and dramatically ameliorated. Increasingly efficient and sensitive tests for micro-deletion disorders are being developed rapidly. Moreover, understanding the long-term development of persons with a variety of micro-deletion syndromes can provide understanding of exactly what to expect, provide ideas as to ameliorative or anticipatory forms of therapy to be implemented, and provide knowledge to families to improve familial adjustment to having children with intellectual disabilities (Crocker, Prokić, Morin, & Reyes, 2014). Ultimately, the goal of research is to develop preventative and curative therapies. Whether prevention or cure is possible for all causes of intellectual disabilities is unlikely. Nonetheless, sophisticated research continues to result in findings that, when interpreted and implemented appropriately, can improve the quality of life for all persons with intellectual disabilities.

Conclusions

Commenting on the massive advances in the understanding of the causes, symptoms, and diagnosis of intellectual disabilities can only be a drop in the ocean. There is a large amount of information coming from multiple sources in this area. Clinical and molecular genetics alone results in hundreds of new studies each year. Many of the studies have profound implications for the types of testing for intellectual disabilities that can be considered.

Despite these advances there is no cure for most genetic causes of intellectual disabilities. Advances may lead to improved treatment of symptoms, preventative medical and behavioural therapies, and understanding of family transmission of genetic disorders. Yet, many parents are looking for a cure for their child's developmental disabilities. At this point, these parents are likely to be disappointed. Most treatments for children with developmental disabilities will depend on their functional impairment rather than the causal mechanisms. Despite the leaps made in understanding the causes of intellectual disabilities, these are only the beginning stages of this research and improve knowledge base. Although breakthroughs and specific treatments based on these findings are possible, direct influence of the knowledge of the causes of intellectual disabilities on educational and psychological interventions is currently limited.

References

Adams, W. G., Deaver, K. A., Cochi, S. L., Plikaytis, B. D., Zell, E. R., Broome, C. V., & Wenger, J. D. (1993). Decline of childhood Haemophilus influenzae type b (Hib) disease in the Hib vaccine era. *Journal of the American Medical Association, 269*, 221–226.

Antoni, S. D., Spatuzza, M., Bonaccorso, C. M., Musumeci, S. A., Ciranna, L., Nicoletti, F., … Catania, M. V. (2014). Dysregulation of group-I metabotropic glutamate (mGlu) receptor mediated signalling in disorders associated with intellectual disability and autism. *Neuroscience & Biobehavioral Reviews, 46*(Pt. 2), 228–241. https://doi.org/10.1016/j.neubiorev.2014.02.003

Atwal, P. S., Brennan, M.-L., Cox, R., Niaki, M., Platt, J., Homeyer, M., … Hudgins, L. (2014). Clinical whole-exome sequencing: Are we there yet? *Genetics in Medicine, 16*(9), 717–719. https://doi.org/10.1038/gim.2014.10

Au, P. Y. B., Argiropoulos, B., Parboosingh, J. S., & Micheil Innes, A. (2014). Refinement of the critical region of 1q41q42 microdeletion syndrome identifies FBXO28 as a candidate causative gene for intellectual disability and seizures. *American Journal of Medical Genetics Part A, 164*(2), 441–448. https://doi.org/10.1002/ajmg.a.36320

Baird, P. A., & Sadovnick, A. D. (1985). Mental retardation in over half-a-million consecutive livebirths: An epidemiological study. *American Journal of Mental Deficiency, 89*, 323–330.

Bassell, G. J., & Warren, S. T. (2008). Fragile X Syndrome: Loss of local mRNA regulation alters synaptic development and function. *Neuron, 60*(2), 201–214. https://doi.org/10.1016/j.neuron.2008.10.004

Battaglia, A., Hoyme, H. E., Dallapiccola, B., Zackai, E., Hudgins, L., McDonald-McGinn, D., … Carey, J. C. (2008). Further delineation of deletion 1p36 syndrome in 60 patients: A recognizable phenotype and common cause of developmental delay and mental retardation. *Pediatrics, 121*(2), 404–410. https://doi.org/10.1542/peds.2007-0929

Bergen, D. C. (2008). Effects of poverty on cognitive function: A hidden neurologic epidemic. *Neurology, 71*, 447–451.

Black, M. (2015). Genetic causes of intellectual disability in a birth cohort: A population-based study. *American Journal of Medical Genetics Part A, 167*(6), 1204–1214. https://doi.org/10.1002/ajmg.a.37011

Boycott, K. M., Vanstone, M. R., Bulman, D. E., & MacKenzie, A. E. (2013). Rare-disease genetics in the era of next-generation sequencing: Discovery to translation. *Nature Reviews Genetics, 14*(10), 681–691. https://doi.org/10.1038/nrg3555

Burnett, L. C., LeDuc, C. A., Sulsona, C. R., Paull, D., Rausch, R., Eddiry, S., … Leibel, R. L. (2017). Deficiency in prohormone convertase PC1 impairs prohormone processing in Prader-Willi syndrome. *The Journal of Clinical Investigation, 127*(1), 293–305. https://doi.org/10.1172/JCI88648

Carvalho, C. M. B., Vasanth, S., Shinawi, M., Russell, C., Ramocki, M. B., Brown, C. W., … Lupski, J. R. (2014). Dosage changes of a segment at 17p13.1 lead to intellectual disability and microcephaly as a result of complex genetic interaction of multiple genes. *The American Journal of Human Genetics, 95*(5), 565–578. https://doi.org/10.1016/j.ajhg.2014.10.006

Clark, D. J., Boer, H., & Webb, T. (1995). General and behavioural aspects of PWS: A review. *Mental Health Research, 8*, 38–49.

Coe, B. P., Witherspoon, K., Rosenfeld, J. A., van Bon, B. W. M., Vulto-van Silfhout, A. T., Bosco, P., … Eichler, E. E. (2014). Refining analyses of copy number variation identifies specific genes associated with developmental delay. *Nature Genetics, 46*(10), 1063–1071. https://doi.org/10.1038/ng.3092

Crocker, A. G., Prokić, A., Morin, D., & Reyes, A. (2014). Intellectual disability and co-occurring mental health and physical disorders in aggressive behaviour. *Journal of Intellectual Disability Research, 58*(11), 1032–1044. https://doi.org/10.1111/jir.12080

de Ligt, J., Willemsen, M. H., van Bon, B. W. M., Kleefstra, T., Yntema, H. G., Kroes, T., … Vissers, L. E. L. M. (2012). Diagnostic exome sequencing in persons with severe intellectual disability. *New England Journal of Medicine, 367*(20), 1921–1929. https://doi.org/10.1056/NEJMoa1206524

Decoufle, F., & Boyle, C. A. (1995). The relationship between maternal education and mental retardation in 10-year-old children. *Annals of Epidemiology, 4*, 347–353.

Donaldson, M. D. C., Gault, E. J., Tan, K. W., & Dunger, D. B. (2006). Optimising management in Turner syndrome: From infancy to adult transfer. *Archives of Disease in Childhood, 91*(6), 513–520. https://doi.org/10.1136/adc.2003.035907

Dufke, A., Seidel, J., Schöning, M., Döbler-Neumann, M., Kelbova, C., Liehr, T., … Enders, H. (2000). Microdeletion 4p16.3 in three unrelated patients with Wolf-Hirschhorn syndrome. *Cytogenetic and Genome Research, 91*(1–4), 81–84. https://doi.org/10.1159/000056823

Emerson, E. (2007). Poverty and people with intellectual disabilities. *Mental Retardation and Developmental Disabilities Research Review, 13*, 107–113. https://doi.org/10.1002/mrdd.20144

Ge, X., Kwok, P.-Y., & Shieh, J. T. C. (2015). Prioritizing genes for X-linked diseases using population exome data. *Human Molecular Genetics, 24*(3), 599–608. https://doi.org/10.1093/hmg/ddu473

Gilissen, C., Hehir-Kwa, J. Y., Thung, D. T., van de Vorst, M., van Bon, B. W. M., Willemsen, M. H., … Veltman, J. A. (2014). Genome sequencing identifies major causes of severe intellectual disability. *Nature, 511*, 344–347. https://doi.org/10.1038/nature13394

Girirajan, S., Vlangos, C. N., Szomju, B. B., Edelman, E., Trevors, C. D., Dupuis, L., … Elsea, S. H. (2006). Genotype–phenotype correlation in Smith-Magenis syndrome: Evidence that multiple genes in 17p11.2 contribute to the clinical spectrum. *Genetics in Medicine, 8*(7), 417–427. https://doi.org/10.1097/01.gim.0000228215.32110.89

Glover, G., Bernard, S., Branford, D., Holland, A., & Strydom, A. (2014). Use of medication for challenging behaviour in people with intellectual disability. *The British Journal of Psychiatry, 205*(1), 6–7. https://doi.org/10.1192/bjp.bp.113.141267

Hardwick, S. A., Reuter, K., Williamson, S. L., Vasudevan, V., Donald, J., Slater, K., … Christodoulou, J. (2007). Delineation of large deletions of the MECP2 gene in Rett syndrome patients, including a familial case with a male proband. *European Journal of Human Genetics, 15*(12), 1218–1229. https://doi.org/10.1038/sj.ejhg.520191

Harripaul, R., Vasli, N., Mikhailov, A., Rafiq, M. A., Mittal, K., Windpassinger, C., … Vincent, J. B. (2017). Mapping autosomal recessive intellectual disability: Combined microarray and exome sequencing identifies 26 novel candidate genes in 192 consanguineous families. *Molecular Psychiatry, 23*(4), 973–984. https://doi.org/10.1038/mp.2017.60

He, W., Sun, X., Liu, L., Li, M., Jin, H., & Wang, W.-H. (2014). The prevalence of chromosomal deletions relating to developmental delay and/or intellectual disability in human euploid blastocysts. *PLoS One, 9*(1), e85207. https://doi.org/10.1371/journal.pone.0085207

Heuvelman, H., Abel, K., Wicks, S., Gardner, R., Johnstone, E., Lee, B., … Rai, D. (2017). Gestational age at birth and risk of intellectual disability without a common genetic cause: Findings from the Stockholm Youth Cohort. *European Journal of Epidemiology*. https://doi.org/10.1101/129049

Huang, J., Zhu, T., Qu, Y., & Mu, D. (2016). Prenatal, perinatal and neonatal risk factors for intellectual disability: A systemic review and meta-analysis. *PLoS One, 11*(4), e0153655. https://doi.org/10.1371/journal.pone.0153655

Janvier, A., Farlow, B., & Wilfond, B. S. (2012). The experience of families with children with Trisomy 13 and 18 in social networks. *Pediatrics, 130*(2), 293–298. https://doi.org/10.1542/peds.2012-0151

Jenkins, D., Seelow, D., Jehee, F. S., Perlyn, C. A., Alonso, L. G., Bueno, D. F., … Wilkie, A. O. M. (2007). RAB23 mutations in Carpenter syndrome imply an unexpected role for hedgehog signaling in cranial-suture development and obesity. *The American Journal of Human Genetics, 80*(6), 1162–1170. https://doi.org/10.1086/518047

Kaasinen, E., Rahikkala, E., Koivunen, P., Miettinen, S., Wamelink, M. M. C., Aavikko, M., … Aaltonen, L. A. (2014). Clinical characterization, genetic mapping and whole-genome sequence analysis of a novel autosomal recessive intellectual disability syndrome. *European Journal of Medical Genetics, 57*(10), 543–551. https://doi.org/10.1016/j.ejmg.2014.07.002

Kahn, J., Koh, A., Luckcuck, R., McNeice, J., Walter, E., Yao, W., … Link, T. (2016). A phenylalanine fiasco: The structure of phenylalanine hydroxylase and its impact on phenylketonuria. *The FASEB Journal, 30*(Suppl. 1), 665.8.

Kaufman, L., Ayub, M., & Vincent, J. B. (2010). The genetic basis of non-syndromic intellectual disability: A review. *Journal of Neurodevelopmental Disorders, 2*(4), 182–209. https://doi.org/10.1007/s11689-010-9055-2

Kerr-Wilson, C. O., Mackay, D. F., Smith, G. C., & Pell, J. P. (2012). Meta-analysis of the association between preterm delivery and intelligence. *Journal of Public Health, 34*, 209–216.

Kobrynski, L. J., & Sullivan, K. E. (2007). Velocardiofacial syndrome, DiGeorge syndrome: The chromosome 22q11.2 deletion syndromes. *The Lancet, 370*(9596), 1443–1452. https://doi.org/10.1016/S0140-6736(07)61601-8

Koolen, D. A., Vissers, L. E. L. M., Pfundt, R., de Leeuw, N., Knight, S. J., Regan, R., … de Vries, B. B. A. (2006). A new chromosome 17q21.31 microdeletion syndrome associated with a common inversion polymorphism. *Nature Genetics, 38*(9), 999–1001. https://doi.org/10.1038/ng1853

Landrigan, P. J., Lambertini, L., & Birnbaum, L. S. (2012). A research strategy to discover the environmental causes of autism and neurodevelopmental disabilities. *Environmental Health Perspectives, 120*(7), a258–a260. https://doi.org/10.1289/ehp.1104285

Langridge, A. T., Glasson, E. J., Nassar, N., Jacoby, P., Pennell, C., Hagan, R., … Stanley, F. J. (2013). Maternal conditions and perinatal characteristics associated with autism spectrum disorder and intellectual disability. *PLoS One, 8*, e50963.

Larson, C. P. (2007). Poverty during pregnancy: Its effects on child health outcomes. *Paediatric Child Health, 12*, 673–677.

Lebel, R. R. (2014). Functional symptoms in medical genetics. In R. D. Anbar (Ed.), *Functional symptoms in pediatric disease* (pp. 191–199). New York, NY: Springer. Retrieved from http://link.springer.com/chapter/10.1007/978-1-4899-8074-8_13

Lee, H., Deignan, J. L., Dorrani, N., Strom, S. P., Kantarci, S., Quintero-Rivera, F., … Nelson, S. F. (2014). Clinical exome sequencing for genetic identification of rare Mendelian disorders. *JAMA, 312*(18), 1880–1887. https://doi.org/10.1001/jama.2014.14604

Lelieveld, S. H., Reijnders, M. R. F., Pfundt, R., Yntema, H. G., Kamsteeg, E.-J., de Vries, P., … Gilissen, C. (2016). Meta-analysis of 2,104 trios provides support for 10 new genes for intellectual disability. *Nature Neuroscience, 19*(9), 1194–1196. https://doi.org/10.1038/nn.4352

Lubs, H. A., Stevenson, R. E., & Schwartz, C. E. (2012). Fragile X and X-Linked intellectual disability: Four decades of discovery. *The American Journal of Human Genetics, 90*(4), 579–590. https://doi.org/10.1016/j.ajhg.2012.02.018

Ludvigsson, J. F. (2017). Extensive shaken baby syndrome review provides a clear signal that more research is needed. *Acta Paediatrica, 106*(7), 1028–1030. https://doi.org/10.1111/apa.13765

Magnin, E., Blagosklonov, O., Sylvestre, G., Minot, D., Thevenon, J., Faivre, L., … Rumbach, L. (2014). Neuropsychological and neuroimaging phenotype induced by a CAMTA1 mutation. *Brain and Development, 36*(8), 711–715. https://doi.org/10.1016/j.braindev.2013.09.008

Makela, N. L., Birch, P. H., Friedman, J. M., & Marra, C. A. (2009). Parental perceived value of a diagnosis for intellectual disability (ID): A qualitative comparison of families with and without a diagnosis for their child's ID. *American Journal of Medical Genetics Part A, 149A*(11), 2393–2402. https://doi.org/10.1002/ajmg.a.33050

Mann, J. R., Mcdermott, S., Barnes, T. L., Hardin, J., Bao, H. K., & Zhou, L. (2009). Trichomoniasis in pregnancy and mental retardation in children. *Annals of Epidemiology, 19*, 891–899.

Maurin, T., Zongaro, S., & Bardoni, B. (2014). Fragile X Syndrome: From molecular pathology to therapy. *Neuroscience & Biobehavioral Reviews, 46*(Pt. 2), 242–255. https://doi.org/10.1016/j.neubiorev.2014.01.006

McLaren, J., & Bryson, S. E. (1992). Review of recent epidemiological studies of mental retardation: Prevalence, associated disorders, and etiology. *American Journal of Mental Retardation, 92*, 243–254.

Meola, G., & Cardani, R. (2015). Myotonic dystrophies: An update on clinical aspects, genetic, pathology, and molecular pathomechanisms. *Biochimica et Biophysica Acta (BBA) – Molecular Basis of Disease, 1852*(4), 594–606. https://doi.org/10.1016/j.bbadis.2014.05.019

Moeschler, J. B., Shevell, M., & AAP Committee on Genetics. (2014). Comprehensive evaluation of the child with intellectual disability or global developmental delays. *Pediatrics, 134*(3), e903–e918. https://doi.org/10.1542/peds.2014-1839

Møller, R. S., Jensen, L. R., Maas, S. M., Filmus, J., Capurro, M., Hansen, C., … Kleefstra, T. (2013). X-linked congenital ptosis and associated intellectual disability, short stature, microcephaly, cleft palate, digital and genital abnormalities define novel Xq25q26 duplication syndrome. *Human Genetics, 133*(5), 625–638. https://doi.org/10.1007/s00439-013-1403-3

Morris, C. A. (2010). Introduction: Williams syndrome. *American Journal of Medical Genetics Part C: Seminars in Medical Genetics, 154C*(2), 203–208. https://doi.org/10.1002/ajmg.c.30266

Murgia, C., & Adamski, M. M. (2017). Translation of nutritional genomics into nutrition practice: The next step. *Nutrients, 9*, 366. https://doi.org/10.3390/nu9040366

Musante, L., & Ropers, H. H. (2014). Genetics of recessive cognitive disorders. *Trends in Genetics, 30*(1), 32–39. https://doi.org/10.1016/j.tig.2013.09.008

North, K., Riccardi, V., Samango-Sprouse, C., Ferner, R., Legius, E., Ratner, N., & Denckla, M. (1997). Cognitive function and academic performance in NF1: Consensus statement from the NF1 cognitive disorders task force. *Neurology, 48*, 1121–1127.

O'Brien, G. (2006). Behavioural phenotypes: Causes and clinical implications. *Advances in Psychiatric Treatment, 12*(5), 338–348. https://doi.org/10.1192/apt.12.5.338

O'Leary, C., Leonard, H., Bourke, J., D'Antoine, H., Bartu, A., & Bower, C. (2013). Intellectual disability: Population-based estimates of the proportion attributable to maternal alcohol use disorder during pregnancy. *Developmental Medicine & Child Neurology, 55*(3), 271–277. https://doi.org/10.1111/dmcn.12029

Palmer, E., Speirs, H., Taylor, P. J., Mullan, G., Turner, G., Einfeld, S., … Mowat, D. (2014). Changing interpretation of chromosomal microarray over time in a community cohort with intellectual disability. *American Journal of Medical Genetics Part A, 164*(2), 377–385. https://doi.org/10.1002/ajmg.a.36279

Papp, C., Ban, Z., Szigeti, Z., Csaba, A., Beke, A., & Papp, Z. (2007). Role of second trimester sonography in detecting trisomy 18: A review of 70 cases. *Journal of Clinical Ultrasound, 35*(2), 68–72. https://doi.org/10.1002/jcu.20290

Patterson, D. (2009). Molecular genetic analysis of Down syndrome. *Human Genetics, 126*(1), 195–214. https://doi.org/10.1007/s00439-009-0696-8

Peça, J., Feliciano, C., Ting, J. T., Wang, W., Wells, M. F., Venkatraman, T. N., … Feng, G. (2011). Shank3 mutant mice display autistic-like behaviours and striatal dysfunction. *Nature, 472*(7344), 437–442. https://doi.org/10.1038/nature09965

Peterson, C., Likang, X., Florence, C., Parks, S. E., Miller, T. R., Barr, R. G., & Steinbeigle, R. (2014). The medical cost of abusive head trauma in the United States. *Pediatrics, 134*(1), 91–99. https://doi.org/10.1542/peds.2014-0117

Phelan, M. C., Rogers, R. C., Everman, D. B., Stapleton, G. A., Powers, N. R., & Shaw, S. R. (2001). Deletion 22q13 syndrome-under-recognized and under-diagnosed. *American Journal of Human Genetics, 69*, 194–194.

Pilozzi-Edmonds, L., Maher, T. A., Basran, R. K., Milunsky, A., Al-Thihli, K., Braverman, N. E., & Alfares, A. (2011). Fraternal twins with Aarskog-Scott syndrome due to maternal germline mosaicism. *American Journal of Medical Genetics A, 155A*, 1987–1990.

Poncela-Casasnovas, J., Gutiérrez-Roig, M., Gracia-Lázaro, C., Vicens, J., Gómez-Gardeñes, J., Perelló, J., … Sánchez, A. (2016). Humans display a reduced set of consistent behavioral phenotypes in dyadic games. *Science Advances, 2*(8), e1600451. https://doi.org/10.1126/sciadv.1600451

Rahib, L., MacLennan, N. K., Horvath, S., Liao, J. C., & Dipple, K. M. (2007). Glycerol kinase deficiency alters expression of genes involved in lipid metabolism, carbohydrate metabolism, and insulin signaling. *European Journal of Human Genetics, 15*(6), 646–657. https://doi.org/10.1038/sj.ejhg.5201801

Redin, C., Gérard, B., Lauer, J., Herenger, Y., Muller, J., Quartier, A., … Piton, A. (2014). Efficient strategy for the molecular diagnosis of intellectual disability using targeted high-throughput sequencing. *Journal of Medical Genetics, 51*, 724–736. https://doi.org/10.1136/jmedgenet-2014-102554

Ridler, K., Suckling, J., Higgins, N. J., de Vries, P. J., Stephenson, C. M. E., Bolton, P. F., & Bullmore, E. T. (2007). Neuroanatomical correlates of memory deficits in tuberous sclerosis complex. *Cerebral Cortex, 17*(2), 261–271. https://doi.org/10.1093/cercor/bhj144

Riggs, E. E., Wain, K. E., Riethmaier, D., Smith-Packard, B., Faucett, W. A., Hoppman, N., … Miller, D. T. (2014). Chromosomal microarray impacts clinical management. *Clinical Genetics, 85*(2), 147–153. https://doi.org/10.1111/cge.12107

Rizzo, T. (2014). Advances in autism spectrum disorders and intellectual disability. *MD Conference Express, 14*(6), 21–23. https://doi.org/10.1177/155989771406012

Rojnueangnit, K., Jones, J. R., Basehore, M. J., & Robin, N. H. (2014). Classic phenotype of Coffin–Lowry syndrome in a female with stimulus-induced drop episodes and a genotype with preserved N-terminal kinase domain. *American Journal of Medical Genetics Part A, 164*(2), 516–521. https://doi.org/10.1002/ajmg.a.36299

Rump, P., Jazayeri, O., van Dijk-Bos, K. K., Johansson, L. F., van Essen, A. J., Verheij, J. B. G. M., … Sikkema-Raddatz, B. (2016). Whole-exome sequencing is a powerful approach for establishing the etiological diagnosis in patients with intellectual disability and microcephaly. *BMC Medical Genomics, 9*, 7. https://doi.org/10.1186/s12920-016-0167-8

Scheepers, M., Kerr, M., O'Hara, D., Bainbridge, D., Cooper, S.-A., Davis, R., … Wehmeyer, M. (2005). Reducing health disparity in people with intellectual disabilities: A Report from Health Issues special interest research group of the international association for the scientific study of intellectual disabilities. *Journal of Policy and Practice in Intellectual Disabilities, 2*, 249–255. https://doi.org/10.1111/j.1741-1130.2005.00037.x

Shah, P. M. (1991). Prevention of mental handicaps in children in primary health care. *Bulletin of the World Health Organization, 69*, 779–789.

Sheth, F., Gohel, N., Liehr, T., Akinde, O., Desai, M., Adeteye, O., & Sheth, J. (2012). Gain of chromosome 4qter and loss of 5pter: An unusual case with features of cri du chat syndrome. *Case Reports in Genetics, 2012*, e153405. https://doi.org/10.1155/2012/153405

Snijders Blok, C., Corsten-Janssen, N., FitzPatrick, D. R., Romano, C., Fichera, M., Vitello, G. A., … Kleefstra, T. (2014). Definition of 5q11.2 microdeletion syndrome reveals overlap with CHARGE syndrome and 22q11 deletion syndrome phenotypes. *American Journal of Medical Genetics Part A, 164*(11), 2843–2848. https://doi.org/10.1002/ajmg.a.36680

Srour, M., & Shevell, M. (2014). Genetics and the investigation of developmental delay/intellectual disability. *Archives of Disease in Childhood, 99*(4), 386–389. https://doi.org/10.1136/archdischild-2013-304063

Stern, A. M. (2012). *Telling genes: The story of genetic counseling in America*. Baltimore, MD: Johns Hopkins University Press.

Strandberg-Larsen, K., Andersen, A.-M. N., & Kesmodel, U. S. (2017). Unreliable estimation of prevalence of fetal alcohol syndrome. *The Lancet Global Health, 5*(6), e573. https://doi.org/10.1016/S2214-109X(17)30172-9

Tan, C. A., Topper, S., del Gaudio, D., Nelakuditi, V., Shchelochkov, O., Nowaczyk, M. J. M., … Das, S. (2015). Characterization of patients referred for non-specific intellectual disability: The importance of autosomal genes for diagnosis. *Clinical Genetics, 89*, 478–483. https://doi.org/10.1111/cge.12575

Tao, Y., Gao, H., Ackerman, B., Guo, W., Saffen, D., & Shugart, Y. Y. (2016). Evidence for contribution of common genetic variants within chromosome 8p21.2-8p21.1 to restricted and repetitive behaviors in autism spectrum disorders. *BMC Genomics, 17*, 163. https://doi.org/10.1186/s12864-016-2475-y

The Deciphering Developmental Disorders Study. (2015). Large-scale discovery of novel genetic causes of developmental disorders. *Nature, 519*(7542), 223–228. https://doi.org/10.1038/nature14135

Tzschach, A., Grasshoff, U., Beck-Woedl, S., Dufke, C., Bauer, C., Kehrer, M., … Bauer, P. (2015). Next-generation sequencing in X-linked intellectual disability. *European Journal of Human Genetics, 23*, 1513–1518. https://doi.org/10.1038/ejhg.2015.5

Valenti, D., de Bari, L., De Filippis, B., Henrion-Caude, A., & Vacca, R. A. (2014). Mitochondrial dysfunction as a central actor in intellectual disability-related diseases: An overview of Down syndrome, autism, Fragile X and Rett syndrome. *Neuroscience & Biobehavioral Reviews, 46*(Pt. 2), 202–217. https://doi.org/10.1016/j.neubiorev.2014.01.012

van Bokhoven, H. (2011). Genetic and epigenetic networks in intellectual disabilities. *Annual Review of Genetics, 45*(1), 81–104. https://doi.org/10.1146/annurev-genet-110410-132512

Van den Veyver, I. B. (2016). Recent advances in prenatal genetic screening and testing. *F1000Research, 5*, 2591. https://doi.org/10.12688/f1000research.9215.1

Van den Veyver, I. B., Patel, A., Shaw, C. A., Pursley, A. N., Kang, S. H., Simovich, M. J., … Beaudet, A. L. (2009). Clinical use of array comparative genomic hybridization (aCGH) for prenatal diagnosis in 300 cases. *Prenatal Diagnistics, 29*, 29–39. https://doi.org/10.1002/pd.2127

Vishnivetskaya, G. B., Skrinskaya, J. A., Seif, I., & Popova, N. K. (2007). Effect of MAO A efficiency on different kinds of aggression and social investigation in mice. *Aggressive Behavior, 33*(1), 1–6. https://doi.org/10.1002/ab.20161

Visootsak, J., Aylstock, M., & Graham, J. M. (2001). Klinefelter syndrome and its variants: An update and review for the primary pediatrician. *Clinical Pediatrics, 40*(12), 639–651. https://doi.org/10.1177/000992280104001201

Vissers, L. E. L. M., Gilissen, C., & Veltman, J. A. (2016). Genetic studies in intellectual disability and related disorders. *Nature Reviews Genetics, 17*(1), 9–18. https://doi.org/10.1038/nrg3999

Wallace, R. A. (2016). Genetic testing of aetiology of intellectual disability in a dedicated physical healthcare outpatient clinic for adults with intellectual disability. *Internal Medicine Journal, 46*(2), 177–185. https://doi.org/10.1111/imj.12946

Willemsen, M. H., & Kleefstra, T. (2014). Making headway with genetic diagnostics of intellectual disabilities. *Clinical Genetics, 85*(2), 101–110. https://doi.org/10.1111/cge.12244

Williams, C. A., Beaudet, A. L., Clayton-Smith, J., Knoll, J. H., Kyllerman, M., Laan, L. A., … Wagstaff, J. (2006). Angelman syndrome 2005: Updated consensus for diagnostic criteria.

American Journal of Medical Genetics Part A, 140A(5), 413–418. https://doi.org/10.1002/ajmg.a.31074

Wilson, H. L., Wong, A. C., Shaw, S. R., Tse, W. Y., Stapleton, G. A., Phelan, M. C., … McDermid, H. E. (2003). Molecular characterisation of the 22q13 deletion syndrome supports the role of haploinsufficiency of *SHANK3/PROSAP2* in the major neurological symptoms. *Journal of Medical Genetics, 40*, 575–584.

Wójcik, C., Volz, K., Ranola, M., Kitch, K., Karim, T., O'Neil, J., … Torres-Martinez, W. (2010). Rubinstein-Taybi syndrome associated with Chiari type I malformation caused by a large 16p13.3 microdeletion: A contiguous gene syndrome? *American Journal of Medical Genetics. Part A, 152A*(2), 479–483. https://doi.org/10.1002/ajmg.a.33303

Wortmann, S. B., Koolen, D. A., Smeitink, J. A., van den Heuvel, L., & Rodenburg, R. J. (2015). Whole exome sequencing of suspected mitochondrial patients in clinical practice. *Journal of Inherited Metabolic Disease, 38*(3), 437–443. https://doi.org/10.1007/s10545-015-9823-y

Yang, Y., Muzny, D. M., Reid, J. G., Bainbridge, M. N., Willis, A., Ward, P. A., … Eng, C. M. (2013). Clinical whole-exome sequencing for the diagnosis of Mendelian disorders. *New England Journal of Medicine, 369*, 1502–1511.

Zarchi, O., Diamond, A., Weinberger, R., Abbott, D., Carmel, M., Frisch, A., … Gothelf, D. (2014). A comparative study of the neuropsychiatric and neurocognitive phenotype in two microdeletion syndromes: Velocardiofacial (22q11.2 deletion) and Williams (7q11.23 deletion) syndromes. *European Psychiatry, 29*(4), 203–210. https://doi.org/10.1016/j.eurpsy.2013.07.001

Chapter 3
Medical Issues, Therapies, and Treatments

Abstract This chapter reviews medication issues, treatments, and therapies for people with intellectual disabilities. Also considered are how commonly concurrent medical issues and their treatments may influence the functioning and development of persons with intellectual disabilities. The spectrum of available treatments from the most widely used to novel and experimental and the research support for each treatment is critically reviewed. Evidence is also weighed concerning unproved and complementary and alternative treatments.

Case Study

James was referred at the age of 13 months to the subspecialty department of developmental pediatrics at a regional hospital due to cleft palate, constipation, sometimes bluish skin secondary to a ventricular septal defect, and a recent non-febrile seizure. The first team that James and his parents saw was the neurodevelopmental genetics team. This diagnostic interdisciplinary team was comprised of a clinical geneticist, neurologist, psychologist, nurse, social worker, speech and language pathologist, and developmental pediatrician. The presenting characteristics led to a rapid consensus that James presented consistent with velocardiofacial syndrome (i.e. 22q11.2 deletion). Diagnosis was confirmed through fluorescence in situ hybridization (FISH) testing (Sarasua et al., 2014), which demonstrated clear deletion at the predicted location. James's next step was to have an additional medical examination and a treatment plan developed by a multidisciplinary treatment team. The treatment team consisted of a cardiologist, plastic surgeon, dentist, neurologist, psychologist, occupational therapist, nurse, genetic counsellor, and speech and language therapist. In addition, the team consulted with nephrology and endocrinology. In this case, the developmental pediatrician served as the case coordinator. The case coordinator communicates diverse findings and treatment plans to parents and to the family's general pediatrician. Treatment was prioritized based on risks for immediate threats to health and well-being. The first part of treatments included surgeries to correct a septal heart defect and cleft palate. Upon completion of surgeries and rehabilitation, James began speech and occupational therapies to improve

S. R. Shaw, A. M. Jankowska, *Pediatric Intellectual Disabilities at School*, Pediatric School Psychology, https://doi.org/10.1007/978-3-030-02992-0_3

speech and language development, chewing and swallowing, fine motor skills, and readiness skills to prepare for social activities and functioning in daycare settings. As James approached school-age, the psychologist and speech and language therapist conducted a joint assessment to determine cognitive function and risks for delays in academic and pre-academic skills. Interventions designed to support the development of social skills in group settings and behaviour management for overactive behaviours were begun at age three. These interventions included his parents and daycare service providers. In addition, James showed intolerance to certain foods that created deficits in important nutrition profiles. The multidomain aspects of James's presentation of velocardiofacial syndrome required a coordinated effort with multiple forms of therapy, medical management of specific and general health and well-being, medication, diet and nutrition, family supports, and daycare/school education. Although the developmental pediatrician served as the point person to the multidisciplinary treatment team, his parents served as the ultimate decision makers. Coordinating the large number of professionals in such a way as to support family systems and provide the best possible combination of therapies for James proved a continuous and daunting challenge.

Introduction

Individuals with intellectual disabilities often require extensive medical support. As a population, they are twice as likely to require medical interventions when compared to typically developing peers yet are quite often without access to medical care (Charlot et al., 2011). Even when access to medical care can be attained, the quality of care specific to the needs of the person with intellectual disabilities is questionable. Yet, there have been significant advances in knowledge concerning overall provision of general healthcare and specific medical treatments to improve wellness, quality of life, and longevity (Ptomey, Goetz, Lee, Donnelly, & Sullivan, 2013). The description of general medical care is divided into three components: general health and wellness, syndrome-specific medical conditions, and risks for persons with intellectual disabilities requiring specialized health care.

General Health

Effective general health practices involve lifestyle, environmental supports, and common health promotion and disease prevention practices. People with intellectual disabilities are at high risk for a host of medical issues secondary to lifestyle and environment (Novak, 2014). For persons requiring less daily living support, there is potential for risky behaviours and the conditions that result from lifestyle choices. Moreover, it is possible that there is an interaction among lifestyle, heredity, and medication factors that can lead to negative outcomes (Dagnan, Masson,

Cavagin, Thwaites, & Hatton, 2015). Persons with intellectual disabilities who live in the general community have high risk for tobacco and substance abuse, violent behaviour, high-risk sexual activity, accidents, victimization and exploitation, sedentary lifestyles, and poor diet (Ouellette-Kuntz, 2005). Specific focus on instruction in the complexities of community-based daily living skills are critical components of improving overall health of people with intellectual disabilities.

Preventative health practices are widely recommended for the general population, but are not routinely taught to people with intellectual disabilities (Persch, Lamb, Metzler, & Fristad, 2015). Instruction in basic community functions such as conflict resolution, fire safety, exercise, nutrition and safe meal preparation, safe sex, avoidance of tobacco and drugs or support for quitting tobacco and drugs, and lifestyle choices to reduce hypertension, diabetes, and coronary artery disease can result in improved longevity and quality of life for people with intellectual disabilities just as these practices are identified as helpful in the general population (Robertson et al., 2000). Routine medical care such as standard immunization schedules, screening for sensory impairment, and many other routine medical screening for early identification of disease states such as cancer, sexually transmitted infections, glaucoma, hypertension, and coronary artery disease are just as important for people with intellectual disabilities as for the general population (van Schrojenstein Lantman-de Valk & Walsh, 2008). However, most evidence show that children and adults with intellectual disabilities do not receive supportive medical care that promotes their general physical health. This places people with intellectual disabilities at risk for common but preventable and treatable medical issues.

Syndrome-Specific Conditions

Genetic syndromes, including micro-deletion syndromes, that lead to intellectual disabilities often affect other organ systems beyond the central nervous system (Hodapp & Dykens, 2012). The great advantage of understanding phenotypes of specific genetic syndromes is that common medical issues can be addressed immediately and, in some cases, prophylactically before presentation of symptoms occurs. This also applies to behavioural phenotypes. For example, Smith-Magenis syndrome frequently results in severe aggression (Greydanus & Merrick, 2016), Prader-Willi syndrome results in overeating and food foraging (Alexander, 2016), and 22q11.2 deletion syndrome (i.e. velocardiofacial syndrome) involves a high risk of schizophrenia and severe mental health issues (Weisman et al., 2017). Understanding the probability of having or developing specific medical and mental health risks allows clinicians to consult and work closely with experts in the specific areas. Among the most common organ systems affected include the stomach, heart, kidneys, mouth and teeth, thyroid, intestinal system, and skin. Involvement of medical specialists at the earliest possible stages, especially preventative, is a critical factor in general health, well-being, and longevity.

Specialized Healthcare

Even when there is no evidence of syndrome-specific medical conditions, healthcare for people with intellectual disabilities remains complex. Among the most challenging issues relate to systemic access to preventative healthcare with medical service providers who are trained, experienced, and willing to work with people with intellectual disabilities (Ouellette-Kuntz, 2005). An important factor in basic healthcare is the importance of listening and responding to the needs of the patient. Although there is evidence that this factor is not widely considered in the general population, for people with intellectual disabilities, it is rare that they are provided with opportunities to contribute to their own healthcare and have their needs heard. This may be most important for persons with intellectual disabilities as even without syndrome-specific medical conditions, this population remains at relatively high risk for a host of medical issues. These issues are, in many cases, preventable or treatable with early diagnosis (Weise, Pollack, Britt, & Trollor, 2016). Effective prevention and early diagnosis require strong levels of communication between medical care provider and patient.

An important component of medical care is to encourage and promote persons with intellectual disabilities to be effective self-advocates for effective medical care. Training and education concerning medical conditions, how to communicate effectively with healthcare providers, making and keeping medical appointments, and awareness of bodily sensations that may indicate warning signs or symptoms for severe medical problems are valuable goals of any treatment plan. The ability to control one's medical status and treatment is a critical part of gaining independence skills. Moreover, improved communication between patient and medical care provider will lead to improved medical care by increasing accuracy of diagnosis and treatment effectiveness.

Central nervous system disease states are extremely common in syndrome-specific conditions but less so for idiopathic or familial intellectual disabilities (van Ool et al., 2016). The gross rule of thumb is that the likelihood of seizures increases as general cognitive ability decreases (Robinson, 2012). In other words, the likelihood of seizure activity, including asymptomatic epileptiform activity, is more likely in lower functioning populations (Dunn, Hughes-McCormack, & Cooper, 2017). Febrile and absence (i.e. petit mal) seizures are common, especially in children (Robinson, 2012). Appropriate monitoring or treatment for these conditions is an important factor in overall cognitive development. Although rare, people with intellectual disabilities are also more likely to have vascular disorders of the brain leading to infarct (Erickson, Spoutz, Dorsch, & Bleske, 2016). The possibility of infarct and pediatric stroke is also common for individuals with sickle cell trait (Adler, Reghunathan, Hutchison, & Kalpatthi, 2016). Therefore, complaints of headaches and nausea need to be taken seriously to either prevent or provide early treatment for vascular disorders within the central nervous system. Cognitive decline can also occur in children, adolescents, and adults, although this is a low-incidence event (McPaul, Walker, Law, & McKenzie, 2016). Yet, this is a relatively common phenomenon seen in young children with intellectual disabilities and autism and then observed later in life with cognitive deterioration and dementia. An important factor in diagnosing cognitive loss is to use absolute levels of skill (McPaul et al., 2016). A common error is examining the results of standardized and norm-referenced intelligence test scores from a previous time, noting that recent scores are lower, then inferring that some level of cognitive loss is taken place. Most typically, reduction in scores is an artefact of a norm-referenced test. In other words, the person's skills may be improving slowly, but the typical person of the same age is improving at a much faster rate; therefore, reducing the standard score yet not indicating an absolute loss of skill. Also, loss of absolute skill is sometimes noticeable during an emotional trauma or crisis, transition, illness, or introduction of a new medical treatment and is not part of a pattern of overall and organic cognitive deterioration. Effectively monitoring brain function and development from childhood through adulthood and old age is an ongoing aspect of medical care for all individuals but is especially important and may lead to intervention for persons with intellectual disabilities.

Cardiac-related disorders and risk factors for coronary artery disease are major factors affecting the quality of life for persons with intellectual disabilities (van Timmeren, van der Putten, van Schrojenstein Lantman-de Valk, van der Schans, & Waninge, 2016). In addition to lifestyle factors such as diet and exercise, atypical antipsychotics (e.g. Risperdal) are the second most prescribed psychiatric medication for children (Cohen et al., 2013). These medications are widely administered to persons with intellectual disabilities for controlling aggressive behaviours. However, nearly all persons prescribed atypical antipsychotic medications gain significant body mass. Weight gains of 10–35% of body weight are commonly observed (de Kuijper, Evenhuis, Mindera, & Hoekstra, 2014). Routine management for persons prescribed atypical antipsychotics include regular measures of blood pressure and blood lipid profile. Although the long-term effects of atypical antipsychotics on risks for coronary artery disease are not clear, high blood pressure and high cholesterol represent major risk factors, and there is an increased likelihood of cardiac-related disorders in this population (Edelsohn, Schuster, Castelnovo, Terhorst, & Parthasarathy, 2014). Many other people with intellectual disabilities are prescribed stimulant medication to control attention and focus. Although these medications are proven safe in most general populations, there is some evidence of stimulants in the amphetamine group that can exacerbate heart arrhythmia (Sawyer, Lake, Lunsky, Liu, & Desarkar, 2014). There is also evidence that arrhythmias related to amphetamine-based stimulant treatment for attention deficit hyperactivity disorder and other attention issues may be more common in persons with intellectual disabilities than in the general population. Baseline electrocardiograms are recommended (Shin, Roughead, Park, & Pratt, 2016). Given how common cardiac-related disorders are in the general population, even persons with intellectual disabilities not prescribed atypical antipsychotics or stimulants require preventative screening and lifestyle education (Segal et al., 2016).

Digestive system issues are challenging for medical care providers in cases where clients are typically developing. Diffuse abdominal pain with no identifiable cause is common in school-aged children and adolescents. Sometimes this pain is a manifestation of anxiety (Huguet et al., 2017). Other times there are challenges with menstrual cramping and related discomfort. People with intellectual disabilities have the same complaints. Issues causing extreme discomfort such as ulcers or hernias are extremely common for persons with intellectual disabilities, but are often overlooked in medical examinations (Segal et al., 2016). Moreover, these issues are complicated by inconsistent or poor dietary practices. Even in cases where there are no syndrome-specific digestive system issues, obesity and concurrent digestive system issues are common (Segal et al., 2016). Moreover, typical screening and diagnostic procedures in primary practice such as colonoscopies for persons older than 50 years are still considered best practices for persons with intellectual disabilities (Ouellette-Kuntz, 2005).

Skeletal muscular development and maintenance is a function of lifestyle factors such as diet and exercise along with common syndrome-specific conditions such as hypotonia (common in many syndromes such as Downs; Basil et al., 2016). Lack of exercise and a low-protein/high-carbohydrate diet leads to lack of lean muscle mass and low-density bone structure (Walsh et al., 2017). Lack of lean muscle mass may contribute to falls and other accidents in this population. Weight-bearing and balance exercises with the cardiovascular training component are extraordinarily beneficial to overall well-being, health, and injury prevention. Group exercises may have a social component that also contributes to well-being. However, many times, people with intellectual disabilities are prescribed medications that can result in overeating, weight loss, and lethargy, making the initiation of physical exercise challenging (Segal et al., 2016).

Vision and hearing impairments are common for people with intellectual disabilities, just as they are for the general population (Dijkhuizen, Hilgenkamp, Krijnen, van der Schans, & Waninge, 2016). Although there are syndrome-specific conditions related to vision and hearing, routine sensory acuity screening is an important part of general healthcare (Brown, Jacobstein, Yoon, Anthony, & Bullock, 2016). The primary challenges are access to regular screenings and communication in cooperation with the screener to ensure the accuracy of the screening process. Sensory acuity screening is recommended for scheduled visits to see the school nurse and for all visits to the primary care physician. The bigger challenge is that people with intellectual disabilities may have difficulties communicating changes in sensory acuity status and have difficulty following the instructions on routine vision and hearing screenings. In cases of infants and people who are unable to effectively understand instructions and communicate responses, auditory and visual evoked potentials can be used. The challenge is that evoked potentials assess nerve conduction from sensory channel to receptive components of the brain, but do not effectively investigate functional sensory acuity (Shen & Morton, 2016). Although evoked potentials may rule out some sensorineural impairment, they do not substitute for functional assessment of hearing and vision functioning.

Dental care is an important and frequently overlooked component of general medical care and well-being (Koch, Poulsen, Espelid, & Haubek, 2016). There are several genetic disorders and conditions that involve midline issues such as cleft palate and lead to dysmorphic small jaw (i.e. micrognathia) and other oral, facial, and dental issues. All require specialized dental treatment including oral and plastic surgery. Other conditions create high risk for dental issues such as thin enamel, wide tooth spacing, or connective tissue problems that affect the strength of dental connections to bone structure. Yet, failure to manage routine dental care such as daily brushing and flossing, identification of early dental problems such as cavities, and regular preventative dental visits affect wellness for many persons with intellectual disabilities (Norderyd, Klingberg, Faulks, & Granlund, 2016). Communication, following directions, and managing the unfamiliarity and discomfort of routine dental care often make dental work an aversive experience for all parties. Most family dentists are unfamiliar or uncomfortable with providing services to persons with intellectual disabilities (Norderyd et al., 2016). Commonly, persons with intellectual disabilities are placed under anaesthesia because of the difficulties in cooperation with the dentist. Monitoring the status of persons on anaesthesia is especially important as there are often cardiac and pulmonary disease risk factors. Providing dental services to individuals with intellectual disabilities is considered a subspecialty of dentistry involving a great deal of experience and training (Norderyd et al., 2016). Most persons do not have access to such specialized professionals (Koch et al., 2016). Without quality preventative dentistry, there is a likelihood of painful cavities and infections that can affect quality of life and long-term health. Having persons with severe intellectual disabilities sometime engage in self-injurious behaviour often by striking the mouth or jaw with the heel of the hand due to painful dental caries and the inability to communicate the source of the pain. The challenge of dental care for persons with intellectual disabilities is not simply access to professionals with the requisite skills and experience but also the expense. Most forms of dental insurance in North America cover basic dental care for typically developing children and adults, but do not cover the extra time, deviations from standard procedures, and intensive forms of therapies for this high-risk population (Koch et al., 2016). Although poorly covered and managed, appropriate and effective dental care is a major component of wellness and overall health for persons with intellectual disabilities.

Common Medications for Treatment of Intellectual Disabilities

Because people with intellectual disabilities have many and varied medical concerns, multiple medications to address these medical issues are common. Ensuring there is a medical case coordinator is an important aspect of medical management. Although multi- and interdisciplinary teams have significant advantages for service delivery, multiple medical subspecialties may prescribe appropriate medications without communication in consideration of possible medication interactions. Often, the pharmacist takes on an increased role with such complex combinations of medications. In addition to the medications to address physical issues, there are often specific medications prescribed to manage psychiatric issues for people with intellectual disabilities.

Nootropics

Nootropics are medications that positively affect cognitive abilities. Some forms of intellectual disabilities are caused by deficient synaptogenesis or impaired synaptic plasticity early in brain development. An interesting field of study is to create medications that enhance synaptogenesis, improve signalling status of synapses, and enhance synaptic plasticity. From animal and simulation studies, some molecular switches such as phosphatases, small G proteins, and kinases may be specific processes to directly enhance synaptic plasticity (Häβler, Thome, & Reis, 2014). There are some medications that have been used for addressing Alzheimer's disease and other forms of dementia, such as acetylcholinesterase inhibitors, yet these are not supported treatments for intellectual disabilities, and clinical trials have not been conducted in children (Grieco et al., 2014). Phosphodiesterase inhibitors enhance cortical plasticity in an animal model of fetal alcohol effects but are several steps from human trials (Prasher, 2004). A potentially constructive nootropic approach is the use of intranasal insulin for the specific case of children with 22q13 deletion syndrome and subsequent haploinsufficiency of SHANK3, which is a structural protein in the post-terminal button of synapses in the brain, especially in the hippocampus (Salameh et al., 2015). The intranasal insulin is suspected to overcome the structural impairment caused by the insufficiency of SHANK3 to improve short-term memory and some language functions (Craft et al., 2012; Zwanenburg et al., 2016). Although a potentially productive area of research, currently there is no evidence of long-term cognitive improvement through use of nootropics.

Stimulants

Stimulants are the most common class of medication prescribed to people with intellectual disabilities. The stimulant class medication is prescribed most typically for children and adults with attention deficit hyperactivity disorder (ADHD; Koegel, Krasno, Taras, Koegel, & Frea, 2013). However, this class of medications addresses attention issues for those without the ADHD diagnosis, such as typically developing persons and those with intellectual disabilities (Lance & Shapiro, 2013). The two major subclasses of central nervous system stimulants are methylphenidate-based products, such as Ritalin and Concerta, and dextroamphetamine sulphate-based products, such as Dexedrine and Adderall. These medications frequently improve attention, reduce impulsiveness, and reduce overactivity. In this regard, stimulants can be thought of as effective nootropic medications. There are limited side effects. Side effects include loss of appetite, sleep problems, headaches, stomach aches, and irritability (Barnard-Brak, Davis, Schmidt, & Richman, 2016). Overall, central nervous system stimulants are an effective class of medications with a relatively minor side effect profile that can approve functioning for people with intellectual disabilities (Simonoff et al., 2013).

Antipsychotic Medications

Neuroleptic medications, predominately atypical antipsychotics, are the second most prescribed class of psychiatric medication for children (Allen et al., 2013). For people with intellectual disabilities, antipsychotic medications are prescribed for aggression, overactivity, and self-injury (Lake, Vogan, Sawyer, Weiss, & Lunsky, 2015). There is significant evidence of effectiveness for antipsychotics in reducing aggressive behaviours (Sharma & Shaw, 2012). Risperidone is a medication in this class that has been approved by the US Food and Drug Administration for children with autism spectrum disorder to reduce aggression. There are several other medications in this class that have not been approved by the FDA but are frequently used off label to address behavioural issues, such as Aripiprazole, Clozapine, Ziprasidone, and others (Deb et al., 2014). The adverse effects of atypical antipsychotics tend to be much less severe than the first generation of antipsychotics, which included Thorazine and Haldol. However, extrapyramidal symptoms such as tremors, pseudoparkinsonism, and tardive dyskinesia may still occur (Deb et al., 2008). As an important reminder to caregivers, medications need to be administered exactly as prescribed, and caution is required when weaning patients off the medication. Rapid or sudden removal of atypical antipsychotics can lead immediately to extrapyramidal symptoms. Another common adverse effect is significant weight gain (de Kuijper et al., 2014). Often individuals who have been prescribed atypical antipsychotics for several years are at risk for gynecomastia, hypertension, cardiovascular disease, type II diabetes, and hypercholesterolemia. Although an effective class of medications for many behavioural symptoms in people with intellectual disabilities, the profile of adverse effects requires continuous monitoring and care in administration (Kurtz, Boelter, Jarmolowicz, Chin, & Hagopian, 2011).

Alpha-Adrenergic Agonists

The effectiveness of alpha-adrenergic agonist class of medications is caused by stimulating alpha-2 adrenergic receptors in the brainstem and activating inhibitory neurons (Mula, 2016). These medications are commonly used to address tics, aggression, overactivity, and sleep problems. Examples of the alpha-adrenergic agonists are Catapres and Tenex. Although these medications can reduce problem behaviours and issues, they are unlikely to be first-line medications. Although the evidence is mixed, Tenex has been associated with decreased academic performance and cognitive function in typically functioning students with mental health issues (Mula, 2016). It is unclear whether this medication may result in changed cognitive functioning in people with intellectual disabilities.

Diet and Nutrition

There is a history of using diet and nutrition as cures or therapies for specific symptoms for people with intellectual disabilities. With few exceptions, diet and nutrition have no major demonstrated therapeutic effects. However, appropriate nutrition provides significant challenges for people with intellectual disabilities and is an important factor in maintaining health, quality of life, and longevity.

General

An appropriate and nutritious diet is a factor in maintaining quality of life for all people. Certainly, people with intellectual disabilities are no different. People with intellectual disabilities often have diets that are deficient in protein, fibre, fruits and vegetables, vitamins and minerals, and other key nutrients. Some of the causes for the deficient diet are financial. Persons with disabilities are often members of families who are of low income (Heller, McCubbin, Drum, & Peterson, 2011). Nutritionally dense food with minimal processing tends to be much more expensive than overly processed foods with high sugar content, high calorie, low fibre, and minimal other nutritive value. Another common reason for poor diet is that people with intellectual disabilities often have restricted food preferences. The restrictions may have to do with sensory issues that affect preferences for foods with certain textures, temperatures, or taste profiles. Sometimes the restricted diet is due to habit formation of specific foods and a personal preference for consistent foods. The result, along with lack of physical activity, is that a large percentage of people with intellectual disabilities experience overweight or obesity. Obesity influences quality of life, opportunities for socialization, community involvement, health, and longevity. Working closely with a nutritionist can significantly support high-quality nutritious foods that can support maintenance of an appropriate weight. Like many issues concerning people with intellectual disabilities, a high-quality nutritious diet can improve readiness to learn and the overall effectiveness of education, social acceptance by others, and overall health.

In addition to overall nutrition, there have been several proposed ideas concerning specialized diet and nutrition for the amelioration of problem and issues specific to people with intellectual disabilities (Ruud, Raanaas, & Bjelland, 2016). In some cases, there is strong research support for specialized diet, and in other cases there is limited data for diet and nutrition interventions to be dangerous and contraindicated by the research literature.

Specialize Dietary Needs

Most genetic disorders that lead to intellectual disabilities do not have a specific set of specialized dietary needs. However, several causes of intellectual disabilities have secondary effects on digestive system functioning that require a modified diet (Scott & Havercamp, 2016). Some common genetic syndromes such as Down syndrome, velocardiofacial syndrome, and Smith-Magenis syndrome have liver, kidney, stomach, heart, and intestinal abnormalities that may require supportive dietary interventions. Examples include low-acid diets for the common secondary characteristic of acid reflux.

Metabolic disorders are a less common, but not insignificant, cause of intellectual disabilities where specialized dietary needs are essential for functioning and management of cognitive and physical symptoms. The two most common examples are phenylketonuria (PKU) and maple syrup urine disease (MSUD). PKU is characterized by the complete or partial absence of phenylalanine hydroxylase (PAH), which is an enzyme essential for converting phenylalanine into tyrosine (Moses, Katz, & Weizman, 2014). With a severe PAH deficiency, phenylalanine reaches high levels in the blood and eventually creates permanent brain damage and intellectual disabilities. Therefore, a lifetime diet that removes high levels of protein is removed from diets. A specialized nutritional substitute that creates nutritionally complete proteins, vitamins, minerals, and the other essential amino acids necessary for growth are included, but phenylalanine is systematically removed from this nutritional formula. Eliminating phenylalanine from the diet is required to maintain appropriate cognitive and physical growth (Kahn et al., 2016). In most cases, introducing phenylalanine into the diet can include lowering of general mental ability, overactivity, tremors, and severe mental health problems. Therefore, the phenylalanine-free diet is recommended to be adhered to throughout the lifespan (Kahn et al., 2016).

MSUD is a metabolic disorder affecting the ability to metabolize the branched-chain amino acids of leucine, isoleucine, and valine. This is caused by a deficit in the enzymes required to break down these amino acids (van Karnebeek et al., 2014). The amino acids and their by-products can become elevated in the blood and create brain damage. Much like the case of PKU, specialized diets are created and must be adhered to for life. Both PKU and MSUD can be life-threatening or cause significant brain damage affecting cognitive development and leading to intellectual disabilities. However, with the diet that is initiated immediately after birth and maintained well, people with these two metabolic disorders can expect near typical development and lifespan.

Supplements

For most people with intellectual disabilities, nutritional supplements have little effect on cognitive development, and there is sparse evidence that nutritional supplements have clinically important outcomes. However, nutritional supplements can serve a valuable role in cases where dietary preferences or other limitations on food intake result in a situation in which some vitamins and minerals are lacking. The general rule is that dietary supplements that increase general health and well-being by assisting in overcoming a minimally nutritious diet will also assist in cognitive development (Koslowski et al., 2016). There is limited evidence that supplements that include polyunsaturated fatty acids (PUFAs), such as omega-3 or omega-6 fatty acids like that found in fish oil, can have a positive effect on behaviour (Posar & Visconti, 2016). PUFAs and docosahexaenoic acid (DHA) are found in heavy concentrations and create the predominant structural fatty acid components of the brain and retina. There is little question that DHA is a critical component and supporter of brain development. However, it is not clear whether supplementation of DHA through ingestion of fish oil, walnuts, and some other seeds will result in positive changes of brain development. D vitamins have also been researched for possible contribution to brain development in persons with intellectual disabilities and ASD (Mazahery et al., 2016). D vitamins do have a small positive affect on general energy, metabolism, and well-being; however, a direct link to improvements in cognitive functioning has yet to be established.

Proposed Dietary Therapies

There are several specialized diets that have been proposed to reduce problematic symptoms that commonly co-occur with intellectual disabilities. To date, there is no substantial evidence that these diets reliably produce improvements in any outcome variable. Many of the proposed therapies are elimination diets that exclude specific substances that are thought to create symptoms or reactions that manifest themselves in behavioural or cognitive problems. One of the most well-known diet programs was developed by Feingold in 1974 (Glanzman & Toomey, 2016). The assumption made in the Feingold diet is that overactive behaviour, other psychiatric issues, and learning disabilities may be caused or exacerbated by allergies to specific substances. Based on his observations, he recommended that tartrazine and salicylate acid and other compounds that are chemically similar be removed from diets (Glanzman & Toomey, 2016). Food colourings, preservatives, artificial sweeteners, and artificial flavours often fall into this category. This diet has many parent and professional adherents. The diet consists of 6 weeks eliminating all artificial colours and flavors; preservatives such as butylated hydroxytoluene, butylated hydroxyanisole, and tertiary butylhydroquinone; and foods that are high in salicylate-related compounds (e.g. peppers, berries, peaches, vinegar, tea). Versions of the Feingold diet include other substances that can be eliminated from the diet as they may cause reactions that affect behaviour (Glanzman & Toomey, 2016). Some of these other substances are nitrates, gluten, and casein. If the targeted symptoms are reduced after elimination, then the foods with the salicylate-related compounds are gradually reintroduced until symptoms return. Although there is a significant amount of anecdotal and case study evidence supporting the Feingold diet for improving overactive symptoms related to attention deficit hyperactivity disorder, the only double-blind, crossover, experimental study on this form of diet demonstrates no significant therapeutic effect (Harner & Foiles, 1980). The evidence for this form of elimination diet based on the idea that food additive allergies are responsible for many problematic behaviours is weak.

The oligoantigenic diet is a related program that focuses on food sensitivities that may cause a variety of neurological and behavioural reactions, especially non-IgE-mediated immunologic reactions (Ly et al., 2017). Although there are many versions of this diet, the general principle is that low allergenic foods create the foundation of a diet. Gradually, foods with artificial colours, dairy, wheat, corn, foods with high concentration of salicylate-like compounds, and other foods known to elicit common allergic reactions are reintroduced. The effects for inattentive and overactive behaviours are mixed. However, there are several strong methodological studies that support this diet in reducing inattentive and overactive behaviours in children diagnosed with ADHD. There are no strong studies focusing on behaviour change in persons with intellectual disabilities. It is possible that allergic responses to food may create general discomfort and therefore increase inattentive behaviours rather than have a direct effect on neurological functioning. For purposes of intervention, the mechanism for improvement does not matter. To some degree, this much of the oligoantigenic diet's effectiveness may be due to a reasonable approach to general nutrition. Caution should be exercised for possible allergic reactions to foods that may directly or indirectly affect behaviour. Because many people with intellectual disabilities may have compromised or otherwise unusual immune systems, additional attention to allergic reactions may be warranted.

There has been increasing attention to the interaction between abnormalities of the digestive system and autism spectrum disorder. The concept is that gluten and casein peptides, which passes through a "leaky gut", and binds to opioid receptors and affects neurotransmitter activity (Ding, Taur, & Walkup, 2017). There is also evidence that people with autism spectrum disorder are more likely to have elevated serum markers for celiac disease. The causal mechanism has yet to be tested and can only be considered conjectural at this point. However, these interesting ideas have led to introduction of a gluten–/casein-free diet as a treatment mechanism for autism spectrum disorders. Like all dietary interventions, the gluten–/casein-free diet has passionate adherents. There have been several small-scale but well-designed studies of the effectiveness of this diet (Hyman et al., 2016). There is a consistent small positive affect on the gluten–/casein-free diet in reducing symptoms of overactivity for children with autism spectrum disorder. A relatively consistent finding is that the effects are small in the beginning and tend to decrease over time (Hyman et al., 2016). Although the mechanism of the gluten–/casein-free diet is speculative, there is enough supportive evidence to suggest this is a reasonable therapy option to address overactive behaviours. Specific studies on samples of people with intellectual disabilities without autism spectrum disorder have yet to be carried out.

Overall, proposed dietary therapies have demonstrated at most a small positive affect on addressing overactive and inattentive behaviours (Glanzman & Toomey, 2016). The primary problems are that these diets can be expensive and difficult to maintain. For many families, mealtime and diet are important parts of family connectedness, ritual, consistency, and bonding (Crnic, Neece, McIntyre, Blacher, & Baker, 2017). Parents and clinicians should consider whether the likely small positive gain is worth the cost of disrupting traditional food preparation and mealtime, the expense, and time intensive inconvenience of adhering to these diets.

Therapeutic Interventions

There are several therapeutic interventions that promote functioning for people with intellectual disabilities that have strong research support. Although there are no therapies that provide anything close to a cure for the multifaceted issues of intellectual disabilities, improving and applying functional skills are valuable components of any comprehensive treatment program for people with intellectual disabilities.

Occupational Therapy

Occupational therapies are heterogeneous activities that are structured to support adaptation to the demands of the environments of clients. The goals are to identify and eliminate barriers to functioning and independence, increase participation in daily activities, improve daily living skills, teaching accident prevention, create positive leisure activities, prepare for work life, and other supportive goals. Although frequently thought of as improving the skills of an individual client, there is also significant energy placed on adapting the environment, increasing support services, and increasing opportunities for participation. Although occupational therapists work with a host of clients, including those with physical injuries, illness, and mental health issues; occupational therapists serve a valuable role for people with intellectual disabilities. Most often, occupational therapy is an important part of a multidisciplinary team providing comprehensive services to people with intellectual disabilities.

Occupational therapy is an essential component of improving adaptive behaviours (Barnett & O'Shaughnessy, 2015). There is strong evidence that consistent occupational therapy can improve quality of life along many domains. By improving the capabilities of people with intellectual disabilities, there is evidence of improved executive functioning, time management, use of leisure time, preparation for employment, and understanding time and organization. Occupational therapy also played a significant role in reducing stereotyped and self-injurious behaviours in people with intellectual disabilities and autism. Occupational therapy is a complex undertaking of teaching specific abilities, such as refining fine motor skills and implementing those skills in real-life environments to improve overall functioning.

Sensory Integration Therapy

Sensory integration therapies are usually administered by occupational therapists but are different from the traditional occupational therapy role. Many people with intellectual disabilities and autism spectrum disorder have challenges in how they respond to sensory input. Sensory integration interventions are intended to assist clients with how they interpret, organize, and make sense of environmental stimuli. The goal is to use various vestibular, auditory, visual, gustatory, and olfactory sensory diets to influence an individual's neurological organization so that they improve orientation in space and time and thus are better able to function in their real environment. There is a logical leap from identifying a neurological basis of sensory integration impairments to determining that sensory diet can change neurology to produce a functional change. Sensory integration therapies are widely used for people with intellectual disabilities and autism spectrum disorder. Despite being a form of therapy that has been developed and widely implemented since the mid-1970s, there are still no high-quality evaluative studies of the effectiveness of sensory integration for improving any important outcome measures for people with intellectual disabilities or autism (Barton, Reichow, Schnitz, Smith, & Sherlock, 2015).

The persistence of sensory integration therapy despite no strong supporting evidence is likely due to the consideration of the oft-ignored and serious issues related to hyper- or hyposensitivity to the environment and the proposed solution; and the neuroscientific foundation of the theory adds an aspect of credibility that is lacking in many complementary and alternative therapies (Case-Smith, Weaver, & Fristad, 2015). There are many methodological and practical challenges to evaluating sensory integration therapies. Among those problems are treatment fidelity, controlling for development (i.e. would individuals with sensory integration disorders improve simply as a function of development?), random assignment of treatment, blind assessment, and other features of a randomized controlled treatment study that make for strong scientific evidence. To be fair, the challenges of designing studies for this form of treatment with specialized populations are daunting. For example, talk therapies involved in counselling were commonly dismissed as having no proof of effectiveness for over 50 years until advances and methodologies made effective evaluation and proof of effectiveness possible. Yet, the current state of the research is that sensory integration therapy is an unproved treatment mechanism without sufficient supporting evidence (Case-Smith et al., 2015).

Physical Therapy

Physical therapy promotes and instructs functional gross motor performance to increase functional activities in daily life. This form of activity involves motor training to improve walking, posture, gait, and other motor issues that are common problems for people with intellectual disabilities. Physical therapy is a heterogeneous field of practice with multiple subspecialties including rehabilitative medicine, cardiovascular physiotherapy, geriatric functioning, palliative care, and sports rehabilitation (Hooking, McNeil, & Campbell, 2016). Physical therapy is commonly used for persons with intellectual disabilities that involve concurrent motor issues. For example, physical therapy is a primary form of intervention for persons with cerebral palsy to improve motor function. However, numerous disorders leading to intellectual disabilities have features such as hypotonia, spasticity, tremors, and other motor issues that need to be addressed before improving functioning can take place. Although not a required form of therapy for every person with intellectual disabilities, evidence is extremely strong that quality of life, motor skills, and daily functioning are significantly enhanced via many forms of physical therapy (Hooking et al., 2016).

Speech and Language Therapy

Language is a keystone variable for people with intellectual disabilities. As such, speech and language pathologists are critical components of multidisciplinary teams. The expertise of speech and language pathologist is wide. Speech and language pathologist for pediatric settings are usually thought of as addressing speech delays and disorders such as articulation, motor speech disorders due to dyspraxia, fluency disorders such as stuttering, and voice disorders with a neurological basis. These are important features of therapy (Schoenbrodt, Kumin, Dautzenberg, & Lynds, 2016). However, speech and language therapists also provide valuable therapies for addressing cognitive and communication disorders, social communication, pragmatic language skills, reasoning, problem-solving, and executive functioning skills (Schoenbrodt et al., 2016). Speech and language therapy has also proved effective in addressing preliteracy and literacy skills that are necessary for phonological awareness, decoding, reading comprehension, and written language. Although a subspecialty area, feeding and swallowing issues are common for children with intellectual and multiple disabilities and are frequently addressed by speech and language pathologist (Williams, Seiverling, & Field, 2014).

The role of developing receptive and expressive communication cannot be overstated in functional improvements for persons with intellectual disabilities. In addition to basic communication skills, improvements and language have important ramifications for multiple domains. For example, individuals with emotional regulation and behaviour problems are reported to have significantly fewer outbursts, aggressive behaviours, and other maladaptive reactions when they learn vocabulary to express their emotions and challenges (Martin, Lee, & Losh, 2017). Language is a keystone variable for people with intellectual disabilities. As such, speech and language pathologists are critical components of multidisciplinary therapies. The expertise of speech and language pathologist is wide. Speech and language pathologist for pediatric settings are usually thought of as addressing speech delays and disorders such as articulation, motor speech disorders due to dyspraxia, fluency disorders such as stuttering, and voice disorders with a neurological basis. These are important features of therapy (Schoenbrodt et al., 2016). However, speech and language therapists also provide valuable therapies for addressing cognitive and communication disorders, social communication, pragmatic language skills, reasoning, problem-solving, and executive functioning skills (Schoenbrodt et al., 2016). Speech and language therapy has also proved effective in addressing preliteracy and literacy skills that are necessary for phonological awareness, decoding, reading comprehension, and written language. Although a subspecialty area, feeding and swallowing issues are common for children with intellectual and multiple disabilities and are frequently addressed by speech and language pathologist (Williams et al., 2014). The role of developing receptive and expressive communication cannot be overstated in functional improvements for persons with intellectual disabilities. In addition to basic communication skills, improvements and language have important ramifications for multiple domains. For example, individuals with emotional regulation and behaviour problems are reported to have significantly fewer outbursts, aggressive behaviours, and other maladaptive reactions when they learn vocabulary to express their emotions and challenges (Martin et al., 2017). And more than simply addressing communications with other people, self-talk is a critical aspect of problem-solving, reasoning, and higher-level cognitive functioning. Therefore, language improvement also has important influence on cognitive functioning. Developing and applying the communication skills addressed by speech and language pathologists are important evidence-based components of improving the functioning of people with intellectual disabilities (Martin et al., 2017). Effective therapy can affect multiple domains and often provide efficient treatment mechanisms for improving the functioning of persons with intellectual disabilities. As with other people, self-talk is a critical aspect of problem-solving, reasoning, and higher-level cognitive functioning. Therefore, language improvement also has important influence on cognitive functioning. Developing and applying the communication skills addressed by speech and language pathologists are important evidence-based components of improving the functioning of people with intellectual disabilities (Martin et al., 2017). Effective therapy can affect multiple domains and often provide efficient treatment mechanisms for improving the functioning of persons with intellectual disabilities.

Complementary and Alternative Therapies

Complementary and alternative therapies are forms of treatment that have yet to be validated through scientific processes. Some therapies represent folk remedies, traditional Chinese medicine, fringe ideas about the nature and development of intellectual disabilities, and entirely novel approaches to treatment of any of the symptoms related to intellectual disabilities. Some forms of diet and sensory integration therapy can still be referred to as complementary and alternative therapies because the state of the science does not support their use in improving symptoms related to intellectual disabilities. Complementary and alternative therapies are extremely common in the treatment of specific medical issues and overall health. To a large degree, this is because intellectual disabilities represent a lifelong impairment of cognitive function, and parents frequently seek out hope in any place they can find it. One of the challenges in the use of complementary and alternative therapies is that they are almost entirely rejected by the traditional medical community. The result is that many families do not report the use of these therapies to their physicians (Travers, 2017). By not reporting all forms of therapies to physicians, there runs a risk of adverse interactions with traditional medicines and symptoms that are difficult to explain without knowledge of the existence of complementary and alternative therapy use. Should parents choose to adopt complementary and alternative therapies, traditional medical and educational professionals must understand the needs for parents and individuals to control their own treatment or provide the best possible advice without judgment or scolding.

Complementary and alternative therapies can be divided into two major forms: one form consists of disproved concepts or theories that have no possibility of working, and the other form consists of therapies that have not gone through a rigorous scientific testing process, yet. The first form may be dangerous, while the second form may provide some level of hope and hold the possibility of effectiveness. Although the adage that "complementary and alternative therapies are a complement and alternative to therapies that actually work" has some validity, an open mind can be helpful and is critical to building trust with parents (Glanzman & Toomey, 2016). Guiding parents towards constructive therapies is not possible if those decision-makers do not trust medical professionals.

Chelation Therapy

Chelation therapy is a chemical process in which ethylenediaminetetraacetic acid (EDTA) is introduced to the bloodstream to bind to heavy metals and minerals such as lead, mercury, arsenic, aluminium, and other toxins and removes them from the body (Travers, 2017). The primary purpose of chelation therapy is for removal of lead in the case of exposure to extremely large levels of heavy metal toxicity. This form of therapy has been used to treat autism spectrum disorders and intellectual disabilities, because some not proved ideas concerning the cause of these developmental disorders have been attributed to heavy metal toxicity. There is no supporting evidence for this use of chelation therapy. Doses of EDTA can lead to severe medical consequences. There have been multiple cases of children with autism treated with EDTA who have died due to its use (Travers, Ayers, Simpson, & Crutchfield, 2016). Given the risk factors for heart and kidney problems that are common in people with intellectual disabilities, EDTA represents a serious health risk with no evidence of success (Travers, 2017).

Herbal Therapies

Herbal medicine is a form of dietary supplement in which a plant or a plant part is used for its underlying chemical makeup, scent, flavour, or some other combination of therapeutic properties. Herbs are typically sold as capsules, powders, oils, extract, or plants. Nearly all medicines that now have a strong evidence base had their origins in some form of folk-based herbal medicine (Liao et al., 2017). As result, it is difficult to dismiss all herbal therapies as not evidence-based or clinical poor practice. The primary danger is that many patients and their families think of herbal remedies as "natural" and therefore not harmful. Yet, many herbal substances can be fatal, present high risk of side effects, or interact with prescription or over-the-counter medications. The second major problems are dosage and purity (Travers, 2017). Most herbal medicines do not have a standard dosage or government oversight to assure purity of the product. Even herbal medicine that has a high likelihood of success is extremely dangerous without clear guidelines as to dosage and purity. Herbal medicines require coordination with traditional healthcare providers to ensure that otherwise innocuous herbal treatments do not interact with prescription or over-the-counter medications. Given the large number of unknowns with potentially serious consequences, and there is limited and often no evidence that most herbal medications have positive treatment outcomes, these products are typically not recommended.

There are no widely used herbal medicines reported in literature that are purported to affect cognitive functioning for people with intellectual disabilities (Travers et al., 2016). However, there are multiple herbal therapies for related issues. The most commonly used herbal therapies are for sleep disorders. Two herbal medications that have been evaluated for improving sleep onset for persons with intellectual disabilities are kava (sometimes referred to as kava-kava) and valerian (Glanzman & Toomey, 2016). There is some evidence that kava and valerian have resulted in significant improvements for cases of insomnia. However, there are questions concerning the methodological rigour of these two studies. There are other studies that demonstrate no positive effects of these two herbal medications. There are also well-known adverse effects of using these herbal remedies, including rash, jaundice, and hepatotoxicity (which has resulted in cases of liver failure and death; Glanzman & Toomey, 2016).

Homeopathy

Homeopathy is a system of alternative medicine involving extremely diluted substances such as minerals, metals, essential oils, and other substances. Although there is nothing wrong about keeping an open mind about complementary and alternative therapies, homeopathy has been entirely debunked as pseudoscience (Foxx & Mulick, 2015). The only positive outcomes are via placebo effects (Dolce Filho, 2006).

Experiential Therapies

There are a host of activities with purported beneficial effects for people with intellectual disabilities. These therapies are guided experiences that are typically physical or tactile in nature and are almost always enjoyable. Some of the examples of these therapies are equine therapy, simulated hippotherapy, animal-assisted therapy, aqua therapy, art therapy, music therapy, and many others. These forms of therapy have elements in common with sensory integration therapy, physical therapy, occupational therapy, and even speech and language therapy. The challenge is that much of the evaluative research does not identify a specific outcome or engage in standard research practices. There are important descriptive studies, case studies, and testimonials that indicate improved language, improved connections with animals, improved motor skills and balance, improved motor strength, and increased energy (Jeng, Chang, Liu, Hou, & Lin, 2017). Whether effective as a therapy or not, most of these activities increase social participation in self-directed or therapist-directed leisure activities that bring enjoyment to people with intellectual disabilities and their families. Given that most of these activities are safe, there are few problems in engaging in these activities. However, expectations for a specific therapeutic effect should be limited. The only specific recommendation and warning is for hippotherapy, and pursuing a certified riding program for individuals with disabilities is recommended to ensure safe procedures, professional instructors, and correct riding techniques are used.

Power of Placebo

Much of the value of complementary and alternative therapies are due to placebo effects. This is not a condemnation of these therapies. Some complementary and alternative therapies will likely prove to be cutting-edge evidence-based treatments yet have not been evaluated effectively. Even those therapies that will not be proven to be effective may have some benefit as a placebo. We often think of the term placebo as a pejorative phrase that connotes fooling or misleading the patient into thinking a nonevidence-based practice is effective. Hype, public relations, marketing, and quackery often come to mind when we think of a treatment as a placebo. These characterizations are unfair and misleading. Placebo effects rely on transmitters and activation of specific, relevant, and observable (via imaging) areas of the brain (Kaptchuk & Miller, 2015). Several evidence-based medications and treatments are known to affect the brain in similar fashion. Although there has been a recent increase in research related to placebo effects, there is still much that is not known about placebo. There are four overall findings in placebo research that are relevant to the use of complementary and alternative treatments:

1. There are many cases in which placebo can provide relief from problematic symptoms but rarely provide more than a temporary fix of a problem, and there are no cases where placebo has resulted in a cure of any complex condition.
2. Often treatments that rely primarily on placebo effects are administered when problems and symptoms are at their worst. The patient identifies improvement of symptoms, which are almost certainly due to regression to the mean, but mistakenly identifies the placebo treatment as a causal factor in the improvement of symptoms.
3. Placebo illustrates the interaction between clinicians' behaviours, symbols of effective treatment (e.g. a degreed clinician in a white coat, formal and official sounding procedures and treatments, clinicians of high status), and outcomes. Clinician behaviours and symbols of effective treatment result in dramatically improved outcomes even when evidence-based practices are used. In other words, clinician confidence or professional stature can provide a boost or increased effectiveness in many types of treatments that are proved to be effective.
4. The same factors that cause placebo effects can have negative consequences as well. Known as "nocebo" effects, if a client or parent is anticipating negative effects or a high degree of side effects, then responses to a medication or treatment are more likely to be interpreted as negative (Carlino, Piedimonte, & Benedetti, 2016). Too often, placebo effects are considered unworthy, illegitimate, and unscientific and caused by bias and prejudice. Placebo effects are a legitimate component of any formal treatment and are worthy of respect and judicious use. Although many treatments labelled as complementary and alternative therapies received their positive results in relatively poorly designed evaluation studies due to placebo effects, caution, judgment, and patient need should be firmly considered by clinicians before dismissing such treatments out of hand.

Future Therapies

Some of the therapies that are referred to as complementary and alternative therapies have the potential to be evidence-based practices. In addition, some of the proposed therapies in diet and nutrition and interventions such as sensory integration therapy may eventually be proved to ameliorate common problems or issues experienced by people with intellectual disabilities and their families. However, there remain significant hurdles before this can take place. There must not only be anecdotal, historical, cultural, or belief system foundations for new therapies; but there must also be sound short- and long-term evaluation of the safety and effectiveness of the intervention. This form of evaluation and testing of potentially useful therapies is a long and tedious process with few shortcuts. Several of the described therapies may be effective, but there is no compelling consensus in the literature supporting effectiveness. The burden of proof is on those wishing to implement an intervention without scientific support. Simply stating that an intervention is worth implementing because there is no literature disproving the effectiveness is illogical and dangerous. An open mind is important for advancing the treatment and therapies for people with intellectual disabilities who have significant and multidomain needs for effective therapies, but there is no substitute for well-designed and scientifically based evaluative studies.

Conclusions

That some complementary and alternative therapies will result in positive outcomes for people with intellectual disabilities is a real possibility. Even placebo effects are not necessarily poor outcomes. The primary risks of adopting alternative and complementary therapies are (1) they may pose a risk by introducing dangerous medical practices or substances to the individual, (2) they introduce an unknown interaction with medications currently being administered, (3) they may be expensive and pose a potential financial hardship to families with little promise of effectiveness, (4) they may take family energy and commitment away from therapies that have been proven to be effective, and (5) they may disrupt family relationships and rituals to the point that they may cause harm to individuals and their familial support system. Should the five primary risks of adopting alternative and complementary therapies be evaluated and determined to be minimal or acceptable in nature, then families or individuals should be encouraged or at least supported in the introduction of these therapies into the treatment plan if this is what they desire. Although the approach of supporting families in implementing complementary and alternative therapies is not consistent with evidence-based practices, there may be additional trust added to the relationship that can be of later clinical value. In addition, professionals can assist parents in evaluating the effectiveness of the evidence-based practice on the outcome variable of interest. This form of practice-based evidence provides some data as to the utility of the alternative and complementary variable.

Summary

There is no cure for autism spectrum disorders or intellectual disabilities, but there are several approaches to improve functioning, health, behaviour, and quality of life. All forms of treatment have advantages and risks. Careful interpretation of the safety and effectiveness of each form of therapy is required before any decisions can be made.

References

Adler, K., Reghunathan, A., Hutchison, L. H., & Kalpatthi, R. (2016). Dural Venous Sinus Diameters in children with sickle cell disease: Correlation with history of stroke in a case-control study. *Southern Medical Journal, 109*(9), 511–515. https://doi.org/10.14423/SMJ.0000000000000513

Alexander, R. C. (2016). Prader-Willi syndrome. In I. L. Rubin, J. Merrick, D. E. Greydanus, & D. R. Patel (Eds.), *Health care for people with intellectual and developmental disabilities across the lifespan* (pp. 779–798). Cham, Switzerland: Springer. https://doi.org/10.1007/978-3-319-18096-0_66

Allen, D., Langthorne, P., Tonge, B., Emerson, E., McGill, P., Fletcher, R., … Kennedy, C. (2013). Towards the prevention of behavioural and psychiatric disorders in people with intellectual disabilities. *Journal of Applied Research in Intellectual Disabilities, 26*(6), 501–514. https://doi.org/10.1111/jar.12050

Barnard-Brak, L., Davis, T. N., Schmidt, M., & Richman, D. M. (2016). Effects associated with on- and off-label stimulant treatment of core autism and ADHD symptoms exhibited by children with autism spectrum disorder. *Developmental Neurorehabilitation, 19*(1), 46–53. https://doi.org/10.3109/17518423.2014.904949

Barnett, J. E. H., & O'Shaughnessy, K. (2015). Enhancing collaboration between occupational therapists and early childhood educators working with children on the autism spectrum. *Early Childhood Education Journal, 43*(6), 467–472. https://doi.org/10.1007/s10643-015-0689-2

Barton, E. E., Reichow, B., Schnitz, A., Smith, I. C., & Sherlock, D. (2015). A systematic review of sensory-based treatments for children with disabilities. *Research in Developmental Disabilities, 37*, 64–80. https://doi.org/10.1016/j.ridd.2014.11.006

Basil, J. S., Santoro, S. L., Martin, L. J., Healy, K. W., Chini, B. A., & Saal, H. M. (2016). Retrospective study of obesity in children with Down Syndrome. *The Journal of Pediatrics, 173*, 143–148. https://doi.org/10.1016/j.jpeds.2016.02.046

Brown, M., Jacobstein, D., Yoon, I. S., Anthony, B., & Bullock, K. (2016). System-wide initiative documents robust health screening for adults with intellectual disability. *Intellectual and Developmental Disabilities, 54*(5), 354–365. https://doi.org/10.1352/1934-9556-54.5.354

Carlino, E., Piedimonte, A., & Benedetti, F. (2016). Nature of the placebo and nocebo effect in relation to functional neurologic disorders. *Handbook of Clinical Neurology, 139*, 597–606. https://doi.org/10.1016/B978-0-12-801772-2.00048-5

Case-Smith, J., Weaver, L. L., & Fristad, M. A. (2015). A systematic review of sensory processing interventions for children with autism spectrum disorders. *Autism, 19*(2), 133–148. https://doi.org/10.1177/1362361313517762

Charlot, L., Abend, S., Ravin, P., Mastis, K., Hunt, A., & Deutsch, C. (2011). Non-psychiatric health problems among psychiatric inpatients with intellectual disabilities. *Journal of Intellectual Disability Research, 55*(2), 199–209. https://doi.org/10.1111/j.1365-2788.2010.01294.x

Cohen, D., Raffin, M., Canitano, R., Bodeau, N., Bonnot, O., Périsse, D., … Laurent, C. (2013). Risperidone or aripiprazole in children and adolescents with autism and/or intellectual disability: A Bayesian meta-analysis of efficacy and secondary effects. *Research in Autism Spectrum Disorders, 7*(1), 167–175. https://doi.org/10.1016/j.rasd.2012.08.001

Craft, S., Baker, L. D., Montine, T. J., Minoshima, S., Watson, G. S., Claxton, A., … Gerton, B. (2012). Intranasal insulin therapy for Alzheimer disease and amnestic mild cognitive impairment: A pilot clinical trial. *Archives of Neurology, 69*(1), 29–38. https://doi.org/10.1001/archneurol.2011.233

Crnic, K. A., Neece, C. L., McIntyre, L. L., Blacher, J., & Baker, B. L. (2017). Intellectual disability and developmental risk: Promoting intervention to improve child and family well-being. *Child Development, 88*(2), 436–445. https://doi.org/10.1111/cdev.12740

Dagnan, D., Masson, J., Cavagin, A., Thwaites, R., & Hatton, C. (2015). The development of a measure of confidence in delivering therapy to people with intellectual disabilities. *Clinical Psychology & Psychotherapy, 22*(5), 392–398. https://doi.org/10.1002/cpp.1898

de Kuijper, G., Evenhuis, H., Minderaa, R. B., & Hoekstra, P. J. (2014). Effects of controlled discontinuation of long-term used antipsychotics for behavioural symptoms in individuals with intellectual disability. *Journal of Intellectual Disability Research, 58*(1), 71–83. https://doi.org/10.1111/j.1365-2788.2012.01631.x

Deb, S., Chaplin, R., Sohanpal, S., Unwin, G., Soni, R., & Lenotre, L. (2008). The effectiveness of mood stabilizers and antiepileptic medication for the management of behaviour problems in adults with intellectual disability: A systematic review. *Journal of Intellectual Disability Research, 52*(2), 107–113. https://doi.org/10.1111/j.1365-2788.2007.00965.x

Deb, S., Farmah, B. K., Arshad, E., Deb, T., Roy, M., & Unwin, G. L. (2014). The effectiveness of aripiprazole in the management of problem behaviour in people with intellectual disabilities, developmental disabilities and/or autistic spectrum disorder – A systematic review. *Research in Developmental Disabilities, 35*(3), 711–725. https://doi.org/10.1016/j.ridd.2013.12.004

Dijkhuizen, A., Hilgenkamp, T. I. M., Krijnen, W. P., van der Schans, C. P., & Waninge, A. (2016). The impact of visual impairment on the ability to perform activities of daily living for persons with severe/profound intellectual disability. *Research in Developmental Disabilities, 48*, 35–42. https://doi.org/10.1016/j.ridd.2015.10.001

Ding, H. T., Taur, Y., & Walkup, J. T. (2017). Gut microbiota and autism: Key concepts and findings. *Journal of Autism and Developmental Disorders, 47*(2), 480–489. https://doi.org/10.1007/s10803-016-2960-9

Dolce Filho, R. (2006). Homeopathic approach in the treatment of patients with mental disability. *Homeopathy: The Journal of the Faculty of Homeopathy, 95*(1), 31–44. https://doi.org/10.1016/j.homp.2005.10.001

Dunn, K., Hughes-McCormack, L., & Cooper, S.-A. (2017). Hospital admissions for physical health conditions for people with intellectual disabilities: Systematic review. *Journal of Applied Research in Intellectual Disabilities, 31*(Suppl 1), 1–10. https://doi.org/10.1111/jar.12360

Edelsohn, G. A., Schuster, J. M., Castelnovo, K., Terhorst, L., & Parthasarathy, M. (2014). Psychotropic prescribing for persons with intellectual disabilities and other psychiatric disorders. *Psychiatric Services, 65*(2), 201–207. https://doi.org/10.1176/appi.ps.201300029

Erickson, S. R., Spoutz, P., Dorsch, M., & Bleske, B. (2016). Cardiovascular risk and treatment for adults with intellectual or developmental disabilities. *International Journal of Cardiology, 221*, 371–375. https://doi.org/10.1016/j.ijcard.2016.07.044

Foxx, R. M., & Mulick, J. A. (2015). *Controversial therapies for autism and intellectual disabilities: Fad, fashion, and science in professional practice*. New York, NY: Routledge.

Glanzman, M. M., & Toomey, M. (2016). Complementary and alternative therapies. In N. N. Singh (Ed.), *Handbook of evidence-based practices in intellectual and developmental disabilities* (pp. 243–282). Cham, Switzerland: Springer.

Greydanus, D. E., & Merrick, J. (2016). Smith-magenis syndrome. In I. L. Rubin, J. Merrick, D. E. Greydanus, & D. R. Patel (Eds.), *Health care for people with intellectual and developmental disabilities across the lifespan* (pp. 821–825). Cham, Switzerland: Springer. https://doi.org/10.1007/978-3-319-18096-0_69

Grieco, J. C., Ciarlone, S. L., Gieron-Korthals, M., Schoenberg, M. R., Smith, A. G., Philpot, R. M., … Weeber, E. J. (2014). An open-label pilot trial of minocycline in children as a treatment for Angelman syndrome. *BMC Neurology, 14*(1), 232. https://doi.org/10.1186/s12883-014-0232-x

Häβler, F., Thome, J., & Reis, O. (2014). Polypharmacy in the treatment of subjects with intellectual disability. *Journal of Neural Transmission, 122*(Suppl. 1), S93–S100. https://doi.org/10.1007/s00702-014-1219-x

Harner, I. C., & Foiles, R. A. (1980). Effect of Feingold's K-P diet on a residential mentally handicapped population. *Journal of the American Dietetic Association, 76*(6), 575–578.

Heller, T., McCubbin, J. A., Drum, C., & Peterson, J. (2011). Physical activity and nutrition health promotion interventions: What is working for people with intellectual disabilities? *Intellectual and Developmental Disabilities, 49*(1), 26–36. https://doi.org/10.1352/1934-9556-49.1.26

Hodapp, R. M., & Dykens, E. M. (2012). Genetic disorders of intellectual disability: Expanding our concepts of phenotypes and of family outcomes. *Journal of Genetic Counseling, 21*(6), 761–769. https://doi.org/10.1007/s10897-012-9536-4

Hooking, J., McNeil, J., & Campbell, J. (2016). Physical therapy interventions for gross motor skills in people with an intellectual disability aged 6 years and over: A systematic review. *International Journal of Evidence-Based Healthcare, 14*, 166–174.

Huguet, A., Olthuis, J., McGrath, P., Tougas, M., Hayden, J., Stinson, J., & Chambers, C. (2017). Systematic review of childhood and adolescent risk and prognostic factors for persistent abdominal pain. *Acta Paediatrica, 106*(4), 545–553. https://doi.org/10.1111/apa.13736

Hyman, S. L., Stewart, P. A., Foley, J., Cain, U., Peck, R., Morris, D. D., … Smith, T. (2016). The gluten-free/casein-free diet: A double-blind challenge trial in children with autism. *Journal of Autism and Developmental Disorders, 46*(1), 205–220. https://doi.org/10.1007/s10803-015-2564-9

Jeng, S.-C., Chang, C.-W., Liu, W.-Y., Hou, Y.-J., & Lin, Y.-H. (2017). Exercise training on skill-related physical fitness in adolescents with intellectual disability: A systematic review and meta-analysis. *Disability and Health Journal, 10*(2), 198–206. https://doi.org/10.1016/j.dhjo.2016.12.003

Kahn, J., Koh, A., Luckcuck, R., McNeice, J., Walter, E., Yao, W., … Link, T. (2016). A phenylalanine fiasco: The structure of phenylalanine hydroxylase and its impact on phenylketonuria. *The FASEB Journal, 30*(1 Suppl), 665.8–665.8.

Kaptchuk, T. J., & Miller, F. G. (2015). Placebo effects in medicine. *New England Journal of Medicine, 373*(1), 8–9. https://doi.org/10.1056/NEJMp1504023

Koch, G., Poulsen, S., Espelid, I., & Haubek, D. (2016). *Pediatric dentistry: A clinical approach*. London, England: Wiley.

Koegel, L. K., Krasno, A. M., Taras, H., Koegel, R. L., & Frea, W. (2013). Is medication information for children with autism spectrum disorder monitored and coordinated across professionals? Findings from a teacher survey. *School Mental Health, 5*(1), 48–57. https://doi.org/10.1007/s12310-012-9098-5

Koslowski, N., Klein, K., Arnold, K., Kösters, M., Schützwohl, M., Salize, H. J., & Puschner, B. (2016). Effectiveness of interventions for adults with mild to moderate intellectual disabilities and mental health problems: Systematic review and meta-analysis. *The British Journal of Psychiatry, 209*(6), 469–474. https://doi.org/10.1192/bjp.bp.114.162313

Kurtz, P. F., Boelter, E. W., Jarmolowicz, D. P., Chin, M. D., & Hagopian, L. P. (2011). An analysis of functional communication training as an empirically supported treatment for problem behavior displayed by individuals with intellectual disabilities. *Research in Developmental Disabilities, 32*(6), 2935–2942. https://doi.org/10.1016/j.ridd.2011.05.009

Lake, J. K., Vogan, V., Sawyer, A., Weiss, J. A., & Lunsky, Y. (2015). Psychotropic medication use among adolescents and young adults with an autism spectrum disorder: Parent views about medication use and healthcare services. *Journal of Child and Adolescent Psychopharmacology, 25*(3), 260–268. https://doi.org/10.1089/cap.2014.0106

Lance, E. I., & Shapiro, B. K. (2013). Confounding diagnoses in the neurodevelopmental disabilities population a child with hearing loss, absence epilepsy, and attention-deficit hyperactivity disorder (ADHD). *Journal of Child Neurology, 28*(5), 645–647. https://doi.org/10.1177/0883073812447980

Liao, H.-H., Yen, H.-R., Muo, C.-H., Lee, Y.-C., Wu, M.-Y., Chou, L.-W., … Chang, T.-T. (2017). Complementary traditional Chinese medicine use in children with cerebral palsy: A nationwide retrospective cohort study in Taiwan. *BMC Complementary and Alternative Medicine, 17*, 155. https://doi.org/10.1186/s12906-017-1668-5

Ly, V., Bottelier, M., Hoekstra, P. J., Vasquez, A. A., Buitelaar, J. K., & Rommelse, N. N. (2017). Elimination diets' efficacy and mechanisms in attention deficit hyperactivity disorder and autism spectrum disorder. *European Child & Adolescent Psychiatry, 26*(9), 1067–1079. https://doi.org/10.1007/s00787-017-0959-1

Martin, G. E., Lee, M., & Losh, M. (2017). Intellectual disability. In L. Cummings (Ed.), *Research in clinical pragmatics* (pp. 109–129). Cham, Switzerland: Springer. https://doi.org/10.1007/978-3-319-47489-2_5

Mazahery, H., Conlon, C., Beck, K. L., Kruger, M. C., Stonehouse, W., Camargo, C. A., … von Hurst, P. R. (2016). Vitamin D and omega-3 fatty acid supplements in children with autism spectrum disorder: A study protocol for a factorial randomised, double-blind, placebo-controlled trial. *Trials, 17*, 295. https://doi.org/10.1186/s13063-016-1428-8

McPaul, A., Walker, B., Law, J., & McKenzie, K. (2016). An exploratory study investigating how adults with intellectual disabilities perform on the Visual Association Test (VAT). *Journal of Applied Research in Intellectual Disabilities, 30*(5), 824–829. https://doi.org/10.1111/jar.12273

Moses, L., Katz, N., & Weizman, A. (2014). Metabolic profiles in adults with autism spectrum disorder and intellectual disabilities. *European Psychiatry, 29*(7), 397–401. https://doi.org/10.1016/j.eurpsy.2013.05.005

Mula, M. (2016). Using anxiolytics in epilepsy: Neurobiological, neuropharmacological and clinical aspects. *Epileptic Disorders, 18*(3), 217–227. https://doi.org/10.1684/epd.2016.0837

Norderyd, J., Klingberg, G., Faulks, D., & Granlund, M. (2016). Specialised dental care for children with complex disabilities focusing on child's functioning and need for general anaesthesia. *Disability and Rehabilitation, 39*(24), 2484–2491. https://doi.org/10.1080/09638288.2016.1236406

Novak, I. (2014). Evidence-based diagnosis, health care, and rehabilitation for children with cerebral palsy. *Journal of Child Neurology, 29*(8), 1141–1156. https://doi.org/10.1177/0883073814535503

Ouellette-Kuntz, H. (2005). Understanding health disparities and inequities faced by individuals with intellectual disabilities. *Journal of Applied Research in Intellectual Disabilities, 18*(2), 113–121. https://doi.org/10.1111/j.1468-3148.2005.00240.x

Persch, A. C., Lamb, A. J., Metzler, C. A., & Fristad, M. A. (2015). Healthy habits for children: Leveraging existing evidence to demonstrate value. *American Journal of Occupational Therapy, 69*(4), 6904090010p1–6904090010p5. https://doi.org/10.5014/ajot.2015.694001

Posar, A., & Visconti, P. (2016). Complementary and alternative medicine in autism: The question of omega-3. *Pediatric Annals, 45*(3), e103–e107. https://doi.org/10.3928/00904481-20160129-01

Prasher, V. P. (2004). Review of donepezil, rivastigmine, galantamine and memantine for the treatment of dementia in Alzheimer's disease in adults with Down syndrome: Implications for the intellectual disability population. *International Journal of Geriatric Psychiatry, 19*(6), 509–515. https://doi.org/10.1002/gps.1077

Ptomey, L., Goetz, J., Lee, J., Donnelly, J., & Sullivan, D. (2013). Diet quality of overweight and obese adults with intellectual and developmental disabilities as measured by the healthy eating index-2005. *Journal of Developmental and Physical Disabilities, 25*(6), 625–636. https://doi.org/10.1007/s10882-013-9339-z

Robertson, J., Emerson, E., Gregory, N., Hatton, C., Turner, S., Kessissoglou, S., & Hallam, A. (2000). Lifestyle related risk factors for poor health in residential settings for people with intellectual disabilities. *Research in Developmental Disabilities, 21*(6), 469–486. https://doi.org/10.1016/S0891-4222(00)00053-6

Robinson, S. J. (2012). Childhood epilepsy and autism spectrum disorders: Psychiatric problems, phenotypic expression, and anticonvulsants. *Neuropsychology Review, 22*(3), 271–279. https://doi.org/10.1007/s11065-012-9212-3

Ruud, M. P., Raanaas, R. K., & Bjelland, M. (2016). Caregivers' perception of factors associated with a healthy diet among people with intellectual disability living in community residences: A concept mapping method. *Research in Developmental Disabilities, 59*, 202–210. https://doi.org/10.1016/j.ridd.2016.09.006

Salameh, T. S., Bullock, K. M., Hujoel, I. A., Niehoff, M. L., Wolden-Hanson, T., Kim, J., … Banks, W. A. (2015). Central nervous system delivery of intranasal insulin: Mechanisms of uptake and effects on cognition. *Journal of Alzheimer's Disease, 47*(3), 715–728. https://doi.org/10.3233/JAD-150307

Sarasua, S. M., Dwivedi, A., Boccuto, L., Chen, C.-F., Sharp, J. L., Rollins, J. D., … DuPont, B. R. (2014). 22q13.2q13.32 genomic regions associated with severity of speech delay, developmen-

tal delay, and physical features in Phelan-McDermid syndrome. *Genetics in Medicine, 16*(4), 318–328. https://doi.org/10.1038/gim.2013.144
Sawyer, A., Lake, J. K., Lunsky, Y., Liu, S.-K., & Desarkar, P. (2014). Psychopharmacological treatment of challenging behaviours in adults with autism and intellectual disabilities: A systematic review. *Research in Autism Spectrum Disorders, 8*(7), 803–813. https://doi.org/10.1016/j.rasd.2014.03.021
Schoenbrodt, L., Kumin, L., Dautzenberg, D., & Lynds, J. (2016). Training parents to enhance narrative language skills in their children with intellectual disability. *International Medical Review on Down Syndrome, 20*(3), 31–38. https://doi.org/10.1016/j.sdeng.2016.09.001
Scott, H. M., & Havercamp, S. M. (2016). Systematic review of health promotion programs focused on behavioral changes for people with intellectual disability. *Intellectual and Developmental Disabilities, 54*(1), 63–76. https://doi.org/10.1352/1934-9556-54.1.63
Segal, M., Eliasziw, M., Phillips, S., Bandini, L., Curtin, C., Kral, T. V. E., … Must, A. (2016). Intellectual disability is associated with increased risk for obesity in a nationally representative sample of U. S. children. *Disability and Health Journal, 9*(3), 392–398. https://doi.org/10.1016/j.dhjo.2015.12.003
Sharma, A., & Shaw, S. R. (2012). Efficacy of risperidone in managing maladaptive behaviors for children with autistic spectrum disorder: A meta-analysis. *Journal of Pediatric Health Care, 26*(4), 291–299. https://doi.org/10.1016/j.pedhc.2011.02.008
Shen, J., & Morton, C. C. (2016). Next-generation newborn hearing screening. *Monographs in Human Genetics, 20*, 30–39. https://doi.org/10.1159/000444598
Shin, J.-Y., Roughead, E. E., Park, B.-J., & Pratt, N. L. (2016). Cardiovascular safety of methylphenidate among children and young people with attention-deficit/hyperactivity disorder (ADHD): Nationwide self-controlled case series study. *BMJ, 353*, i2550. https://doi.org/10.1136/bmj.i2550
Simonoff, E., Taylor, E., Baird, G., Bernard, S., Chadwick, O., Liang, H., … Jichi, F. (2013). Randomized controlled double-blind trial of optimal dose methylphenidate in children and adolescents with severe attention deficit hyperactivity disorder and intellectual disability. *Journal of Child Psychology and Psychiatry, 54*(5), 527–535. https://doi.org/10.1111/j.1469-7610.2012.02569.x
Travers, J. C. (2017). Evaluating claims to avoid pseudoscientific and unproven practices in special education. *Intervention in School and Clinic, 52*(4), 195–203. https://doi.org/10.1177/1053451216659466
Travers, J. C., Ayers, K., Simpson, R. L., & Crutchfield, S. (2016). Fad, pseudoscientific, and controversial interventions. In R. Lang, T. B. Hancock, & N. N. Singh (Eds.), *Early intervention for young children with autism spectrum disorder* (pp. 257–293). Cham, Switzerland: Springer.
van Karnebeek, C. D. M., Stockler-Ipsiroglu, S., Jaggumantri, S., Assmann, B., Baxter, P., Buhas, D., … Hartmann, H. (2014). Lysine-restricted diet as adjunct therapy for pyridoxine-dependent epilepsy: The PDE consortium consensus recommendations. In J. Zschocke, K. M. Gibson, G. Brown, E. Morava, & V. Peters (Eds.), *JIMD reports* (Vol. 15, pp. 47–57). Berlin Heidelberg: Springer. Retrieved from http://link.springer.com/chapter/10.1007/8904_2014_296
van Ool, J. S., Snoeijen-Schouwenaars, F. M., Schelhaas, H. J., Tan, I. Y., Aldenkamp, A. P., & Hendriksen, J. G. M. (2016). A systematic review of neuropsychiatric comorbidities in patients with both epilepsy and intellectual disability. *Epilepsy & Behavior, 60*, 130–137. https://doi.org/10.1016/j.yebeh.2016.04.018
van Schrojenstein Lantman-de Valk, H. M., & Walsh, P. N. (2008). Managing health problems in people with intellectual disabilities. *BMJ, 337*, a2507. https://doi.org/10.1136/bmj.a2507
van Timmeren, E. A., van der Putten, A. a. J., van Schrojenstein Lantman-de Valk, H. M. J., van der Schans, C. P., & Waninge, A. (2016). Prevalence of reported physical health problems in people with severe or profound intellectual and motor disabilities: A cross-sectional study of medical records and care plans. *Journal of Intellectual Disability Research, 60*(11), 1109–1118. https://doi.org/10.1111/jir.12298

Walsh, D., Belton, S., Meegan, S., Bowers, K., Corby, D., Staines, A., … Sweeney, M. R. (2017). A comparison of physical activity, physical fitness levels, BMI and blood pressure of adults with intellectual disability, who do and do not take part in Special Olympics Ireland programmes: Results from the SOPHIE study. *Journal of Intellectual Disabilities, 22*(2), 154–170. https://doi.org/10.1177/1744629516688773

Weise, J., Pollack, A., Britt, H., & Trollor, J. N. (2016). Primary health care for people with an intellectual disability: An exploration of demographic characteristics and reasons for encounters from the BEACH programme. *Journal of Intellectual Disability Research, 60*(11), 1119–1127. https://doi.org/10.1111/jir.12301

Weisman, O., Guri, Y., Gur, R. E., McDonald-McGinn, D. M., Calkins, M. E., Tang, S. X., … Gothelf, D. (2017). Subthreshold psychosis in 22q11.2 deletion syndrome: Multisite naturalistic study. *Schizophrenia Bulletin, 43*(5), 1079–1089. https://doi.org/10.1093/schbul/sbx005

Williams, K. E., Seiverling, L. J., & Field, D. G. (2014). Feeding problems. In P. Sturmey & R. Didden (Eds.), *Evidence-based practice and intellectual disabilities* (pp. 198–218). London, England: Wiley.

Zwanenburg, R. J., Bocca, G., Ruiter, S. A. J., Dillingh, J. H., Flapper, B. C. T., van den Heuvel, E. R., & van Ravenswaaij-Arts, C. M. A. (2016). Is there an effect of intranasal insulin on development and behaviour in Phelan-McDermid syndrome? A randomized, double-blind, placebo-controlled trial. *European Journal of Human Genetics, 24*(12), 1696–1701. https://doi.org/10.1038/ejhg.2016.109

Chapter 4
Impacts on Learning and Development

Abstract This chapter discusses how intellectual disabilities influence children's psychological development and developmental milestones in cognitive, language, and emotional-social domains. Furthermore, it examines the influence of intellectual disabilities on learning abilities, educational attainment, and social school adaptation. The chapter also includes strategies for educational teams on how to address certain developmental and educational concerns.

Case Study

Adam is a 5-year-old diagnosed with Prader-Willi syndrome. His physical and psychological development are significantly delayed. His gross and fine motor skills are below age level as are his receptive and expressive language abilities. He has a confirmed diagnosis of mild intellectual disability. Additionally, Adam's parents reported that he experiences serious sleep difficulties and obstructive sleep apnea, which cause his excessive daytime sleepiness. Due to obesity, low muscle tone, and motor control, classroom activities that require motor skills are difficult for him to perform. Teachers describe Adam as underactive, lethargic, and unenthusiastic about classroom activities. However, teachers also claim that he is sensitive to schedule changes and report frequent behaviour issues, such as throwing tantrums, stubbornness, and compulsions (e.g. picking at the skin, repeated engagement in solo play). Furthermore, Adam's inability to control excessive appetite and constant search for food, including eating nonfood items, are difficult for teachers to manage. Consequently, Adam's behaviour often disrupts learning activities in the classroom, and teachers describe his adaptation to school requirements as poor. Due to difficulties in controlling behaviour and speech delay, including speech articulation defects, his kindergarten peer group rejected Adam. The multiplicity of Adam's behavioural and social difficulties required management and several adjustments.

Primarily, positive behavioural strategies were implemented. These focused on providing positive reinforcement through a reward system and short-term goals and ignoring undesirable behaviours. Furthermore, strict food management strategies were introduced including maintenance of adequate and appropriate nutrition

S. R. Shaw, A. M. Jankowska, *Pediatric Intellectual Disabilities at School*, Pediatric School Psychology, https://doi.org/10.1007/978-3-030-02992-0_4

provided in kindergarten, controlling access to food, and maintaining mealtime routines. These strategies were established in collaboration with parents in order to ensure that both home and school support same rules for food management. Teachers were instructed to develop and maintain a predictable daily routine and strategies to signal upcoming changes to respond to Adam's sensitivity to change. Twice per week Adam attended speech therapy and physical therapy. He was also enrolled in an intervention program addressing his socialization needs with an intense social skills training, while teachers were responsible for creating opportunities for him to socialize with peers. This was also crucial in establishing flexible, yet effective, channels of communication with parents who were already involved, cooperating with several other specialists. Adam's health and development were under the control of various specialists like dietitian, pediatric ophthalmologist, pediatric orthopaedist, pediatric dentist, and pulmonary specialist. Despite the detail of the program set up for Adam, three times per year evaluation of all programs were conducted because Adam's needs and issues will change over time.

Introduction

Human development is a universal and lifelong process. This means that all people, over the course of their lives and regardless of their age, gender, health, or cultural background, continue to grow, change, and learn to better adapt to changing life circumstances. This development occurs across dimensions; we grow and change physically, we progress in our cognitive abilities, and we gradually become emotionally and socially mature. However, these changes do not necessarily occur in a linear fashion, nor simultaneously. Therefore, the process of development is different for every child and follows a unique path marked with acceleration and delay in various areas.

The child's individual trajectory of development, including its course, tempo, and plasticity, is determined by a diversity of interacting biological and environmental factors. These factors and the interplay between them either enhance the child's progress or compromise reaching developmental milestones. Severe developmental delays are a distinctive characteristic of children with intellectual disabilities. The deficits present in this population have an early onset, are permanent, and prevent the child from reaching developmental milestones at a typical rate. With time, this delay becomes more apparent. Although children with intellectual disabilities are progressing in their development significantly slower than their peers, they still develop, change, and learn at their own pace.

Limitations in cognitive functioning and low adaptive behaviours are major characteristics of children with intellectual disabilities (American Psychiatric Association, 2013); however, the delay concerns also other domains of their functioning (Amiet et al., 2008; Williams et al., 2006; Zoghbi & Bear, 2012). Intellectual disability is mainly a result of various pathogenic biological processes, including prenatal genetic disorders; students with intellectual disabilities present an array of heterogeneous deficits and abilities (Gates & Barr, 2009). Persons with intellectual disabilities also often struggle with health problems that require medical attention, regular treatment, or even hospitalization (Robinson & Richdale, 2004; Slevin, Truesdale-Kennedy, McConkey, Livingstone, & Fleming, 2014). The symptoms of a disease and side effects of the treatment are not indifferent to a child's developmental and educational path. To be able to reach educational standards and adapt to the academic and social demands of school, certain levels of development in physical, cognitive, and socio-emotional domains are required. Reaching specific developmental and educational milestones may be affected in a negative manner by symptoms of diseases as well as medical treatments.

The following chapter is dedicated to review the most vital aspects of development and education of children with intellectual disabilities. The text is divided into four sections that correspond with four developmental and educational stages: from preschool to postsecondary education. Each stage has unique developmental issues and specific milestones to be achieved that consequently influences the child's ability to learn and to successfully function in schools.

Preschool

The preschool years are exciting for most children. This is the time of incredible growth and learning. Multiple psychological and motor abilities, which developed through infancy and toddlerhood, enable children to explore independently and experience new forms of activities and relationships with both adults (i.e. preschool teacher) and peers. It is also the critical time of further expansive psychological growth and the development of new motor abilities that are crucial for achieving school readiness.

Preschool education presents several learning opportunities. The central activity for the preschool children is play, and through play they learn and develop multiple skills in all areas of development. Their vocabulary and grammar expands rapidly, general knowledge grows, and their cognitive abilities advance (i.e. attention, memory, understanding of similarities and differences between objects, awareness of cause and effect). Self-regulation improves, along with socially appropriate forms of expressing feelings, sharing, and abilities to develop friendships. Improvements in coordination and gross and fine motor skills will allow a level of self-care (Berk, 2015). Consequently, children are gradually becoming prepared for independent functioning and effective learning.

The development of preschool children with intellectual disabilities occurs in an atypical manner and is characterized by significant delays and deficits both in physical and psychological domains. One of the most noticeable characteristics of preschool children with intellectual disabilities is a significant delay in attainment of motor skills, along with deficits in sensorimotor and perceptual functioning (Batshaw & Shapiro, 2002; Burack, Hodapp, & Zigler, 1998; Hogan, Rogers, & Msall, 2000). Difficulties in initiating and executing goal-directed movements

(Savelsbergh, van der Kamp, Ledebt, & Planinsek, 2000), perceptual-motor slowness (Elliott & Bunn, 2004), limb control problems (Anson & Mawston, 2000), and decreased motor proficiency (Wuang & Su, 2009) may impede their daily activities and integration into social life (e.g. spontaneous play with a peer group) (Dolva, Coster, & Lilja, 2004; Pivik, McComas, & Laflamme, 2002). Most of forms of play, which is the main social activity of preschoolers, require high levels of gross and fine motor skills. Thus, motor proficiency determines the level of participation in social activities in preschool among children with intellectual disabilities (Egilson & Coster, 2004; Leung, Chan, Chung, & Pang, 2011). Nonetheless, the importance of motor proficiency expands beyond simple play activities.

Motor development is coupled with cognitive development both in children with and without developmental delays and intellectual disability (Houwen, Visser, van der Putten, & Vlaskamp, 2016). Brain structures responsible for motor functioning and cognition are mutually activated when performing motor and cognitive tasks (Abe & Hanakawa, 2009; Diamond, 2000; Hanakawa, 2011). Although fine motor skills are strongly associated with higher-order cognitive skills in a general population of typically developing individuals (Van der Fels et al., 2015), a significant relationship was found between gross motor skills and planning (and other higher-order executive functions) among students with borderline intellectual functioning (Hartman, Houwen, Scherder, & Visscher, 2010). There is a strong relationship between motor proficiency and cognitive development among children with typical and atypical development (Marlow, Hennessy, Bracewell, & Wolke, 2007; Piek, Dawson, Smith, & Gasson, 2008; Rigoli et al., 2013), which also demonstrates the association between motor and language development (Alcock & Krawczyk, 2010; Cheng, Chen, Tsai, Chen, & Cherng, 2009; Wang, Lekhal, Aarø, & Schjølberg, 2014; Willems & Hagoort, 2007). Brain areas responsible for language functions (e.g. Broca's area) were activated while performing motor tasks (Nishitani, Schürmann, Amunts, & Hari, 2005), and performing language tasks activated the motor cortex (Hauk, Johnsrude, & Pulvermüller, 2004; Pulvermüller, 2005). Furthermore, for children with developmental delays, this relationship may be greater than for typically developing children (Houwen et al., 2016; Roebers & Kauer, 2009) and that this relationship may be a result of atypical patterns of neurocognitive processes (Dyck, Piek, Hay, Smith, & Hallmayer, 2006; Martin, Tigera, Denckla, & Mahone, 2010). Supporting the development of fine and gross motor control in children with intellectual disabilities is of importance not only for the improvement of their motor skills and social integration, but also for the development of language and cognitive skills. Thus, the delays in cognitive development in children with intellectual disabilities in some cases may be partial, in which only specific cognitive abilities are impaired, or global, concerning all areas of cognitive functioning.

For example, preschool boys with Fragile X syndrome (FXS) show higher levels of performance on tasks requiring short-term memory than boys with Down syndrome; however, no differences were found on nonverbal reasoning tasks between the groups (Valencia-Naranjo & Robles-Bello, 2017). Nonetheless, preschoolers with FXS present impairments in inhibitory control and attention. As inhibitory control plays a crucial role in preschool social and learning activities (e.g. taking turns in games, listening to a whole question before answering, delaying gratification), children with FXS may struggle with being a part of social group and completing academic tasks (Blair & Razza, 2007; Kochanska, Murray, & Coy, 1997). Furthermore, working memory deficits among boys with FXS are mainly pronounced when they are engaged in tasks requiring high demands on inhibitory control (Lanfranchi, Cornoldi, Drigo, & Vianello, 2009). Deficits in inhibitory control improve over time in children with FXS, unlike their attention deficits that are stable over time (Tonnsen, Grefer, Hatton, & Roberts, 2015). Attention problems are pronounced among individuals with FXS since early childhood (e.g. Roberts, Hatton, Long, Anello, & Colombo, 2012) and have a negative impact on their further neurocognitive development, academic learning, and social adaptation (Cornish, Cole, Longhi, Karmiloff-Smith, & Scerif, 2012). Early interventions and treatment of attention difficulties in children with FXS can bring positive outcomes and improve their cognition and behaviour (Halperin, Bédard, & Curchack-Lichtin, 2012). Children with Down syndrome present deficits in verbal working memory that contribute to poor language and learning outcomes (Jarrold, Baddeley, & Phillips, 1999; Miolo, Chapman, & Sindberg, 2005). Yet, these children show relative strengths in visuospatial memory and visuospatial processing (Klein & Mervis, 1999).

Deficits in cognitive abilities are associated with the delay in language development among children with intellectual disabilities (Van der Schuit, Peeters, Segers, Van Balkom, & Verhoeven, 2009). Nonverbal IQ predicted phonological working memory, vocabulary, and syntax. Children with intellectual disabilities experience difficulties performing tasks requiring phonological working memory (Henry & Maclean, 2002; Van der Molen, Van Luit, Jongmans, & Van der Molen, 2007), and weak phonological working memory is linked to possible delays in vocabulary growth. In typically developing children, the relationship between the development of lexical and syntactic skills in early childhood is strong (Dionne, Dale, Boivin, & Plomin, 2003). However, in preschool these skills become less interdependent (Bates & Goodman, 1997; Moyle, Weismer, Evans, & Lindstrom, 2007). In children with intellectual disabilities, the relationship between lexicon and syntax is maintained much longer, and thus they require more time and a more intensive development of syntax to simultaneously develop their syntactic skills (Jarrold, Baddeley, Hewes, Leeke, & Phillips, 2004; van der Schuit, Segers, van Balkom, & Verhoeven, 2011).

The delay in the language development process in children with intellectual disabilities does not concern all language components and is often asynchronous. For example, children with intellectual disabilities show delays in language development in comparison to their chronological age group (i.e. their phonological working memory and syntax level are below their mental level; van der Schuit et al., 2011). However, the level of vocabulary development, including receptive and expressive vocabulary, corresponds to mental age (Facon, Facon-Bollengier, & Grubar, 2002; Miolo et al., 2005; Roberts, Price, & Malkin, 2007).

For children with FXS, the delayed development of syntax and speech difficulties (e.g. articulation, fluency, oral motor skills) are accompanied by strengths in vocabulary and language comprehension (Roberts, Hennon, & Anderson, 2003). Children with Down syndrome experience deficits in syntactic skills, speech production, and speech intelligibility but have relatively strong lexical abilities (Berglund, Eriksson, & Johansson, 2001; Roberts et al., 2007). They also experience difficulties in complex pragmatic skills (e.g. using language for different purposes, staying on topic, taking turns in conversation, using verbal and nonverbal signals; Kumin, 1994), which are also an issue among children with FXS (Abbeduto & Sterling, 2011).

Consequently, typically developing children may have difficulties in understanding attempts of verbal and nonverbal communication of preschoolers with intellectual disabilities (Guralnick, Connor, Neville, & Hammond, 2006). Therefore, language is closely associated with an ability to function effectively in a social network. Delays in language development may limit the child's abilities to fully participate in social preschool activities and maintain individual relationships with peers. Language comprehension and expressive language are crucial components of such social competences as initiating and maintaining friendships, solving peer conflicts, and participating in group academic and nonacademic activities and in social adaptation to their peer group (Tzouriadou, Barbas, Vouyoukas, & Anagnostopoulou, 2013). For children with FXS, difficulties in social behaviour were also associated with impairments in language acquisition (Abbeduto, Brady, & Kover, 2007) and the delayed development of their expressive and receptive language (Hatton et al., 2009; Mirrett, Bailey Jr, Roberts, & Hatton, 2004; Roberts et al., 2008). Additionally, their social functioning, especially social and communication joint engagements, is due to deficits in early gesture communication, joint attention behaviours, and maintaining and shifting eye gaze (Flenthrope & Brady, 2010; Marschik et al., 2014; Murphy, Abbeduto, Schroeder, & Serlin, 2007; Roberts, Mirrett, Anderson, Burchinal, & Neebe, 2002; Scerif, Cornish, Wilding, Driver, & Karmiloff-Smith, 2004). Children with FXS who used joint engagement were found to have better developed expressive language than children with FXS who used it less often (Hahn, Brady, Fleming, & Warren, 2016).

Preschoolers with intellectual disability are frequently rejected and excluded from social activities, not only because of their delayed language acquisition but also due to their social impairments. To adapt to the preschool social context and to collaborate with peers and follow the teacher's instructions, a child must have sufficient self-control and the ability to withhold impulsive reactions (e.g. waiting patiently when taking turns; Lynne Lane, Stanton-Chapman, Roorbach Jamison, & Phillips, 2007; Mancini & Coster, 2004). Children with intellectual disabilities often lack such competences (e.g. peer conflict resolution) and fail to adapt to various social situations (Guralnick, 1997; Guralnick et al., 1998). Thus, preschoolers with intellectual disabilities may not keep up with the pace of play and do not respond flexibly to the constantly changing forms and rhythm of formal and informal preschool activities, which may be the reason for exclusion from group play (Kemp & Carter, 2002). Therefore, they are more often engaged in solitary play (Guralnick et al., 2006). Moreover, as children with intellectual disabilities usually require more assistance, they interact more frequently with their teachers rather than their typically developing peers (Guralnick et al., 2006). Adults were also found to often make decisions about types of social interactions in which a child with intellectual disabilities should be involved. Consequently, children with intellectual disabilities are endorsed by teachers to interact with peers during structured activities rather than during free play (Luttropp & Granlund, 2010).

Play develops from infancy and is stimulated by gradual development of cognitive, social, and motor skills. Although play level is positively correlated with mental age, children with intellectual disabilities may not differ from their typically developing peers regarding types of objects they use for play. Differences emerge, however, in the frequency and length of a play; children with intellectual disabilities play less often and for shorter periods of time than their peers (Gowen, Johnson-Martin, Goldman, & Hussey, 1992). If the intellectual disability is not accompanied by physical incapacities, then children with intellectual disabilities are keen on sensorimotor play experiences and perform relatively well in recreations that involve gross and fine motor abilities (Messier, Ferland, & Majnemer, 2008). In typical development, pretend play appears; however, it is only when a child turns 4 that symbolic play becomes more social and interactive (e.g. they assign roles themselves and others while throwing an imaginary tea party). The development of symbolic play may be delayed in children with intellectual disabilities. However, symbolic play depends rather on language and cognitive levels than on the type of developmental disability such as autism (DeLoache, 2002; Thiemann-Bourque, Brady, & Fleming, 2012). Furthermore, play is significantly linked to self-regulation skills (Nader-Grosbois & Vieillevoye, 2012). Children with intellectual disabilities do not differ from their peers matched on mental age in terms of pretend play; nonetheless, they have significantly more difficulties in self-regulation when involved in symbolic play (Vieillevoye & Nader-Grosbois, 2008). Poor self-regulation is a common feature in children with intellectual disabilities (Glenn & Cunningham, 2008; Whitman, 1990). Children with intellectual disabilities have deficits in regulating their attention (Paparella & Kasari, 2004), persisting on a task (Glenn & Cunningham, 2008), planning, monitoring, and flexibly solving problems (Gilmore, Cuskelly, & Hayes, 2003). Self-regulation is an ability that advances intensively during preschool years and is an important developmental milestone (Bronson, 2000; Gilmore et al., 2003) that allows children to guide behaviour, solve goal-oriented problems, follow social rules, and successfully learn (Kopp, 1982). Self-regulation is a more important predictor of school readiness than IQ (Blair, 2002). The development of self-regulation is aligned with language development, and language was identified as an important tool in the self-regulating process, which serves as self-instruction to plan, guide, and monitor behaviours (Bronson, 2000; Whitman, 1990).

Difficulties with self-regulation in children with intellectual disabilities result in frequent behaviour difficulties reported by their parents and teachers. For example, preschoolers with autism and cerebral palsy present more behavioural difficulties in comparison to children with Down syndrome or typically developing peers (Eisenhower, Baker, & Blacher, 2005). Furthermore, children with Down syndrome display higher levels of adjustment than children with other types of intellectual disabilities (Bieberich & Morgan, 1998; Hodapp, Ly, Fidler, & Ricci, 2001). Although it is a typical developmental pattern for most children under the age of 5 to present some level of difficulties in regulating their behaviour, problems presented by children with intellectual disabilities tend to be more intense and may occur in atypical conduct, such as stereotyped behaviours and aggressive and autoaggressive outbursts (Cooper, Smiley, Morrison, Williamson, & Allan, 2007). Self-biting, self-scratching, self-pinching, and self-hair pulling are common (Rojahn, Schroeder, & Hoch, 2007). Repetitive and restrictive behaviours, including rituals, mannerisms, and exaggerated preoccupation with objects, are also manifested by many children in this population, and many individuals present inflexibility to changes in their routines (APA, 2013; Lam & Aman, 2007). Children with PWS and autism spectrum disorder are sensitive to unexpected interruptions in their routine. They often react to such situations with tantrum outbursts and aggression (Tunnicliffe, Woodcock, Bull, Oliver, & Penhallow, 2014; Woodcock, Oliver, & Humphreys, 2009). Tantrums in this population can be produced by frustration caused by constant food-seeking (Dimitropoulos, Feurer, Butler, & Thompson, 2001). As children with PWS experience difficulties in regulating their appetite and struggle with the constant feeling of not being full after consuming a meal, they are constantly preoccupied with searching for more food. Due to the elevated risk of obesity and diabetes, this behaviour requires careful management, to which children with PWS may react with anger outbursts. Tantrums, however, are not only specific to children with PWS but are a common behaviour issue among children with intellectual disabilities (Chadwick, Walker, Bernard, & Taylor, 2000; Lowe et al., 2007).

Low social and language competences have further negative consequences for children with intellectual disabilities when they transfer to primary school (Guralnick, 2010). To decrease the risk of behavioural problems and increase their chances for successful school adaptation, the problems are best addressed during preschool years (Donovan & Cross, 2002; Shonkoff & Phillips, 2000). As the preschool curriculum is flexible, this is a perfect time for introducing an individualized plan for supporting each child with intellectual disabilities and adjusting the curriculum to their distinctive needs and developmental strengths (Tzouriadou et al., 2013). The interventions are most effective when focused on developing social and functional communication skills, as well as motor skills to increase the chances of children with intellectual disabilities to participate in social activities in preschool (Leung et al., 2011), which are a great opportunity for further social, language, emotional, and cognitive growth, as well as practicing the generalisation of new skills on new spheres of activity.

Difficulty in transferring skills from therapy and individual instructions into everyday life situations is one major problem for children with intellectual disability (Kaiser & Trent, 2007). Interventions that focus on physical activity programs and interactive play, including attention training, were beneficial for children with developmental delays (Tanta, Deitz, White, & Billingsley, 2005; Verschuren et al., 2007) as they boost the development of competences that allow children with intellectual disabilities to participate in the free peer play and other typical preschool social activities. Various interventions aimed at the improvement of academic performance and cognitive functioning of children with Fragile X syndrome and Down syndrome (Valencia-Naranjo & Robles-Bello, 2017) and literacy skills (Kaiser, Hester, & McDuffie, 2001; Koppenhaver & Erickson, 2003; van der Schuit, Segers, van Balkom, Stoep, & Verhoeven, 2010), and interventions for language and social communication (Hahn et al., 2016). The neurodevelopmental group interventions for preschoolers with Angelman syndrome (AS) based on applied behaviour analysis (ABA) on neurodevelopmental were found to bring positive outcomes in both cognitive and adaptive aspects of their functioning (Summers, 2012). Early interventions requiring parental involvement contributed significantly to the improvement of phonological awareness, letter name, and sound knowledge in preschoolers with Down syndrome (van Bysterveldt, Gillon, & Moran, 2006). Successful interventions for children with intellectual disabilities include facilitation and generalization of the skills, as transferring skills from therapy or individual instructions into everyday life situations is one of the most significant problems of children with intellectual disability (Kaiser & Trent, 2007). Interventions are most effective when involving a multiple strategies that allow applying and practicing skills across settings and therefore improving generalization (Snell et al., 2010).

Primary School

Entering primary school imposes new challenges on all students, both those who develop typically and those whose development is delayed. Children have to meet several requirements regarding new ways of teaching and learning, entering a new group of peers, as well as higher expectations concerning independence and self-regulation. The key factor for effective and successful functioning in this new educational setting is school readiness. This concept pertains to a certain level of psychological and motor development that allows a child to respond independently and adequately to the academic and social demands of a primary school setting (Carlton & Winsler, 1999). School readiness concerns such areas of development as cognition (e.g. attention, memory, reasoning), expressive and receptive language abilities, gross and fine motor skills, emotional self-regulation, and social competences. Children with a developed school readiness at the moment of commencing education in primary school have improved chances of acquiring basic academic skills (i.e. reading, writing, and mathematics) and the ability to cope with learning demands in an independent manner.

School Readiness

Children with intellectual disabilities achieve a sufficient level of school readiness with significant delay, compared to their chronological-age peers (Sadock, Sadock, & Kaplan, 2009). Deficits and impairments in cognitive, language, and socio-emotional domains of their development limit the ability to cope effectively with academic and social challenges of primary school. Their learning abilities are significantly reduced by general and domain-specific deficits in their cognitive abilities. The profiles of cognitive development deficits among children with intellectual disabilities are varied and depend on the predispositions of the child as well as on the characteristics of the disorder which accompanies the intellectual disability. For instance, students with FXS experience problems with attention (Ornstein et al., 2008) and poor inhibition in tasks that require sustaining and switching attention (Cornish, Scerif, & Karmiloff-Smith, 2007; Scerif et al., 2004). These difficulties are more severe than students with other neurodevelopmental disorders, such as children with Down syndrome (Cornish et al., 2007), Williams syndrome (Cornish et al., 2007), and Prader-Willi syndrome (Woodcock et al., 2009). Inhibitory control deficits in children with FXS emerge early in their development, are pervasive, and significantly contribute to academic underachievement and social disadvantages later in school-aged childhood and adolescence (Cornish et al., 2012). Students with FXS also have low working memory (Baker et al., 2011), especially when high control over the task is required (Gallagher & Hallahan, 2012; Lanfranchi et al., 2009). Despite significant delays and lower general IQ (Kover, Pierpont, Kim, Brown, & Abbeduto, 2013), both cognitive attention and working memory in boys with FXS improve over the course of development; however, the progress in working memory was found to be significantly greater compared to attention skills (Cornish, Cole, Longhi, Karmiloff-Smith, & Scerif, 2013). Longitudinal studies on the level of cognitive development among children with FXS show that the delays in their verbal comprehension, perceptual organization, and processing speed were becoming greater, compared to their typically developing peers. The the study group with mature verbal skills improved compared to visuospatial skills, whereas the difference between poor working memory and strong processing speed diminished in adolescence, working memory was developing rapidly (Quintin et al., 2016).

Students with PWS also experience developmental impairments that impact negatively their learning abilities and social school adaptation, such as delays in motor development (hypotonia), poor social competences and behavioural problems, and cognitive development. Impairments in cognitive development may be affected indirectly through treatment with human growth hormone (GH) in children with PWS (Festen et al., 2008; Siemensma et al., 2012). Furthermore, the growth hormone treatment also introduced improvements in body composition and growth, psychomotor development, and adaptive functioning (Bakker et al., 2013; Bakker et al., 2015; Carrel, Myers, Whitman, Eickhoff, & Allen, 2010; Lo, Festen, Tummers-de Lind van Wijngaarden, Collin, & Hokken-Koelega, 2015). Pharmacotherapy also yield positive results in cognitive and social abilities of children with Angelman syndrome (Peters et al., 2004), who also experience several deficits including profound cognitive and speech impairments, movements and balance disorders, dimorphic facial features, hyperactivity, and difficulties in sleep; these children also struggle with epilepsy quite often (Clayton-Smith & Laan, 2003; Kyllerman, 2013).

Reading Skills

Cognitive impairments delay the development of literacy skills (i.e. phonological awareness, letter knowledge, and word decoding; Van Tilborg, Segers, Van Balkom, & Verhoeven, 2014) and reading skills among students with intellectual disability. Improving functional reading skills is one of the main factors for supporting autonomy of children with intellectual disability (Klusek, Roberts, & Losh, 2015). For instance, only 19% of adults with FXS were reading books, 44% of which read basic picture books, and 59% were familiar with letter sounds (Bailey Jr, Raspa, Holiday, Bishop, & Olmsted, 2009). Although in early and middle childhood children with FXS may steadily gain literacy skills (Bailey et al., 2009), around late childhood the acquisition of letters, word recognition (Roberts et al., 2005), and phonological awareness (Adlof, Klusek, Shinkareva, Robinson, & Roberts, 2015) significantly slow down. Nonetheless, phonological decoding skills (word identification skills) are relatively well developed in this population and on a similar level as in age-matched healthy peers (Johnson-Glenberg, 2008). Furthermore, despite some phonological skill deficits, reading abilities and letter-word recognition of children with FXS are also comparable to typically developing children, when the match is based on their mental age (Klusek et al., 2015). Reading skills in children with Down syndrome depend on their phoneme awareness and letter-sound knowledge, and their reading accuracy was stronger than reading comprehension skills (Van Bysterveldt & Gillon, 2014). Phonological awareness and listening comprehension predict reading comprehension among children with DS (Laws, Brown, & Main, 2016). Students with DS, in comparison to children with Williams syndrome who have relatively stronger verbal short-term memory and language abilities, showed phonological recording abilities (Danielsson, Henry, Messer, Carney, & Rönnberg, 2016).

School Adaptation

Students with intellectual disabilities were found to interact less with other children in both structured academic activities or during recess (Eriksson, Welander, & Granlund, 2007). Therefore, the successful transition and adaptation of children with intellectual disabilities to primary school environment require limiting the risk of excluding them from participating in social and educational activities (Egilson & Coster, 2004; Wong, 2002). Students with disorders, including cognitive impairments, were found to present numerous difficulties in social situations both in a classroom and on the playground (Egilson & Coster, 2004).

Difficulties in initiating and maintaining interpersonal relationships concern also their relationship with teachers. Students with intellectual disabilities have less warm and satisfactory and more dependent relationship with a teacher than their typically developing peers (Eisenhower, Baker, & Blacher, 2007). A poor relationship with teachers may be caused by modest social communication skills with adults as well as by behaviour issues arising from poor self-regulation. Self-regulation is a factor that influences the level of school adaptation and has impact on the way in which parents and teachers assess the student's level of social skills (McIntyre, Blacher, & Baker, 2006).

Self-regulation is not the sole cause of behavioural and adaptation problems present in children with intellectual disabilities. The variety of issues can be as follows: (a) a symptom of a disorder (e.g. compulsive behaviours in autism spectrum disorder), (b) caused by treatment side effects (e.g. sleep-related breathing disorders in children with PWS caused by growth hormone treatment; Festen et al., 2006), or (c) triggered by the environment's response to the child's symptoms (e.g. aggression in students with PWS whose food-seeking behaviour was interrupted). Constant cravings for food, eating inedible items, or their frustration caused by not being able to wait for the next meal, which is common for individuals with PWS, can seriously disrupt classroom order and activities; thus, specific behaviour management is required. However, food intake management in a school setting requires preparation, focus, and engagement from the teachers. Behavioural issues among school children can be also caused by sleep deficiencies (Sadeh, Gruber, & Raviv, 2002). Daytime challenging behaviours, such as aggression, defiance, arousal and agitation, or drowsiness and exhaustion, are frequently observed among children with intellectual disabilities who also experience sleep difficulties. The severity of sleep difficulties was linked to the intellectual disabilities' level, the use of medication, and greater likelihood of epilepsy (Didden, Korzilius, Aperlo, Overloop, & Vries, 2002).

Despite cognitive and behavioural difficulties, students with intellectual disabilities can be successfully educated (Turnbull, Turnbull, Wehmeyer, & Shank, 2004). Current inclusive education should focus on the third-generation inclusive practices that primarily emphasize what the students are being taught, not where, and promote the self-determination of students (Agran, Wehmeyer, Cavin, & Palmer, 2010). The third-generation inclusive practices lead to empowering students and increasing quality of life, independence, and success. This approach also includes a universally designed curriculum and flexible instructions and employing interventions and preventive programs that include and benefit all students. For instance, positive behaviour supports improve the school climate to minimize the risk of misconduct among students by providing instructions and modelling appropriate and prosocial behaviours (Carr, 2000). Interventions that involve all students, typically developing and with developmental delays, were proved to lead to more engagement of students with cognitive impairments (Carter & Kennedy, 2006). Their aim is to include actively all students in intervention programs and create a strong social group that leads to not only learning but also to socialization, emotional maturity, and learning activities and behaviours.

Universal design for learning increases the involvement and educational progress of students with cognitive impairments (Wehmeyer, Smith, & Davies, 2005; Wehmeyer, Smith, Palmer, & Davies, 2004). Introducing a flexible approach to presenting and organizing classroom content by means of digital technology are key factors of facilitating achievement of learning goals among students with intellectual disabilities (Orkwis & McLane, 1998). This flexibility is especially appreciated when the child experiences side effects of a medical treatment that affects the child's physical and mental abilities.

Improving self-determination among students with intellectual disabilities is beneficial (Lee, Wehmeyer, Palmer, Soukup, & Little, 2008). Increasing self-regulation and teaching to set goals and make decisions regarding academic activities and learning in return will encourage the students' involvement and increase their motivation. Consequently, students were found to have greater knowledge and skills (Agran et al., 2010), were better prepared for classes, became engaged in group activities, and initiated tasks more frequently (Agran, Wehmeyer, Cavin, & Palmer, 2008).

Teaching self-determination among students with intellectual impairments should start with changing the mindset of many professional who, due to many reasons, may not be supportive of this idea (Powers, 2005). For instance, some school personnel may believe they should not include the child in the decision-making process regarding the given child, simply because they assume they know better than the child what is best learning and growth.

High School

Transitioning to high school is a challenging time for all students. Educational and social requirements of a high school setting differ from what a student is familiar with in primary school. The transition is especially difficult as it coincides with the beginning of adolescence (Schneider, Wedgewood, Llewellyn, & McConnell, 2006). The transitional stage between childhood and adulthood is characterized by emotional tensions and internal conflicts and for many turns out to be turbulent. During puberty, physical changes and various psychological transformations may cause anxiety. Issues of independence and interdependence, identity, peer group acceptance and pressure, romantic and sexual interests, as well as intense preoccupation on external appearance become pronounced and overlap with numerous demands regarding schoolwork, further education, and adaptation to the unknown context of high school.

Self-Concept and Self-Perception

Adolescence is a twofold challenge for persons with intellectual disabilities for which typical developmental tasks associated with adolescence are combined with symptoms of disability and medical treatments (Schneider et al., 2006). For many persons with intellectual and developmental disabilities, it is during their adolescent years that they begin to recognize differences between themselves and their typically developing peers. This recognition may lead to feelings of inadequacy, frustration, or isolation (Evans, 1998; Levy-Shiff, Kedem, & Sevillia, 1990) and influences further psychological development (Harter, 1999). For instance, recognition of differences affects the level of self-concept among students with intellectual disabilities, which is a set of beliefs about oneself and answers the question "Who am I?". Adolescents with intellectual disability reported a less positive self-concept than their typically developing peers (Levy-Shiff et al., 1990). Furthermore, adolescents with intellectual disabilities may have realistic self-esteem (Evans, 1998) based on performance in different activity areas (e.g. appearance, school attainments, peer group acceptance; Harter, 1999). In terms of self-perception, adolescents with intellectual disabilities do not differ from the typically developing peers, matched for mental age. Nonetheless, groups vary in self-regulation, metacognition, and self-perception of competences in specific domains which depend on mental age and verbal comprehension (Nader-Grosbois, 2014).

Social Skills and Social Acceptance

Self-concept in adolescents with disabilities is linked to the level of their social acceptance (Rothman & Cosden, 1995). Social acceptance is a group's perception of an individual and has significant meaning in adolescence. Adolescents who are accepted by a peer group enjoy better social adjustment, more meaningful interpersonal relations (Pedersen, Vitaro, Barker, & Borge, 2007), and acceptance is associated with better social competences (Berk, 2015). Those accepted by peer groups also present enhanced social information processing skills and more positive behaviour (Crick & Dodge, 1994).

Adolescents with intellectual disabilities often lack sufficient social skills, and behaviour problems often interfere with development of friendships (Tipton, Christensen, & Blacher, 2013). Poor social skills are associated with a lower IQ level (Nota, Ferrari, Soresi, & Wehmeyer, 2007), and, in youth with high-functioning autism spectrum disorder, age and IQ were best predictors of poor self-perceived social competences, which consequently produced higher levels of depressive symptoms (Vickerstaff, Heriot, Wong, Lopes, & Dossetor, 2007). Vulnerability of peer rejection for adolescents with intellectual disabilities (Kock et al., 2012) is also caused by their limitations in adaptive functioning (Duvdevany, 2002), poor language development and communication (Hartley & Sikora, 2010; Lancioni, O'Reilly, & Basili, 2001), externalizing behaviours (Kleinert, Miracle, & Sheppard-Jones, 2007; Orsmond, Krauss, & Seltzer, 2004), as well as psychiatric disorders (e.g. conduct, anxiety, and emotional disorders and ADHD; Emerson & Hatton, 2007).

As in adolescence, peers become particularly important; typically developing adolescents are seeking opportunities for socialization and mainly prefer informal, unorganized interactions. A group of close friends provides opportunities to improve social skills, comprehend and internalize norms and values, receive social support and companionship, and fulfil the need of belonging (Rubin, Bukowski, & Parker,

1998). These social opportunities to interact with others and learn through these interactions have great influence on their further development (Hartup & Stevens, 1997). Therefore, they spend more time with people their age than parents and family members. Adolescents with intellectual disabilities are no different in that respect, and they usually prefer to engage with their peers instead of spending time with parents or siblings (Helsen, Vollebergh, & Meeus, 2000). However, due to their disability symptoms, most of them are usually not included in social and recreational activities with their colleagues (Braun, Yeargin-Allsopp, & Lollar, 2006; Poulsen, Ziviani, & Cuskelly, 2007). Adolescents with intellectual disabilities have few opportunities for spontaneous socialization, and their peer interactions are limited to organized and planned peer activities, like sports (Abells, Burbidge, & Minnes, 2008). Adolescents with intellectual disabilities usually do not have a group of close friends and rarely spend time outside of school with peers (Tipton et al., 2013). Therefore, most of these students are more likely to spend time with family or alone (Pretty, Rapley, & Bramston, 2002; Solish, Minnes, & Kupferschmidt, 2003) or engage in solidarity leisure activities that lead to the feeling of isolation and loneliness (Kleinert et al., 2007; Orsmond et al., 2004).

Adolescents with intellectual disabilities benefit from interacting with peers, which plays a positive role in the attainment of academic goals, progress in functional development, and improvement in social skills and competences (Goldstein, Kaczmarek, & English, 2002). Although adolescents with intellectual disabilities are prone to interacting with others, forming and maintaining close relationships with peers is a challenging task. They are required to invest extensive effort to establish friendships and require constant support to make relationships last (Sigstad, 2016). Individuals with intellectual disabilities may have troubles in understanding and adapting to new social situations as their ability to decode social cues is limited, just as the range of other social skills, like engaging in reciprocal social interactions (Carter & Hughes, 2005). These limitations in social functioning have a particularly negative outcome in adolescence when it becomes challenging to navigate peer interactions, as they become more complex and intense. For instance, to establish a close relationship with a peer, an adolescent must also be able to reach the communication level and language typically used among peers (e.g. figurative speech) and monitor their social behaviour (Carter & Hughes, 2005)—both of which are subtle and cognitively advanced social skills. Thus, a high school setting might be particularly challenging for the socialization of adolescents with intellectual disabilities.

High school students no longer spend most their time in one classroom among the same peers who they have already known for years. As they can choose courses, they attend classes with different cohorts (Carter & Hughes, 2005). For persons with intellectual disabilities, this is an uncomfortable situation to initiate and maintain relationship with many colleagues at different classroom settings. Typically developing students also find initiating acquaintanceships with classmates with intellectual disabilities to be difficult. These students may not have adequate knowledge or previous experience to feel sufficiently comfortable (Copeland et al., 2004).

Autonomy and Self-Determination

Being engaged in peer activities is also essential for the development of autonomy. Adolescents are taking first steps towards becoming responsible and capable of independently making healthy, positive decisions. Through interactions with peers, they engage in various situations that provide opportunities to make choices in which they must act without parental control. Most parents carefully and gradually reduce levels of parent supervision, allowing their children to learn from the consequences of their decisions.

Gaining autonomy means behaving in the most preferable manner and in compliance with one's own interests or abilities (Wehmeyer, Kelchner, & Richards, 1996), while fostering self-determination and independence. Due to cognitive impairments, individuals with intellectual disability are often perceived as incapable of developing autonomy and self-determination (Wehmeyer & Schwartz, 1998). Many adults who provide them with care and education, and who acquired a similar mindset, may unintentionally limit their opportunities to develop independence. Contrary to this false belief, many individuals with intellectual disabilities can achieve levels of autonomy and self-determination, as both were found independent of the level of cognitive abilities. Furthermore, providing this population with occasions to make decisions strengthens the development of both capabilities (Palmer & Wehmeyer, 2003).

Environment sensitivity and responsiveness to the needs of adolescents with intellectual disabilities play a significant role in enhancing their self-determination (Wehmeyer & Garner, 2003). Allowing this population to actively engage in the decision-making process regarding their further education and vocational training increases their proactive attitude and empowers them (Wehmeyer & Garner, 2003).

Promoting independent functioning and self-determination is crucial for the health and well-being of this population (Wullink, Widdershoven, Van Schrojenstein Lantman-de Valk, Metsemakers, & Dinant, 2009) because self-determination is important in preparing adolescents with intellectual disabilities for the transition into adulthood (Field, Martin, Miller, Ward, & Wehmeyer, 1998), determining their self-worth and social acceptance, and improving their chances for independence and employment (Palmer & Wehmeyer, 2003) and for better quality of life (Lachapelle et al., 2005). Promoting autonomy and independence is not possible without developing daily living skills in individuals with intellectual disabilities. Variability in personal living skills (e.g. eating, toileting and hygiene, communication) is observed among adolescents with intellectual disabilities (Brun Gasca et al., 2010). In individuals with FXS, the level of living skills was linked to reasoning abilities and the number of co-occurring disorders (e.g. hyperactivity, autism, anxiety; Bailey et al., 2009). Their independent living skills, which require initiative, maintaining rules, personal care, home management, and social and community skills, were also associated with age and executive functions (Martin, Quintin, Hall, & Reiss, 2016). Therefore, interventions aiming at expediting adaptive behaviours and independence ought to promote equal opportunities for skills training (Santos & Morato, 2012). The interventions should target various symptoms of a disorder

(Hustyi et al., 2015) and should be meticulously planned, taking into consideration individual needs, strengths, and deficits (Fu, 2015).

Transition from High School to Further Postsecondary Education or Vocational Setting

Ensuring that adolescents with disabilities receive adequate and sufficient support and training to secure their chances for employment should be the key goal for all specialists involved in this population. High rates of unemployment and underemployment are still a critical issue in this population, and they often endure social isolation, dependence, and limited opportunities to improve quality of life. Successful employment, however, increases their chances for social inclusion, economic self-sufficiency, and life satisfaction (Carter, Austin, & Trainor, 2012). Thus, the process of transition to adulthood and independence must be meticulously planned and carefully executed (e.g. enrollment in vocational education or employment-related programs in high school) (Carter et al., 2012; Shandra & Hogan, 2008). Hart Barnett and Crippen (2014) proposed eight tasks vital for implementing and improving employment training programs:

1. Enhance collaboration with other schools and professionals in order to achieve support and the exchange of knowledge and best practices.
2. Ensure that the vocational training is functional and result-oriented.
3. Consider students as equal partners, consider their preferences and interests, and apply a student-directed approach.
4. Immerse the program into the school community that will simulate real-world challenges in a similar context.
5. Ensure the program reflects/resembles a realistic vocational setting. Thus, skills acquired during the training will be transferable into real employment situations (e.g. greeting customers, taking orders, accepting directions, maintaining hygiene and cleanness of the uniform).
6. Additionally prepare training materials as realistic as possible to imitate the real vocational setting (e.g. employee manuals).
7. Similarly with feedback and reinforcement provided to students during the training, use social praise and approbation common for the employment context.
8. Apply training methods whose efficacy was already proved in research.

Postsecondary

Young adults with intellectual disabilities, like their typically developing peers, desire opportunities to further develop their independence, establish meaningful social relationships, and become respected members of their community (Moon, Grigal, & Neubert, 2001). However, unlike their typically developing peers, they face additional obstacles to achieving their developmental goals. Thus, many students with intellectual disabilities who are older than 18 years are interested in taking further steps in education and preparation for an independent adult life. For instance, they become interested in attending postsecondary education (PSE) programs.

As students with intellectual disabilities do not meet typical college entrance criteria, traditional PSE programs do not offer sufficient support required for youth with intellectual disabilities to achieve positive academic outcomes successfully. In the past students with intellectual disabilities had few opportunities to enter postsecondary education, and they were the smallest group of students with developmental disabilities attending postsecondary education institutions (Wagner, Newman, Cameto, Garza, & Levine, 2005). Typical education for these students focused on developing functional life skills, community-based instruction, and job training (Grigal, Neubert, Moon, & Reed, 2001), and, as they needed pervasive support, they typically attended special education schools until they were ineligible to do so (until the age of 21), exceeding the typical age of high school students (Wagner et al., 2005), even though high school was not best fit for their needs. Currently, students in the United States can choose from over 220 postsecondary education programs designed for persons with disabilities (PSE, Mazzoni, 2013), and most of the PSE programs have become available only in the last 10 years. As higher education institutions recognize the need for providing inclusive education and vocational opportunities for students with intellectual disabilities, inequalities in the access to postsecondary education programs have been systematically reduced since the 1970s.

Through the introduction of the Individuals with Disabilities Education Act (IDEA) of 1990 and IDEA Amendments of 1997 and 2004, procedures for transitioning students with intellectual disabilities from high school to adult living, as well as access to postsecondary education, have been established and guaranteed. Further postsecondary education opportunities for students with intellectual disabilities were founded in 2008 with Higher Education Opportunity Act (HEOA), namely, (a) providing financial aid for students with intellectual disabilities who wish to continue their education on the postsecondary level, (b) developing model programs designed specifically for providing comprehensive transition to postsecondary education for students with intellectual disabilities (Transition and Postsecondary Education Programs for Students with Intellectual Disabilities, TPSID), and (c) funding the National Coordinating Centre that provides support and coordinating the above mentioned postsecondary programs.

Consequently, the enrollment of students with intellectual disabilities into PSE programs in colleges has significantly increased, and currently students with intellectual disabilities participate in college courses and activities alongside their healthy peers (Papay & Bambara, 2011). These postsecondary education programs provide a wide range of educational opportunities, as they are offered at technical schools, colleges, and universities. Furthermore, students with intellectual disabilities who are 18–21 years old are also permitted to attend colleges and to simultaneously continue their high school education (Grigal, Hart, & Weir, 2012;

Mazzoni, 2013). Participation in both postsecondary education and vocational rehabilitation has positive employment outcomes; in comparison to persons who received only vocational training, students who participated in both had almost 30% higher chances of becoming employed and received a significantly higher income (Migliore, Butterworth, & Hart, 2009).

Three types of PSE programs are available for students with intellectual disabilities: mixed, separate, and individual (Grigal, Dwyre, & Davis, 2006). Within the mixed (or hybrid) model, students with intellectual disabilities participate in college classes and social activities with their peers without disabilities (inclusive academic coursework) but attend additional classes that focus on improving their life skills and providing vocational training along with other students with ID. Separate programs do not offer inclusive classes with typical peers, although they still take place at college campuses. Hence, students with intellectual disabilities may join other students in enjoying social activities held on campus. The curriculum of this program is mainly focused on providing life skills instructions, community-based instruction, and vocational training.

The individual program models provide students with intellectual disabilities with individualized services (e.g. tutors, educational coaches) in college courses, certificate programs, and degree programs. This individualized training is planned flexibly accordingly to the student's individual career goals, which directs the course of the study and vocational experience (e.g. internships). Students with intellectual disabilities in this model may be enrolled in college classes, if it is related to an individual plan of professional development. Creating and developing these three types of programs provide much-needed flexibility in providing education to students with ID. Various options for types of postsecondary education allow to choose the best options for the abilities and needs of certain individuals, their personal and professional goals. Most college lecturers are supportive of these PSE models (Plotner & Marshall, 2015).

PSE offers a unique opportunity for students with intellectual disabilities to not only increase their chances for employment and career development but also empower them by expanding the network of their social support and become a valuable member of the local community (Thoma et al., 2011), which later translates itself into positive outcomes in adulthood (Lynch & Getzel, 2013). Students with intellectual disabilities who have participated in inclusive postsecondary education reported increased satisfaction across several life domains, including emotional well-being, interpersonal relationships, personal development, self-determination, and social inclusion. Furthermore, becoming an active and engaged member of the college community, enrolled in one of the educational or vocational trainings, brings the students with intellectual disabilities a sense of self-determination (Farley, Gibbons, & Cihak, 2014; Grigal et al., 2012). Shogren and Shaw (2016) found that self-determination elements, such as autonomy, self-realization, and psychological empowerment, have significant influence on the quality of life of persons with intellectual disabilities; autonomy was positively linked to enrollment to PSE, greater chances for employment and financial independence, as well as a more satisfactory social network and independent living.

Although the offer of PSE for students with intellectual disabilities is constantly expanding and improving, both researchers and practitioners pay attention to factors that could pose barriers to the full implementation of a program into a college or university (institutions of higher education, IHE) or limit the students' possibility to fully participate in it. Creating a positive inclusive IHE setting primarily requires a clearly defined definition and awareness of what inclusion is and how to achieve it (Folk, Yamamoto, & Stodden, 2012). Barriers can occur in various areas, such as the matriculation process and policies, financial aid and housing options, access to various courses and social activities, acceptance of other students, and the faculty's readiness to teach courses that are attended by students with intellectual disabilities (Plotner & Marshall, 2015; Thoma et al., 2011).

The lack of acceptance and support from peers, together with the reluctance of the faculty, is one of the greatest concerns (Neubert & Redd, 2008). However, research shows that the majority of students and faculty support the idea of inclusive college education for students with intellectual. Although some lecturers may feel not sufficiently prepared for teaching students with intellectual disabilities (Causton-Theoharis, Ashby, & DeClouette, 2009), most faculty are willing to introduce flexibility to delivered courses to accommodate the needs of this student population, as well as advocate for their social justice and inclusion within the college community (O'Connor, Kubiak, Espiner, & O'Brien, 2012). Furthermore, students who have already had experiences with persons with intellectual disabilities in PSE programs presented a more positive and accepting attitude towards them (Westling, Kelley, Cain, & Prohn, 2013).

Admission criteria can also pose a barrier for some students to enrol to PSE programs. Apart from obvious reasons for matriculation, such as motivation to become a college student, the school district in which the child attends a high school plays an important role. PSE programs may be open solely to students who enrolled in those school districts that fund and operate these programs. Furthermore, especially mixed and separate programs may favour students who are not struggling with behaviour issues and who have skills to independently function in the campus. Students who present such issues may have better chances for admission in individualized programs which can provide them with more adequate and appropriate forms of support.

Students with intellectual disabilities identified the need for greater inclusion, financial issues, and concerns regarding the validity of nonacademic diplomas for access to further academic courses/education. Most students with intellectual disabilities who enrolled in PSE programs attended noncredit classes and are mainly enrolled to health and fitness classes; a few participated in computing or remedial reading and math classes (Neubert, Moon, & Grigal, 2004). Mixed and separate models were more popular than individualized programs (Papay & Bambara, 2011). Furthermore, more students were enrolled in classes for credit or audit in 2-year programs in colleges (as opposed to 4-year university programs) that were primarily vocational and remedial classes (and students had sufficient skills to participate in those with no modification of the curriculum of the course). However, students with intellectual disabilities were likely to take informal classes (i.e. health and fitness) in which modification to curriculum and assessment are easily introduced. PSE programs for students with intellectual disabilities serve for increasing their employment chances and vocational training, developing life skills, and participating in activities with typically developing peers without intellectual disabilities. Therefore, meaningful involvement in campus life, such as engaging in campus events, joining clubs, volunteering, helping with a collegiate sports team, as well as engaging in informal social activities, are excellent methods to develop their communication and collaboration skills, which are much needed both in vocational settings and in everyday life situations. Furthermore, through informal contact and common activities, the barriers created by historical biases and misinformation can be effectively dismantled.

One of the most crucial aspects of overcoming the barriers is helping students with intellectual disabilities in the transition process. Several institutions and programs have been created to support and facilitate this process. In 2004, the Individuals with Disabilities Education Act (IDEA) obliged schools across the United States to launch the summary of performance (SOP), which is a document that contains sensitive information regarding academic achievements and the current level of functioning, information that is essential for developing a plan and strategies to guide students when transitioning from high school to postschool life or postsecondary educational settings (e.g. higher education, vocational training, or further employment). This document, which is prepared when a student is attending high school, contains information regarding the best policies and strategies to support and guide students in achieving their postsecondary goals and help other professionals in the process of vocational training evaluation as well as postsecondary institutions in adjusting their offer to the special needs of students with intellectual disabilities. It is recommended that it is coupled with the Individual Educational Plan (IEP) and students ought to be endorsed to actively participate in creating this document.

In 2010, the US Department of Education established the Transition and Postsecondary Programs for Students with Intellectual Disabilities (TPSID) program. The goal of TPSID is to ensure that students with intellectual disabilities receive adequate and sufficient support and guidance when transitioning to PSE. TPSID is successful in facilitating admission and entering the PSE programs and highly effective in enhancing motivation and socialization of students with intellectual disabilities, preparing them to become engaged members of the college community (Folk et al., 2012).

Self-advocacy among students with intellectual disabilities considering the continuation of their education in a postsecondary educational setting could also be endorsed through the implementation of the person-centred planning (PCP). PCP is an individualized approach to a person with disability, also applicable to adolescents with intellectual disabilities in high school, which is a process that is aimed to support these individuals, in collaboration with them, their future goals. Therefore, it is especially helpful during any transition period (Claes, Van Hove, Vandevelde, van Loon, & Schalock, 2010). This is a flexible planning tool that is useful for any type of transition: to postsecondary educational programs, employment and vocational training, or independent living. As the PCP is a collaborative process, it empowers the individual's independence while considering his or her individual preferences. Through this involvement in the decision-making process of the PCP, self-determination and involvement in all aspects of life increase among students with intellectual disabilities (Michaels & Ferrara, 2006). Self-determination among students with intellectual disabilities can be also enhanced through such tools as the self-directed summary of performance (SD-SOP). This is another process that helps students with intellectual disabilities in transitioning from high school to a postsecondary educational setting or postschool life, providing students with intellectual disabilities with training in recognizing their strengths and limitations, identifying their needs, and, therefore, formulating their goals for adult life (Martin, Van Dycke, D'Ottavio, & Nickerson, 2007). Mazzotti, Kelley, and Coco (2015) found the SD-SOP has a significantly positive impact on students with intellectual disabilities who have participated in PCP, and students applied SD-SOP strategies to employment settings.

Peer mentoring is a valuable strategy for guiding and supporting students with intellectual disabilities who are transitioning to postschool life. The mentorship programs are led by typically developing college students. The goal of peer mentoring programs is to increase the inclusion of students with intellectual disabilities into the college community and improve their interpersonal skills (O'Brien et al., 2009), academic outcome (Hafner, Moffatt, & Kisa, 2011), professional development (Canter, Kessler, Odar, Aylward, & Roberts, 2011), and employment (McDonald, Erickson, Johnson, & Elder, 2007). Apart from the obvious benefits for students with intellectual disabilities, mentoring programs are also valuable experience for mentors. For instance, students who served as mentors appreciated their experience of mentoring students with intellectual disabilities and stated that it was valuable in terms of their career choices, or they even made them consider a new path of career that they had not considered before (Farley et al., 2014). The mentors also identified five areas in which they feel they benefited: friendships, personal growth, community involvement, experiences with people with disabilities, and future careers related to people with disabilities (Griffin, Mello, Glover, Carter, & Hodapp, 2016).

The success of students with intellectual disabilities in PSE programs depends on various factors, including the quality of the PSE program itself, the support received through transitioning programs, and guidance in peer mentoring programs. However, parents of students with intellectual disabilities should not be overlooked, as support received by these students at home is the most crucial. Parents of students with intellectual disabilities may have limited knowledge on PSE programs available for their children and do not always fully comprehend the transitioning process. Parental expectations for PSE and their involvement in the transitioning process were found to moderate the student's inclusion (Martinez, Conroy, & Cerreto, 2012).

Conclusions

Developing educational and psychological interventions for people with intellectual disabilities requires significant expertise and specialized knowledge in the specific constellation of behaviours typical for the specific cause of the intellectual disability. However, understanding the individual, interpersonal, and systemic (e.g. school and community) needs requires an understanding of the developmental progression of the child with intellectual disabilities. There is a requirement that professionals be prepared to alter programming as the individual develops, transitions take place, and the functional needs of the environment change.

References

Abbeduto, L., Brady, N., & Kover, S. T. (2007). Language development and fragile X syndrome: Profiles, syndrome-specificity, and within-syndrome differences. *Developmental Disabilities Research Reviews, 13*(1), 36–46.

Abbeduto, L., & Sterling, A. (2011). Language development and fragile X syndrome. *SIG 1 Perspectives on Language Learning and Education, 18*(3), 87–97.

Abe, M., & Hanakawa, T. (2009). Functional coupling underlying motor and cognitive functions of the dorsal premotor cortex. *Behavioural Brain Research, 198*(1), 13–23.

Abells, D., Burbidge, J., & Minnes, P. (2008). Involvement of adolescents with intellectual disabilities in social and recreational activities. *Journal on Developmental Disabilities, 14*(2), 88–94.

Adlof, S. M., Klusek, J., Shinkareva, S. V., Robinson, M. L., & Roberts, J. E. (2015). Phonological awareness and reading in boys with fragile X syndrome. *Journal of Child Psychology and Psychiatry, 56*(1), 30–39.

Agran, M., Wehmeyer, M., Cavin, M., & Palmer, S. (2010). Promoting active engagement in the general education classroom and access to the general education curriculum for students with cognitive disabilities. *Education and Training in Autism and Developmental Disabilities, 45*(2), 163–174.

Agran, M., Wehmeyer, M. L., Cavin, M., & Palmer, S. (2008). Promoting student active classroom participation skills through instruction to promote self-regulated learning and self-determination. *Career Development for Exceptional Individuals, 31*(2), 106–114.

Alcock, K. J., & Krawczyk, K. (2010). Individual differences in language development: Relationship with motor skill at 21 months. *Developmental Science, 13*(5), 677–691.

American Psychiatric Association. (2013). *Diagnostic and statistical manual of mental disorders* (5th ed.). Washington, DC: Author.

Amiet, C., Gourfinkel-An, I., Bouzamondo, A., Tordjman, S., Baulac, M., Lechat, P., … Cohen, D. (2008). Epilepsy in autism is associated with intellectual disability and gender: Evidence from a meta-analysis. *Biological Psychiatry, 64*(7), 577–582.

Anson, J. G., & Mawston, G. A. (2000). Patterns of muscle activation in simple reaction-time tasks. In D. J. Weeks, R. Chua, & D. Elliot (Eds.), *Perceptual-motor behavior in Down syndrome*. Champaign, IL: Human Kinetics.

Bailey, D. B., Jr., Raspa, M., Holiday, D., Bishop, E., & Olmsted, M. (2009). Functional skills of individuals with fragile X syndrome: A lifespan cross-sectional analysis. *American Journal on Intellectual and Developmental Disabilities, 114*(4), 289–303.

Baker, S., Hooper, S., Skinner, M., Hatton, D., Schaaf, J., Ornstein, P., & Bailey, D. (2011). Working memory subsystems and task complexity in young boys with fragile X syndrome. *Journal of Intellectual Disability Research, 55*(1), 19–29.

Bakker, N. E., Kuppens, R. J., Siemensma, E. P. C., Tummers-de Lind van Wijngaarden, R. F. A., Festen, D. A. M., Bindels-de Heus, G. C. B., … Jira, P. E. (2013). Eight years of growth hormone treatment in children with Prader-Willi syndrome: Maintaining the positive effects. *The Journal of Clinical Endocrinology & Metabolism, 98*(10), 4013–4022.

Bakker, N. E., Kuppens, R. J., Siemensma, E. P. C., Tummers-de Lind van Wijngaarden, R. F. A., Festen, D. A. M., Bindels-de Heus, G. C. B., … Jira, P. E. (2015). Bone mineral density in children and adolescents with Prader-Willi syndrome: A longitudinal study during puberty and 9 years of growth hormone treatment. *The Journal of Clinical Endocrinology & Metabolism, 100*(4), 1609–1618.

Bates, E., & Goodman, J. (1997). On the inseparability of grammar and the lexicon: Evidence from acquisition, aphasia and real-time processing. *Language and Cognitive Processes, 12*(5–6), 507–584.

Batshaw, M. L., & Shapiro, B. (2002). Mental retardation. In M. L. Batshaw (Ed.), *Children with disabilities* (5th ed.). Baltimore, MD: Paul H. Brookes.

Berglund, E., Eriksson, M., & Johansson, I. (2001). Parental reports of spoken language skills in children with down syndrome. *Journal of Speech, Language, and Hearing Research, 44*(1), 179–191.

Berk, L. (2015). *Child development*. New York, NY: Pearson Higher Education.

Bieberich, A. A., & Morgan, S. B. (1998). Brief report: Affective expression in children with autism or down syndrome. *Journal of Autism and Developmental Disorders, 28*(4), 333–338.

Blair, C. (2002). School readiness: Integrating cognition and emotion in a neurobiological conceptualization of children's functioning at school entry. *American Psychologist, 57*(2), 111.

Blair, C., & Razza, R. P. (2007). Relating effortful control, executive function, and false belief understanding to emerging math and literacy ability in kindergarten. *Child Development, 78*(2), 647–663.

Braun, K. V. N., Yeargin-Allsopp, M., & Lollar, D. (2006). Factors associated with leisure activity among young adults with developmental disabilities. *Research in Developmental Disabilities, 27*(5), 567–583.

Bronson, M. (2000). *Self-regulation in early childhood: Nature and nurture*. New York, NY: Guilford Press.

Brun Gasca, C., Obiols, J. E., Bonillo, A., Artigas, J., Lorente, I., Gabau, E., … Turk, J. (2010). Adaptive behaviour in Angelman syndrome: Its profile and relationship to age. *Journal of Intellectual Disability Research, 54*(11), 1024–1029.

Burack, J. A., Hodapp, R. M., & Zigler, E. (1998). *Handbook of mental retardation and development*. Cambridge, England: Cambridge University Press.

Canter, K. S., Kessler, E. D., Odar, C., Aylward, B. S., & Roberts, M. C. (2011). Perceived benefits of mentoring in pediatric psychology: A qualitative approach. *Journal of Pediatric Psychology, 37*(2), 158–165.

Carlton, M. P., & Winsler, A. (1999). School readiness: The need for a paradigm shift. *School Psychology Review, 28*(3), 338.

Carr, S. (2000). As distance education comes of age, the challenge is keeping the students. *The Chronicle of Higher Education, 46*(23), 39–41.

Carrel, A. L., Myers, S. E., Whitman, B. Y., Eickhoff, J., & Allen, D. B. (2010). Long-term growth hormone therapy changes the natural history of body composition and motor function in children with Prader-Willi syndrome. *The Journal of Clinical Endocrinology & Metabolism, 95*(3), 1131–1136.

Carter, E. W., Austin, D., & Trainor, A. A. (2012). Predictors of postschool employment outcomes for young adults with severe disabilities. *Journal of Disability Policy Studies, 23*(1), 50–63.

Carter, E. W., & Hughes, C. (2005). Increasing social interaction among adolescents with intellectual disabilities and their general education peers: Effective interventions. *Research and Practice for Persons with Severe Disabilities, 30*(4), 179–193.

Carter, E. W., & Kennedy, C. H. (2006). Promoting access to the general curriculum using peer support strategies. *Research and Practice for Persons with Severe Disabilities, 31*(4), 284–292.

Causton-Theoharis, J., Ashby, C., & DeClouette, N. (2009). Relentless optimism: Inclusive postsecondary opportunities for students with significant disabilities. *Journal of Postsecondary Education and Disability, 22*(2), 88–105.

Chadwick, O., Walker, N., Bernard, S., & Taylor, E. (2000). Factors affecting the risk of behaviour problems in children with severe intellectual disability. *Journal of Intellectual Disability Research, 44*(2), 108–123.

Cheng, H. C., Chen, H. Y., Tsai, C. L., Chen, Y. J., & Cherng, R. J. (2009). Comorbidity of motor and language impairments in preschool children of Taiwan. *Research in Developmental Disabilities, 30*(5), 1054–1061.

Claes, C., Van Hove, G., Vandevelde, S., van Loon, J., & Schalock, R. L. (2010). Person-centered planning: Analysis of research and effectiveness. *Intellectual and Developmental Disabilities, 48*(6), 432–453.

Clayton-Smith, J., & Laan, L. A. E. M. (2003). Angelman syndrome: A review of the clinical and genetic aspects. *Journal of Medical Genetics, 40*(2), 87–95.

Cooper, S. A., Smiley, E., Morrison, J., Williamson, A., & Allan, L. (2007). Mental ill-health in adults with intellectual disabilities: Prevalence and associated factors. *The British Journal of Psychiatry, 190*(1), 27–35.

Copeland, S. R., Hughes, C., Carter, E. W., Guth, C., Presley, J., Williams, C. R., & Fowler, S. E. (2004). Increasing access to general education: Perspectives of participants in a high school peer support program. *Remedial and Special Education, 25*(6), 342–352.

Cornish, K., Cole, V., Longhi, E., Karmiloff-Smith, A., & Scerif, G. (2012). Does attention constrain developmental trajectories in fragile X syndrome? A 3-year prospective longitudinal study. *American Journal on Intellectual and Developmental Disabilities, 117*(2), 103–120.

Cornish, K., Cole, V., Longhi, E., Karmiloff-Smith, A., & Scerif, G. (2013). Mapping developmental trajectories of attention and working memory in fragile X syndrome: Developmental freeze or developmental change? *Development and Psychopathology, 25*(2), 365–376.

Cornish, K., Scerif, G., & Karmiloff-Smith, A. (2007). Tracing syndrome-specific trajectories of attention across the lifespan. *Cortex, 43*(6), 672–685.

Crick, N. R., & Dodge, K. A. (1994). A review and reformulation of social information-processing mechanisms in children's social adjustment. *Psychological Bulletin, 115*(1), 74.

Danielsson, H., Henry, L., Messer, D., Carney, D. P., & Rönnberg, J. (2016). Developmental delays in phonological recoding among children and adolescents with Down syndrome and Williams syndrome. *Research in Developmental Disabilities, 55*, 64–76.

DeLoache, J. S. (2002). *The symbol-mindedness of young children. Child psychology in retrospect and prospect: In celebration of the 75th anniversary of the Institute of Child Development* (Vol. 32, pp. 73–101). London, England: L. Erlbaum Associates.

Diamond, A. (2000). Close interrelation of motor development and cognitive development and of the cerebellum and prefrontal cortex. *Child Development, 71*(1), 44–56.

Didden, R., Korzilius, H. P. L. M., Aperlo, B. V., Overloop, C. V., & Vries, M. D. (2002). Sleep problems and daytime problem behaviours in children with intellectual disability. *Journal of Intellectual Disability Research, 46*(7), 537–547.

Dimitropoulos, A., Feurer, I. D., Butler, M. G., & Thompson, T. (2001). Emergence of compulsive behavior and tantrums in children with Prader-Willi syndrome. *American Journal on Mental Retardation, 106*(1), 39–51.

Dionne, G., Dale, P. S., Boivin, M., & Plomin, R. (2003). Genetic evidence for bidirectional effects of early lexical and grammatical development. *Child Development, 74*(2), 394–412.

Dolva, A. S., Coster, W., & Lilja, M. (2004). Functional performance in children with Down syndrome. *American Journal of Occupational Therapy, 58*(6), 621–629.

Donovan, M. S., & Cross, C. T. (2002). *Minority students in special and gifted education, committee on minority representation in special education*. Washington, DC: National Academy of Education.

Duvdevany, I. (2002). Self-concept and adaptive behaviour of people with intellectual disability in integrated and segregated recreation activities. *Journal of Intellectual Disability Research, 46*(5), 419–429.

Dyck, M. J., Piek, J. P., Hay, D., Smith, L., & Hallmayer, J. (2006). Are abilities abnormally interdependent in children with autism? *Journal of Clinical Child and Adolescent Psychology, 35*(1), 20–33.

Egilson, S. T., & Coster, W. J. (2004). School function assessment: Performance of Icelandic students with special needs. *Scandinavian Journal of Occupational Therapy, 11*(4), 163–170.

Eisenhower, A. S., Baker, B. L., & Blacher, J. (2005). Preschool children with intellectual disability: Syndrome specificity, behaviour problems, and maternal well-being. *Journal of Intellectual Disability Research, 49*(9), 657–671.

Eisenhower, A. S., Baker, B. L., & Blacher, J. (2007). Early student–teacher relationships of children with and without intellectual disability: Contributions of behavioral, social, and self-regulatory competence. *Journal of School Psychology, 45*(4), 363–383.

Elliott, D., & Bunn, L. (2004). Motor disorders in children with intellectual disabilities. In D. Dewey & D. E. Tupper (Eds.), *The science and practice of neuropsychology. Developmental motor disorders: A neuropsychological perspective* (pp. 137–151). New York, NY: Guilford Press.

Emerson, E., & Hatton, C. (2007). Mental health of children and adolescents with intellectual disabilities in Britain. *The British Journal of Psychiatry, 191*(6), 493–499.

Eriksson, L., Welander, J., & Granlund, M. (2007). Participation in everyday school activities for children with and without disabilities. *Journal of Developmental and Physical Disabilities, 19*(5), 485–502.

Evans, D. W. (1998). Development of the self-concept in children with mental retardation: Organismic and contextual factors. In J. A. Burack, R. M. Hodapp, & E. Zigler (Eds.), *Handbook of mental retardation and development*. New York, NY: Cambridge University Press.

Facon, B., Facon-Bollengier, T., & Grubar, J. C. (2002). Chronological age, receptive vocabulary, and syntax comprehension in children and adolescents with mental retardation. *American Journal on Mental Retardation, 107*(2), 91–98.

Farley, J. A., Gibbons, M. M., & Cihak, D. F. (2014). Peer mentors in a postsecondary education program for students with intellectual disabilities. *College Student Journal, 48*(4), 651–660.

Festen, D. A. M., De Weerd, A. W., Van Den Bossche, R. A. S., Joosten, K., Hoeve, H., & Hokken-Koelega, A. C. S. (2006). Sleep-related breathing disorders in prepubertal children with Prader-Willi syndrome and effects of growth hormone treatment. *The Journal of Clinical Endocrinology & Metabolism, 91*(12), 4911–4915.

Festen, D. A. M., Wevers, M., Lindgren, A. C., Böhm, B., Otten, B. J., Wit, J. M., … Hokken-Koelega, A. C. S. (2008). Mental and motor development before and during growth hormone treatment in infants and toddlers with Prader–Willi syndrome. *Clinical Endocrinology, 68*(6), 919–925.

Field, S., Martin, J., Miller, R., Ward, M., & Wehmeyer, M. (1998). Self-determination for persons with disabilities: A position statement of me division on career development and transition. *Career Development for Exceptional Individuals, 21*(2), 113–128.

Flenthrope, J. L., & Brady, N. C. (2010). Relationships between early gestures and later language in children with fragile X syndrome. *American Journal of Speech-Language Pathology, 19*(2), 135–142.

Folk, E. D., Yamamoto, K. K., & Stodden, R. A. (2012). Implementing inclusion and collaborative teaming in a model program of postsecondary education for young adults with intellectual disabilities. *Journal of Policy and Practice in Intellectual Disabilities, 9*(4), 257–269.

Fu, T. (2015). Profiles and development of adaptive behavior in adolescents and adults with Williams syndrome. *International Journal of Information and Education Technology, 5*(12), 931–935.

Gallagher, A., & Hallahan, B. (2012). Fragile X-associated disorders: A clinical overview. *Journal of Neurology, 259*(3), 401–413.

Gates, B., & Barr, O. (2009). *Oxford handbook of learning and intellectual disability nursing*. Oxford, England: Oxford University Press.
Gilmore, L., Cuskelly, M., & Hayes, A. (2003). Self-regulatory behaviors in children with Down syndrome and typically developing children measured using the Goodman Lock Box. *Research in Developmental Disabilities, 24*(2), 95–108.
Glenn, S., & Cunningham, C. (2008). Self-regulation in children and young people with Down. In M. Cuskelly, A. Jobling, & S. Buckley (Eds.), *Down syndrome across the life span*. London, England: Whurr.
Goldstein, H., Kaczmarek, L., & English, K. (2002). *Promoting social communication: Children with developmental disabilities from birth to adolescence*. Baltimore, MD: Brookes.
Gowen, J. W., Johnson-Martin, N., Goldman, B. D., & Hussey, B. (1992). Object play and exploration in children with and without disabilities: A longitudinal study. *American Journal of Mental Retardation, 97*(1), 21–38.
Griffin, M. M., Mello, M. P., Glover, C. A., Carter, E. W., & Hodapp, R. M. (2016). Supporting students with intellectual and developmental disabilities in postsecondary education: The motivations and experiences of peer mentors. *Inclusion, 4*(2), 75–88.
Grigal, M., Dwyre, A., & Davis, H. (2006). *Transition services for students aged 18–21 with intellectual disabilities in college and community settings: Models and implications of success* (NCSET Information Brief No. 5). Minneapolis, MN: Institute for Community Integration, University of Minnesota.
Grigal, M., Hart, D., & Weir, C. (2012). A survey of postsecondary education programs for students with intellectual disabilities in the United States. *Journal of Policy and Practice in Intellectual Disabilities, 9*(4), 223–233.
Grigal, M., Neubert, D. A., & Moon, S. S. (2001). Public school programs for students with significant disabilities in postsecondary settings. *Education and Training in Mental Retardation and Developmental Disabilities, 36*, 244–254.
Guralnick, M. J. (1997). Effectiveness of early intervention for vulnerable children: A developmental perspective. *American Journal on Mental Retardation, 102*(4), 319–345.
Guralnick, M. J. (2010). Early intervention approaches to enhance the peer-related social competence of young children with developmental delays: A historical perspective. *Infants and Young Children, 23*(2), 73.
Guralnick, M. J., Connor, R. T., Neville, B., & Hammond, M. A. (2006). Promoting the peer-related social development of young children with mild developmental delays: Effectiveness of a comprehensive intervention. *American Journal on Mental Retardation, 111*(5), 336–356.
Guralnick, M. J., Paul-Brown, D., Groom, J. M., Booth, C. L., Hammond, M. A., Tupper, D. B., & Gelenter, A. (1998). Conflict resolution patterns of preschool children with and without developmental delays in heterogeneous playgroups. *Early Education and Development, 9*(1), 49–77.
Hafner, D., Moffatt, C., & Kisa, N. (2011). Cutting-edge: Integrating students with intellectual and developmental disabilities into a 4-year liberal arts college. *Career Development for Exceptional Individuals, 34*(1), 18–30.
Hahn, L. J., Brady, N. C., Fleming, K. K., & Warren, S. F. (2016). Joint engagement and early language in young children with fragile X syndrome. *Journal of Speech, Language, and Hearing Research, 59*(5), 1087–1098.
Halperin, J. M., Bédard, A. C. V., & Curchack-Lichtin, J. T. (2012). Preventive interventions for ADHD: A neurodevelopmental perspective. *Neurotherapeutics, 9*(3), 531–541.
Hanakawa, T. (2011). Rostral premotor cortex as a gateway between motor and cognitive networks. *Neuroscience Research, 70*(2), 144–154.
Hart Barnett, J. E., & Crippen, R. (2014). Eight steps to school-based employment training for adolescents with autism spectrum disorder and intellectual disability. *Physical Disabilities: Education and Related Services, 33*(2), 1–15.
Harter, S. (1999). *The construction of the self: A developmental perspective*. New York, NY: Guilford Press.

Hartley, S. L., & Sikora, D. M. (2010). Detecting autism spectrum disorder in children with intellectual disability: Which DSM-IV-TR criteria are most useful? *Focus on Autism and Other Developmental Disabilities, 25*(2), 85–97.

Hartman, E., Houwen, S., Scherder, E., & Visscher, C. (2010). On the relationship between motor performance and executive functioning in children with intellectual disabilities. *Journal of Intellectual Disability Research, 54*(5), 468–477.

Hartup, W. W., & Stevens, N. (1997). Friendships and adaptation in the life course. *Psychological Bulletin, 121*(3), 355.

Hatton, D. D., Wheeler, A., Sideris, J., Sullivan, K., Reichardt, A., Roberts, J., … Bailey, D. B., Jr. (2009). Developmental trajectories of young girls with fragile X syndrome. *American Journal on Intellectual and Developmental Disabilities, 114*(3), 161–171.

Hauk, O., Johnsrude, I., & Pulvermüller, F. (2004). Somatotopic representation of action words in human motor and premotor cortex. *Neuron, 41*(2), 301–307.

Helsen, M., Vollebergh, W., & Meeus, W. (2000). Social support from parents and friends and emotional problems in adolescence. *Journal of Youth and Adolescence, 29*(3), 319–335.

Henry, L. A., & MacLean, M. (2002). Working memory performance in children with and without intellectual disabilities. *American Journal on Mental Retardation, 107*(6), 421–432.

Hodapp, R. M., Ly, T. M., Fidler, D. J., & Ricci, L. A. (2001). Less stress, more rewarding: Parenting children with Down syndrome. *Parenting: Science and practice, 1*(4), 317–337.

Hogan, D. P., Rogers, M. L., & Msall, M. E. (2000). Functional limitations and key indicators of well-being in children with disability. *Archives of Pediatrics & Adolescent Medicine, 154*(10), 1042–1048.

Houwen, S., Visser, L., van der Putten, A., & Vlaskamp, C. (2016). The interrelationships between motor, cognitive, and language development in children with and without intellectual and developmental disabilities. *Research in Developmental Disabilities, 53*, 19–31.

Hustyi, K. M., Hall, S. S., Quintin, E. M., Chromik, L. C., Lightbody, A. A., & Reiss, A. L. (2015). The relationship between autistic symptomatology and independent living skills in adolescents and young adults with fragile X syndrome. *Journal of Autism and Developmental Disorders, 45*(6), 1836.

Jarrold, C., Baddeley, A., & Phillips, C. (1999). Down syndrome and the phonological loop: The evidence for, and importance of, a specific verbal short-term memory deficit. *Down Syndrome Research and Practice, 6*(2), 61–75.

Jarrold, C., Baddeley, A. D., Hewes, A. K., Leeke, T. C., & Phillips, C. E. (2004). What links verbal short-term memory performance and vocabulary level? Evidence of changing relationships among individuals with learning disability. *Journal of Memory and Language, 50*(2), 134–148.

Johnson-Glenberg, M. C. (2008). Fragile X syndrome: Neural network models of sequencing and memory. *Cognitive Systems Research, 9*(4), 274–292.

Kaiser, A. P., Hester, P. P., & McDuffie, A. S. (2001). Supporting communication in young children with developmental disabilities. *Developmental Disabilities Research Reviews, 7*(2), 143–150.

Kaiser, A. P., & Trent, J. A. (2007). Communication intervention for young children with disabilities: Naturalistic approaches to promoting development. In S. L. Odom, R. H. Horner, M. E. Snell, & J. Blacher (Eds.), *Handbook of developmental disabilities*. New York, NY: Guildford Press.

Kemp, C., & Carter, M. (2002). The social skills and social status of mainstreamed students with intellectual disabilities. *Educational Psychology, 22*(4), 391–411.

Klein, B. P., & Mervis, C. B. (1999). Contrasting patterns of cognitive abilities of 9- and 10-year-olds with Williams syndrome or Down syndrome. *Developmental Neuropsychology, 16*(2), 177–196.

Kleinert, H. L., Miracle, S., & Sheppard-Jones, K. (2007). Including students with moderate and severe intellectual disabilities in school extracurricular and community recreation activities. *Intellectual and Developmental Disabilities, 45*(1), 46–55.

Klusek, J., Roberts, J. E., & Losh, M. (2015). Cardiac autonomic regulation in autism and Fragile X syndrome: A review. *Psychological Bulletin, 141*(1), 141.

Kochanska, G., Murray, K., & Coy, K. C. (1997). Inhibitory control as a contributor to conscience in childhood: From toddler to early school age. *Child Development, 68*(2), 263–277.

Kock, E., Molteno, C., Mfiki, N., Kidd, M., Ali, A., King, M., & Strydom, A. (2012). Cross-cultural validation of a measure of felt stigma in people with intellectual disabilities. *Journal of Applied Research in Intellectual Disabilities, 25*(1), 11–19.

Kopp, C. B. (1982). Antecedents of self-regulation: A developmental perspective. *Developmental Psychology, 18*(2), 199–214.

Koppenhaver, D. A., & Erickson, K. A. (2003). Natural emergent literacy supports for preschoolers with autism and severe communication impairments. *Topics in Language Disorders, 23*(4), 283–292.

Kover, S. T., Pierpont, E. I., Kim, J. S., Brown, W. T., & Abbeduto, L. (2013). A neurodevelopmental perspective on the acquisition of nonverbal cognitive skills in adolescents with fragile X syndrome. *Developmental Neuropsychology, 38*(7), 445–460.

Kumin, L. (1994). A longitudinal study of the emergence of phonemes in children with Down Syndrome. *Journal of Communication Disorders, 27*(4), 293–304.

Kyllerman, M. (2013). Angelman syndrome. *Handbook of Clinical Neurology, 111*, 287–290.

Lachapelle, Y., Wehmeyer, M. L., Haelewyck, M. C., Courbois, Y., Keith, K. D., Schalock, R., … Walsh, P. N. (2005). The relationship between quality of life and self-determination: An international study. *Journal of Intellectual Disability Research, 49*(10), 740–744.

Lam, K. S., & Aman, M. G. (2007). The repetitive behavior scale-revised: Independent validation in individuals with autism spectrum disorders. *Journal of Autism and Developmental Disorders, 37*(5), 855–866.

Lancioni, G. E., O'Reilly, M. F., & Basili, G. (2001). Use of microswitches and speech output systems with people with severe/profound intellectual or multiple disabilities: A literature review. *Research in Developmental Disabilities, 22*(1), 21–40.

Lanfranchi, S., Cornoldi, C., Drigo, S., & Vianello, R. (2009). Working memory in individuals with fragile X syndrome. *Child Neuropsychology, 15*(2), 105–119.

Laws, G., Brown, H., & Main, E. (2016). Reading comprehension in children with Down syndrome. *Reading and Writing, 29*(1), 21–45.

Lee, S. H., Wehmeyer, M. L., Palmer, S. B., Soukup, J. H., & Little, T. D. (2008). Self-determination and access to the general education curriculum. *The Journal of Special Education, 42*(2), 91–107.

Leung, G. P., Chan, C. C., Chung, R. C., & Pang, M. Y. (2011). Determinants of activity and participation in preschoolers with developmental delay. *Research in Developmental Disabilities, 32*(1), 289–296.

Levy-Shiff, R., Kedem, P., & Sevillia, Z. (1990). Ego identity in mentally retarded adolescents. *American Journal on Mental Retardation, 94*, 541–549.

Lo, S. T., Festen, D. A., Tummers-de Lind van Wijngaarden, R. F., Collin, P. J., & Hokken-Koelega, A. C. (2015). Beneficial effects of long-term growth hormone treatment on adaptive functioning in infants with Prader-Willi syndrome. *American Journal on Intellectual and Developmental Disabilities, 120*(4), 315–327.

Lowe, K., Allen, D., Jones, E., Brophy, S., Moore, K., & James, W. (2007). Challenging behaviours: Prevalence and topographies. *Journal of Intellectual Disability Research, 51*(8), 625–636.

Luttropp, A., & Granlund, M. (2010). Interaction–it depends–a comparative study of interaction in preschools between children with intellectual disability and children with typical development. *Scandinavian Journal of Disability Research, 12*(3), 151–164.

Lynch, K. B., & Getzel, E. E. (2013). Practice brief: Assessing impact of inclusive postsecondary education using the think college standards. *Journal of Postsecondary Education and Disability, 26*(4), 385–393.

Lynne Lane, K., Stanton-Chapman, T., Roorbach Jamison, K., & Phillips, A. (2007). Teacher and parent expectations of preschoolers' behavior: Social skills necessary for success. *Topics in Early Childhood Special Education, 27*(2), 86–97.

Mancini, M. C., & Coster, W. J. (2004). Functional predictors of school participation by children with disabilities. *Occupational Therapy International, 11*(1), 12–25.

Marlow, N., Hennessy, E. M., Bracewell, M. A., & Wolke, D. (2007). Motor and executive function at 6 years of age after extremely preterm birth. *Pediatrics, 120*(4), 793–804.

Marschik, P. B., Bartl-Pokorny, K. D., Sigafoos, J., Urlesberger, L., Pokorny, F., Didden, R., … Kaufmann, W. E. (2014). Development of socio-communicative skills in 9- to 12-month-old individuals with fragile X syndrome. *Research in Developmental Disabilities, 35*(3), 597–602.

Martin, J., Van Dycke, J., D'Ottavio, M., & Nickerson, K. (2007). The student-directed summary of performance. *Career Development for Exceptional Individuals, 30*(1), 13–26.

Martin, A., Quintin, E. M., Hall, S. S., & Reiss, A. L. (2016). The role of executive function in independent living skills in female adolescents and young adults with fragile X syndrome. *American Journal on Intellectual and Developmental Disabilities, 121*(5), 448–460.

Martin, R., Tigera, C., Denckla, M. B., & Mahone, M. E. (2010). Factor structure of paediatric timed motor examination and its relationship with IQ. *Developmental Medicine & Child Neurology, 52*(8), 188–194.

Martinez, D. C., Conroy, J. W., & Cerreto, M. C. (2012). Parent involvement in the transition process of children with intellectual disabilities: The influence of inclusion on parent desires and expectations for postsecondary education. *Journal of Policy and Practice in Intellectual Disabilities, 9*(4), 279–288.

Mazzoni, M. (2013). College options for students with intellectual disabilities. *Think College!* Retrieved November 27, 2018, from http://lifeafterieps.com/college-options-for-students-with-intellectual-disabilities-think-college/

Mazzotti, V. L., Kelley, K. R., & Coco, C. M. (2015). Effects of self-directed summary of performance on postsecondary education students' participation in person-centered planning meetings. *The Journal of Special Education, 48*(4), 243–255.

McDonald, S., Erickson, L. D., Johnson, M. K., & Elder, G. H. (2007). Informal mentoring and young adult employment. *Social Science Research, 36*(4), 1328–1347.

McIntyre, L. L., Blacher, J., & Baker, B. L. (2006). The transition to school: Adaptation in young children with and without intellectual disability. *Journal of Intellectual Disability Research, 50*(5), 349–361.

Messier, J., Ferland, F., & Majnemer, A. (2008). Play behavior of school age children with intellectual disability: Their capacities, interests and attitude. *Journal of Developmental and Physical Disabilities, 20*(2), 193–207.

Michaels, C. A., & Ferrara, D. L. (2006). Promoting post-school success for all: The role of collaboration in person-centered transition planning. *Journal of Educational and Psychological Consultation, 16*(4), 287–313.

Migliore, A., Butterworth, J., & Hart, D. (2009). Postsecondary education and employment outcomes for youth with intellectual disabilities. *Think College Fast Facts*, Issue No. 1. Boston, MA: University of Massachusetts Boston, Institute for Community Inclusion.

Miolo, G., Chapman, R. S., & Sindberg, H. A. (2005). Sentence comprehension in adolescents with down syndrome and typically developing children's role of sentence voice, visual context, and auditory-verbal short-term memory. *Journal of Speech, Language, and Hearing Research, 48*(1), 172–188.

Mirrett, P. L., Bailey, D. B., Jr., Roberts, J. E., & Hatton, D. D. (2004). Developmental screening and detection of developmental delays in infants and toddlers with fragile X syndrome. *Journal of Developmental & Behavioral Pediatrics, 25*(1), 21–27.

Moon, M. S., Grigal, M., & Neubert, D. (2001). High school and beyond. *Exceptional Parent, 31*(7), 52–57.

Moyle, M. J., Weismer, S. E., Evans, J. L., & Lindstrom, M. J. (2007). Longitudinal relationships between lexical and grammatical development in typical and late-talking children. *Journal of Speech, Language, and Hearing Research, 50*(2), 508–528.

Murphy, M. M., Abbeduto, L., Schroeder, S., & Serlin, R. (2007). Contribution of social and information-processing factors to eye-gaze avoidance in fragile X syndrome. *American Journal on Mental Retardation, 112*(5), 349–360.

Nader-Grosbois, N. (2014). Self-perception, self-regulation and metacognition in adolescents with intellectual disability. *Research in Developmental Disabilities, 35*(6), 1334–1348.

Nader-Grosbois, N., & Vieillevoye, S. (2012). Variability of self-regulatory strategies in children with intellectual disability and typically developing children in pretend play situations. *Journal of Intellectual Disability Research, 56*(2), 140–156.

Neubert, D. A., Moon, M. S., & Grigal, M. (2004). Activities of students with significant disabilities receiving services in postsecondary settings. *Education and Training in Developmental Disabilities, 39*(1), 16–25.

Neubert, D. A., & Redd, V. A. (2008). Transition services for students with intellectual disabilities: A case study of a public school program on a community college campus. *Exceptionality, 16*(4), 220–234.

Nishitani, N., Schürmann, M., Amunts, K., & Hari, R. (2005). Broca's region: From action to language. *Physiology, 20*(1), 60–69.

Nota, L., Ferrari, L., Soresi, S., & Wehmeyer, M. (2007). Self-determination, social abilities and the quality of life of people with intellectual disability. *Journal of Intellectual Disability Research, 51*(11), 850–865.

O'Brien, P., Shevlin, M., O'Keefe, M., Fitzgerald, S., Curtis, S., & Kenny, M. (2009). Opening up a whole new world for students with intellectual disabilities within a third level setting. *British Journal of Learning Disabilities, 37*(4), 285–292.

O'Connor, B., Kubiak, J., Espiner, D., & O'Brien, P. (2012). Lecturer responses to the inclusion of students with intellectual disabilities auditing undergraduate classes. *Journal of Policy and Practice in Intellectual Disabilities, 9*(4), 247–256.

Orkwis, R., & McLane, K. (1998). *A curriculum every student can use: Design principles for student access* (ERIC/OSEP Topical Brief).

Ornstein, P. A., Schaaf, J. M., Hooper, S. R., Hatton, D. D., Mirrett, P., & Bailey, D. B., Jr. (2008). Memory skills of boys with fragile X syndrome. *American Journal on Mental Retardation, 113*(6), 453–465.

Orsmond, G. I., Krauss, M., & Seltzer, M. (2004). Peer relationships and social and recreational activities among adolescents and adults with autism. *Journal of Autism and Developmental Disorders, 34*(3), 245–256.

Palmer, S. B., & Wehmeyer, M. L. (2003). Promoting self-determination in early elementary school: Teaching self-regulated problem-solving and goal-setting skills. *Remedial and Special Education, 24*(2), 115–126.

Paparella, T., & Kasari, C. (2004). Joint attention skills and language development in special needs populations: Translating research to practice. *Infants & Young Children, 17*(3), 269–280.

Papay, C. K., & Bambara, L. M. (2011). Postsecondary education for transition-age students with intellectual and other developmental disabilities: A national survey. *Education and Training in Autism and Developmental Disabilities, 46*(1), 78–93.

Pedersen, S., Vitaro, F., Barker, E. D., & Borge, A. I. (2007). The timing of middle-childhood peer rejection and friendship: Linking early behavior to early-adolescent adjustment. *Child Development, 78*(4), 1037–1051.

Peters, S. U., Goddard-Finegold, J., Beaudet, A. L., Madduri, N., Turcich, M., & Bacino, C. (2004). Cognitive and adaptive behavior profiles of children with Angelman syndrome. *American Journal of Medical Genetics Part A, 128*(2), 110–113.

Piek, J. P., Dawson, L., Smith, L. M., & Gasson, N. (2008). The role of early fine and gross motor development on later motor and cognitive ability. *Human Movement Science, 27*(5), 668–681.

Pivik, J., McComas, J., & Laflamme, M. (2002). Barriers and facilitators to inclusive education. *Exceptional Children, 69*(1), 97–107.

Plotner, A. J., & Marshall, K. J. (2015). Postsecondary education programs for students with an intellectual disability: Facilitators and barriers to implementation. *Intellectual and Developmental Disabilities, 53*(1), 58–69.

Poulsen, A. A., Ziviani, J. M., & Cuskelly, M. (2007). Perceived freedom in leisure and physical co-ordination ability: Impact on out-of-school activity participation and life satisfaction. *Child: Care, Health and Development, 33*(4), 432–440.

Powers, L. E. (2005). Self-determination by individuals with severe disabilities: Limitations or excuses? *Research and Practice for Persons with Severe Disabilities, 30*(3), 168–172.

Pretty, G., Rapley, M., & Bramston, P. (2002). Neighbourhood and community experience, and the quality of life of rural adolescents with and without an intellectual disability. *Journal of Intellectual and Developmental Disability, 27*(2), 106–116.

Pulvermüller, F. (2005). Brain mechanisms linking language and action. *Nature Reviews Neuroscience, 6*(7), 576–582.

Quintin, E. M., Jo, B., Hall, S. S., Bruno, J. L., Chromik, L. C., Raman, M. M., … Reiss, A. L. (2016). The cognitive developmental profile associated with fragile X syndrome: A longitudinal investigation of cognitive strengths and weaknesses through childhood and adolescence. *Development and Psychopathology, 28*(4), 1457–1469.

Rigoli, D., Piek, J. P., Kane, R., Whillier, A., Baxter, C., & Wilson, P. (2013). An 18-month follow-up investigation of motor coordination and working memory in primary school children. *Human Movement Science, 32*(5), 1116–1126.

Roberts, J., Hennon, E. A., & Anderson, K. (2003). Fragile X syndrome and speech and language. *The ASHA Leader, 8*(19), 6–7.

Roberts, J., Long, S. H., Malkin, C., Barnes, E., Skinner, M., Hennon, E. A., & Anderson, K. (2005). A comparison of phonological skills of boys with fragile X syndrome and Down syndrome. *Journal of Speech, Language, and Hearing Research, 48*(5), 980–995.

Roberts, J. E., Hatton, D. D., Long, A. C., Anello, V., & Colombo, J. (2012). Visual attention and autistic behavior in infants with fragile X syndrome. *Journal of Autism and Developmental Disorders, 42*(6), 937–946.

Roberts, J. E., Mankowski, J. B., Sideris, J., Goldman, B. D., Hatton, D. D., Mirrett, P. L., … Bailey, D. B., Jr. (2008). Trajectories and predictors of the development of very young boys with fragile X syndrome. *Journal of Pediatric Psychology, 34*(8), 827–836.

Roberts, J. E., Mirrett, P., Anderson, K., Burchinal, M., & Neebe, E. (2002). Early communication, symbolic behavior, and social profiles of young males with fragile X syndrome. *American Journal of Speech-Language Pathology, 11*(3), 295–304.

Roberts, J. E., Price, J., & Malkin, C. (2007). Language and communication development in Down syndrome. *Developmental Disabilities Research Reviews, 13*(1), 26–35.

Robinson, A. M., & Richdale, A. L. (2004). Sleep problems in children with an intellectual disability: Parental perceptions of sleep problems, and views of treatment effectiveness. *Child: Care, Health and Development, 30*(2), 139–150.

Roebers, C. M., & Kauer, M. (2009). Motor and cognitive control in a normative sample of 7-year-olds. *Developmental Science, 12*(1), 175–181.

Rojahn, J., Schroeder, S. R., & Hoch, T. A. (2007). *Self-injurious behavior in intellectual disabilities* (Vol. 2). Oxford, England: Elsevier.

Rothman, H. R., & Cosden, M. (1995). The relationship between self-perception of a learning disability and achievement, self-concept and social support. *Learning Disability Quarterly, 18*(3), 203–212.

Rubin, K. H., Bukowski, W. M., & Parker, J. G. (1998). *Peer interactions, relationships, and groups. Handbook of child psychology*. New York, NY: Wiley.

Sadeh, A., Gruber, R., & Raviv, A. (2002). Sleep, neurobehavioral functioning, and behavior problems in school-age children. *Child Development, 73*(2), 405–417.

Sadock, B. J., Sadock, V. A., & Kaplan, H. I. (2009). *Kaplan and Sadock's concise textbook of child and adolescent psychiatry*. New York, NY: Lippincott Williams & Wilkins.

Santos, S., & Morato, P. (2012). Acertando o passo! Falar de deficiência mental é um erro: deve falar-se de dificuldade intelectual e desenvolvimental (DID). *Por quê? A Revista Brasileira de Educação Especial, 18*(1), 3–16.

Savelsbergh, G., van der Kamp, J., Ledebt, A., & Planinsek, T. (2000). Information coupling in children with Down syndrome. In D. J. Weeks, R. Chua, & D. Elliott (Eds.), *Perceptual-motor behavior in Down syndrome*. Champaign, IL: Human Kinetics.

Scerif, G., Cornish, K., Wilding, J., Driver, J., & Karmiloff-Smith, A. (2004). Visual search in typically developing toddlers and toddlers with Fragile X or Williams syndrome. *Developmental Science, 7*(1), 116–130.

Schneider, J., Wedgewood, N., Llewellyn, G., & McConnell, D. (2006). Families challenged by and accommodating to the adolescent years. *Journal of Intellectual Disability Research, 50*(12), 926–936.

Shandra, C. L., & Hogan, D. P. (2008). School-to-work program participation and the post-high school employment of young adults with disabilities. *Journal of Vocational Rehabilitation, 29*(2), 117–130.

Shogren, K. A., & Shaw, L. A. (2016). The role of autonomy, self-realization, and psychological empowerment in predicting outcomes for youth with disabilities. *Remedial and Special Education, 37*(1), 55–62.

Shonkoff, J. P., & Phillips, D. A. (2000). *From neurons to neighborhoods: The science of early childhood development.* Washington, DC: National Academy Press.

Siemensma, E. P., Tummers-de Lind van Wijngaarden, R. F., Festen, D. A., Troeman, Z. C., Van Alfen-van Der Velden, A. A. E. M., Otten, B. J., … Haring, D. A. (2012). Beneficial effects of growth hormone treatment on cognition in children with Prader-Willi syndrome: A randomized controlled trial and longitudinal study. *The Journal of Clinical Endocrinology & Metabolism, 97*(7), 2307–2314.

Sigstad, H. M. H. (2016). Significance of friendship for quality of life in adolescents with mild intellectual disability: A parental perspective. *Journal of Intellectual & Developmental Disability, 41*(4), 289–298.

Slevin, E., Truesdale-Kennedy, M., McConkey, R., Livingstone, B., & Fleming, P. (2014). Obesity and overweight in intellectual and non-intellectually disabled children. *Journal of Intellectual Disability Research, 58*(3), 211–220.

Snell, M. E., Brady, N., McLean, L., Ogletree, B. T., Siegel, E., Sylvester, L., … Sevcik, R. (2010). Twenty years of communication intervention research with individuals who have severe intellectual and developmental disabilities. *American Journal on Intellectual and Developmental Disabilities, 115*(5), 364–380.

Solish, A., Minnes, P., & Kupferschmidt, A. (2003). Integration of children with developmental disabilities in social activities. *Journal on Developmental Disabilities, 10*(1), 115–121.

Summers, J. (2012). Neurodevelopmental outcomes in children with Angelman syndrome after 1 year of behavioural intervention. *Developmental Neurorehabilitation, 15*(4), 239–252.

Tanta, K. J., Deitz, J. C., White, O., & Billingsley, F. (2005). The effects of peer-play level on initiations and responses of preschool children with delayed play skills. *American Journal of Occupational Therapy, 59*(4), 437–445.

Thiemann-Bourque, K. S., Brady, N. C., & Fleming, K. K. (2012). Symbolic play of preschoolers with severe communication impairments with autism and other developmental delays: More similarities than differences. *Journal of Autism and Developmental Disorders, 42*(5), 863–873.

Thoma, C. A., Lakin, K. C., Carlson, D., Domzal, C., Austin, K., & Boyd, K. (2011). Participation in postsecondary education for students with intellectual disabilities: A review of the literature 2001–2010. *Journal of Postsecondary Education and Disability, 24*(3), 175–191.

Tipton, L. A., Christensen, L., & Blacher, J. (2013). Friendship quality in adolescents with and without an intellectual disability. *Journal of Applied Research in Intellectual Disabilities, 26*(6), 522–532.

Tonnsen, B. L., Grefer, M. L., Hatton, D. D., & Roberts, J. E. (2015). Developmental trajectories of attentional control in preschool males with fragile X syndrome. *Research in Developmental Disabilities, 36*, 62–71.

Tunnicliffe, P., Woodcock, K., Bull, L., Oliver, C., & Penhallow, J. (2014). Temper outbursts in Prader–Willi syndrome: Causes, behavioural and emotional sequence and responses by carers. *Journal of Intellectual Disability Research, 58*(2), 134–150.

Turnbull, H. R., Turnbull, A. P., Wehmeyer, M. L., & Shank, M. (2004). *Exwceptional lives.* Columbus, OH: Merrill.

Tzouriadou, M., Barbas, G., Vouyoukas, C., & Anagnostopoulou, E. (2013). The relationship between language and social competence in high-risk preschoolers. *Advances in Mental Health and Intellectual Disabilities, 7*(4), 232–244.

Valencia-Naranjo, N., & Robles-Bello, M. A. (2017). Learning potential and cognitive abilities in preschool boys with fragile X and Down syndrome. *Research in Developmental Disabilities, 60*, 153–161.

Van Bysterveldt, A., & Gillon, G. (2014). A descriptive study examining phonological awareness and literacy development in children with Down syndrome. *Folia Phoniatrica et Logopaedica, 66*(1–2), 48–57.

van Bysterveldt, A. K., Gillon, G. T., & Moran, C. (2006). Enhancing phonological awareness and letter knowledge in preschool children with Down syndrome. *International Journal of Disability, Development and Education, 53*(3), 301–329.

van der Fels, I. M., te Wierike, S. C., Hartman, E., Elferink-Gemser, M. T., Smith, J., & Visscher, C. (2015). The relationship between motor skills and cognitive skills in 4–16 year old typically developing children: A systematic review. *Journal of Science and Medicine in Sport, 18*(6), 697–703.

Van der Molen, M. J., Van Luit, J. E. H., Jongmans, M. J., & Van der Molen, M. W. (2007). Verbal working memory in children with mild intellectual disabilities. *Journal of Intellectual Disability Research, 51*(2), 162–169.

Van der Schuit, M., Peeters, M., Segers, E., Van Balkom, H., & Verhoeven, L. (2009). Home literacy environment of pre-school children with intellectual disabilities. *Journal of Intellectual Disability Research, 53*(12), 1024–1037.

van der Schuit, M., Segers, E., van Balkom, H., Stoep, J., & Verhoeven, L. (2010). Immersive communication intervention for speaking and non-speaking children with intellectual disabilities. *Augmentative and Alternative Communication, 26*(3), 203–218.

van der Schuit, M., Segers, E., van Balkom, H., & Verhoeven, L. (2011). How cognitive factors affect language development in children with intellectual disabilities. *Research in Developmental Disabilities, 32*(5), 1884–1894.

van Tilborg, A., Segers, E., van Balkom, H., & Verhoeven, L. (2014). Predictors of early literacy skills in children with intellectual disabilities: A clinical perspective. *Research in Developmental Disabilities, 35*(7), 1674–1685.

Verschuren, O., Ketelaar, M., Gorter, J. W., Helders, P. J., Uiterwaal, C. S., & Takken, T. (2007). Exercise training program in children and adolescents with cerebral palsy: A randomized controlled trial. *Archives of Pediatrics & Adolescent Medicine, 161*(11), 1075–1081.

Vickerstaff, S., Heriot, S., Wong, M., Lopes, A., & Dossetor, D. (2007). Intellectual ability, self-perceived social competence, and depressive symptomatology in children with high-functioning autistic spectrum disorders. *Journal of Autism and Developmental Disorders, 37*(9), 1647–1664.

Vieillevoye, S., & Nader-Grosbois, N. (2008). Self-regulation during pretend play in children with intellectual disability and in normally developing children. *Research in Developmental Disabilities, 29*(3), 256–272.

Wagner, M., Newman, L., Cameto, R., Garza, N., & Levine, P. (2005). *After high school: A first look at the postschool experiences of youth with disabilities. A Report from the National Longitudinal Transition Study-2 (NLTS2)*. Online submission.

Wang, M. V., Lekhal, R., Aarø, L. E., & Schjølberg, S. (2014). Cooccurring development of early childhood communication and motor skills: Results from a population-based longitudinal study. *Child: Care, Health and Development, 40*(1), 77–84.

Wehmeyer, M., & Schwartz, M. (1998). The relationship between self-determination and quality of life for adults with mental retardation. *Education and Training in Mental Retardation and Developmental Disabilities, 33*(1), 3–12.

Wehmeyer, M. L., & Garner, N. W. (2003). The impact of personal characteristics of people with intellectual and developmental disability on self-determination and autonomous functioning. *Journal of Applied Research in Intellectual Disabilities, 16*(4), 255–265.

Wehmeyer, M. L., Kelchner, K., & Richards, S. (1996). Essential characteristics of self-determined behavior of individuals with mental retardation. *American Journal on Mental Retardation, 100*, 632–642.

Wehmeyer, M. L., Smith, S. J., & Davies, D. K. (2005). Technology use and students with intellectual disability: Universal design for all students. In D. Edyburn, K. Higgins, & R. Boone (Eds.), *Handbook of special education technology research and practice* (pp. 309–323). Whitefish Bay, WI: Knowledge by Design.

Wehmeyer, M. L., Smith, S. J., Palmer, S. B., & Davies, D. K. (2004). Technology use by students with intellectual disabilities: An overview. *Journal of Special Education Technology, 19*(4), 7–21.

Westling, D. L., Kelley, K. R., Cain, B., & Prohn, S. (2013). College students' attitudes about an inclusive postsecondary education program for individuals with intellectual disability. *Education and Training in Autism and Developmental Disabilities, 48*(3), 306–319.

Whitman, T. L. (1990). Self-regulation and intellectual disability. *American Journal on Intellectual Disability, 94*, 347–362.

Willems, R. M., & Hagoort, P. (2007). Neural evidence for the interplay between language, gesture, and action: A review. *Brain and Language, 101*(3), 278–289.

Williams, C. A., Beaudet, A. L., Clayton-Smith, J., Knoll, J. H., Kyllerman, M., Laan, L. A., … Wagstaff, J. (2006). Angelman syndrome 2005: Updated consensus for diagnostic criteria. *American Journal of Medical Genetics Part A, 140*(5), 413–418.

Wong, S. I. (2002). At home with Down syndrome and gender. *Hypatia, 17*(3), 89–117.

Woodcock, K. A., Oliver, C., & Humphreys, G. W. (2009). Task-switching deficits and repetitive behaviour in genetic neurodevelopmental disorders: Data from children with Prader–Willi syndrome chromosome 15 q11–q13 deletion and boys with Fragile X syndrome. *Cognitive Neuropsychology, 26*(2), 172–194.

Wuang, Y. P., & Su, C. Y. (2009). Reliability and responsiveness of the Bruininks–Oseretsky test of motor proficiency-in children with intellectual disability. *Research in Developmental Disabilities, 30*(5), 847–855.

Wullink, M., Widdershoven, G., Van Schrojenstein Lantman-de Valk, H., Metsemakers, J., & Dinant, G. J. (2009). Autonomy in relation to health among people with intellectual disability: A literature review. *Journal of Intellectual Disability Research, 53*(9), 816–826.

Zoghbi, H. Y., & Bear, M. F. (2012). Synaptic dysfunction in neurodevelopmental disorders associated with autism and intellectual disabilities. *Cold Spring Harbor Perspectives in Biology, 4*(3), 1–25.

Chapter 5
Bridging the Divides Among Healthcare Delivery, Family, and Educational Settings

Abstract There is gulf between initial diagnosis of intellectual disabilities, treatment, and intersystem approaches to education, treatment, and service delivery. Often physicians are not informed regarding how well a child integrates into school or how medical treatments affect learning and behaviour. Likewise, educators are often unaware of treatment regimens, changes to treatment, medications and their side effects, and prognosis and course of disease and disorders. The family is often equally uninformed of what physicians or schools are doing. The school psychologist and educational team can connect all these important individuals into a collaborative problem-solving unit, where information can be easily shared and treatment strategies can be best tailored to each person's unique challenges. In this chapter, strategies unique to families with people with intellectual disabilities are shared that help streamline services and optimize treatments.

Case Study

Angelique was diagnosed with Down syndrome soon after birth. She did not experience the common medical complications associated with trisomy 21. Upon entry into an early intervention program at age 24 months, a multidisciplinary team convened to create a comprehensive intervention plan for Angelique. Angelique's mother was extremely helpful in assisting to design speech and language therapy, occupational therapy, physical therapy, and pre-academic programming. However, when the discussion shifted to Angelique's behaviours at home, her mother became emotional and tearful. The conversation at the team meeting began to change to community and family issues. Most importantly, issues related to the well-being of Angelique's mother were discussed. The team learned that Angelique's parents were recently separated. Because of the time and energy required to parent Angelique, her mother was unable to continue her bookkeeping job. The result is that household income was far lower after the birth of Angelique. Angelique and her family were having a difficulty paying bills, rent, and food. Angelique's mother was extremely concerned that some of the therapies and specialized assistance would

S. R. Shaw, A. M. Jankowska, *Pediatric Intellectual Disabilities at School*, Pediatric School Psychology, https://doi.org/10.1007/978-3-030-02992-0_5

cost money that the household does not have. Moreover, Angelique's mother has recently found out that she is expecting another child. These events have created family stress. Although parenting Angelique has been a challenge, Angelique's mother has been an attentive and supportive parent. The family has been involved in a host of early childhood enrichment activities, and Angelique's mother is actively involved in parenting groups for families of children with Down syndrome. Angelique's mother reports that she feels supported by professionals and the other parents in the support groups. However, the stress has been rising. Angelique's mother believes that Angelique's behaviour has become increasingly oppositional and she even begun to demonstrate aggressiveness towards her peers at a play group. Angelique's mother feels guilty because she believes that her own stress is a major contributor to Angelique's behaviour. She is also worried that the family's income problems will only become worse. Angelique's mother expressed concern that both financial resources and her own energy and patience will wear thin with the birth of Angelique's sibling. The multidisciplinary team began developing a plan for Angelique's mother as well. The team was insistent that continuing support for Angelique's mother will be a key factor in Angelique's outcome and preparation for school.

Introduction

Families are critical in the provision of lifelong support to individuals with intellectual disabilities. A large percentage of people with intellectual disabilities receive long-term services and supports while living with their families (Floyd, Harter, Costigan, & MacLean, 2004). Thus, for expertise to be useful, researchers, practitioners, and policymakers are required to understand how to best support families who provide at-home support to children and adults with intellectual disabilities. This article summarizes (a) the status of research regarding the support of families who provide support at home to individuals with intellectual disabilities, (b) present points of concern regarding supports for these families, and (c) associated future research priorities related to supporting families.

Effective programming for individuals with intellectual disabilities involves intersystem collaboration. The core component for any successful intersystem collaboration is the family system. Families differ dramatically in terms of their resources, constellations, abilities, dynamics, and beliefs about intellectual disabilities (Hewitt, Agosta, Heller, Williams, & Reinke, 2013). How the family communicates and coordinates with education, medical, mental health community, employment, or other systems often determines how effective multisystem interventions are. A major goal of professional support is to encourage, involve, and increase family resources so that they can be valuable and effective components of effective programming. Without strong family support, persons with intellectual disabilities often do not profit from even the most well-planned and implemented interventions (Kuo et al., 2011).

Communication with Medical and Educational Professionals

Family Communications

Communicating with families who have children with intellectual disabilities is among the most important professional considerations in creating an integrated program to improve the outcomes of persons with intellectual disabilities. Parents frequently complain that professionals do not understand the challenges of parenting and do not listen (McIntyre, Blacher, & Baker, 2006). Professionals are frequently referred to as arrogant, out of touch, and judgmental. The result is that parents shut down and do not contribute to work for the benefit of the child with intellectual disabilities (Vohra, Madhavan, Sambamoorthi, & Peter, 2014). Building relationships with parents that indicate respect is far more likely to result in positive interaction and problem-solving than when parents are treated as customers or recipients of a service.

Effective Listening

Active listening skills are critical to building an interdependent relationship among parents and professionals. The principles of humble inquiry are effective for developing these relationships (Schein, 2016). Humble inquiry is the skill and art of drawing someone out, of asking questions to which you do not already know the answer, and of building a relationship based on curiosity and interest in the other person. Asking, rather than telling, parents about appropriate actions to be taken leads to an interdependent relationship that empowers families, improves the accuracy of information that parents have, improves the probability of parental acceptance of information coming from the multidisciplinary team, and creates an environment of respect and shared investment in the problem-solving process. Professionals frequently wish to establish their credibility and professionalism by providing sophisticated and detailed professional information to parents, often communicated with jargon. However, when professionals ask questions with humility, parents typically value the openness and professionalism of the individuals asking the question. Most importantly, working with families is about building relationships that are productive and lead to a problem-solving process that results in effective solutions.

Communicating Assessment Results

One of the difficult aspects of communicating with parents is in the provision of results of psychoeducational assessment (Harnett et al., 2013). Effective communication of assessment results in large part depends on how the assessment was conducted (Tuffrey-Wijne, 2013). If parents had a great deal of input, the assessment process was transparent, and parents were carefully and respectfully interviewed concerning their needs and expectations of the assessment; then the communication of the results has a high probability of effectiveness. The second major issue is that the purpose of communicating assessment results is to provide information and not simply data. Focusing on test numbers is rarely an effective method of communication (Samuel, Hobden, LeRoy, & Lacey, 2012). Most professionals begin to doze off when a blizzard of numbers is presented and parents do the same. The best way to begin communication of assessment results is to answer the primary presenting questions. Some of the common questions are: is the child eligible to meet program criteria? What is the appropriate diagnosis? Is there evidence of a secondary mental health problem? Is there evidence that interventions have been successful in improving functioning? Directly answering the question is what most parents want to hear. Sometimes the assessment data do not effectively converge or create a situation in which interpretation is ambiguous. Telling parents that you do not know an answer to a question because information is inconsistent or ambiguous is completely acceptable if there is a plan to further clarify the answer to the question. After answering the question, the next step is to identify any caveats, concerns, or sources of error that may mitigate the response to the question. This is a part of being transparent in an assessment. At some point, it may be necessary to tell parents how you reached the answer to the questions, and this would be the only appropriate opportunity to present detailed assessment data. Finally, communication needs to answer the question, "What do we do next?" This can be a discussion of short- and long-term planning, developing an individualized education plan, or deferring an action plan to a later date to be determined. Making assessment transparent, answering the important questions, and carefully describing the consequences based on assessment results are the primary issues involving communicating to parents (Carter, 2013).

Psychoeducational assessment and communicating the results to parents frequently lead to an emotional response. This is especially true when parents are hearing for the first time that their child meets criteria for a diagnosis of intellectual disabilities. The most common response is relief (Carter et al., 2013). Parents usually know that something is a problem and are happy to be able to put a label or explanation to the problem. Some parents are angry, sad, frustrated, tearful, guilty, or incredulous. All assessment results have potential to elicit an emotional response from parents. Those conducting psychoeducational assessments need to remember that emotional responses are to be expected because we are providing answers to difficult questions concerning the most important person in their lives. Although each parent has their own specific requirements, there are some general rules and providing communication of challenging assessment results.

- Ask parents whether anything has changed since the date of conducting the assessment. Sometime psychoeducational reports make statements about information, such as developmental milestones or living arrangements, that can quickly become out of date. This also allows parent input.

- If providing a written psychological report, then tell parents that the report is a draft. They can review the report or have other people review the report as they wish. You expect them to have questions or input. Make yourself clearly available to answer these questions or respond to any concerns they may have. This does two major things: Shows parents that you respect their input and information and takes a bit of pressure from preparing a perfect report (i.e. typos and grammatical errors and reports are easy to make yet detract dramatically from credibility).
- Remind parents of what the primary questions were that lead to the psychological report and that you attempted to answer.
- Provide information in short sentences or statements, and leave time for parents to process and respond. Communicating with parents is not a social conversation in which time must be filled. Pauses may seem long and awkward, but that is often productive for purposes of communication.
- Do not judge. There is no such thing as a good or a bad score on a test of intellectual ability. Scores may be high or low, above or below average, but not better or worse, good or bad.
- Do not minimize results. Psychologists frequently do not want to make a diagnosis of intellectual disabilities because of the stigma that is often attached to this diagnosis. Many psychologists make statements such as, "intelligence tests don't measure anything particularly important and I wouldn't worry about it". Minimizing these results detracts from credibility and is not true. If there is a reason to believe there were problems in the administration of the test instruments that reduced the validity of the measures, then do not report numbers, as those results are inaccurate. If there is no reason to doubt the validity of the measures, then acknowledge that all measures have statistical error, yet the results accurately estimate current functioning. As a side note, measures of blood pressure, cholesterol, body fat, and nearly every medical measurement that we use and trust contain error. Sometimes these measures contain a lot of error, and most times there is more error in medical measurements than there is in intelligence tests. But rarely does the physician place a major emphasis on error in measurement.
- Use the appropriate words. If a child's assessment results are consistent with intellectual disabilities, then you must say the words "intellectual disabilities". If the parent seems confused, then it is completely appropriate to use the words "mental retardation" if that phrase clarifies the results to parents.
- Save the diagnosis for last. Once parents hear emotionally laden words such as "autistic spectrum disorder" or "intellectual disabilities," they often do not hear anything that you will say after that. The answer to the question concerning diagnosis often is saved to the end of the meeting.
- Have a next plan. Giving parents difficult information requires listening skills (including reading nonverbal communications), empathy, gentleness, and an authoritative approach. Having tissues and water available is usually a good idea. No matter how challenging information presented may be to parents, having the next step prepared often helps. For example, "I know it is hard to hear that your child has a diagnosis of intellectual disabilities. Now it is time to figure out what

we are going to do about it to improve all aspects of her functioning". Presenting a problem without making efforts to work toward a solution can increase feelings of hopelessness in parents. Although some parents will not be ready to hear about a solution or a plan, professionals need to have a plan prepared. Assessment that does not lead to effective problem-solving is not particularly productive and parents understand that.
- Be willing to reschedule or make a second meeting. Some parents may be distraught or unable to continue a meeting after hearing difficult information. Scheduling a follow-up meeting later is perfectly okay. Many parents simply require time to process all the information presented at the meeting and to read over the written psychoeducational report. Be prepared and ready to schedule a second or third meeting with parents. This may seem inconvenient as most professionals are overburdened with their caseload. However, this is an excellent investment of time for developing trust with parents and respect for their involvement and ensuring that information is accurately communicated.

Negotiating Interventions

Developing a plan to address educational, social, daily living, and other skills is necessary to improve the quality of functioning for people with intellectual disabilities, which requires team involvement (Crnic, Neece, McIntyre, Blacher, & Baker, 2017). Interventions are most likely to be carried out with integrity by families if the families have control over the presenting problems to be solved. Parents with a perceived need to address a specific problem are far more likely to adhere to the plans developed (De Ruiter, Dekker, Verhulst, & Koot, 2007) than when problems are not perceived as disruptive or serious. Treating parents with respect is not sufficient, and as members of the team developing any form of intervention, teams can be most effective when parents lead the direction of interventions. This form of respect is far more likely to lead to improved interventions and improved adherence to implementing these interventions (Dunlap & Fox, 2007). Although professionals have expertise, no one is as expert on the child and the home environment as the parents.

Communicating with Parents Who also Have Intellectual Disabilities

A challenging situation is when the parents of children with intellectual disabilities themselves have intellectual disabilities (Anderson & Lakin, 1998). Parents with intellectual disabilities can provide adequate childcare and be successful parents (Meppelder, Hodes, Kef, & Schuengel, 2014). However, there may be some limitations for delivery and understanding of complex information (Chadwick, Wesson, & Fullwood, 2013). Factors leading to effective parenting are being married, having significant support from extended family, having only one or two children, receiving appropriate parenting models during childhood, good physical and mental health, adequate finances, low stress and effective stress management strategies, and adequate education and reading skills (Baker et al., 2003). Although these below strategies are effective for all families, for families with parents who have intellectual disabilities, these four strategies are especially important: (1) all services must be responsive and focus on the entire family to ensure that the interest of both the parents and the children is served; (2) services include long-term, ongoing supports of the family because the needs of the children change and parenting skills must change along with them; (3) communication with parents includes parents learning needs including minimizing written material and instruction via a demonstration in the home environment with repetition to ensure generalization of the skill; and (4) services must assist parents to become part of the community and benefit from community services (Haven, Manangan, Sparrow, & Wilson, 2013). Although parents with intellectual disabilities provide challenges and risk factors for problematic outcomes for their children, there are protective factors that can foster resilience for entire families (Guralnick, 2011). Some of these protective factors are responsiveness to instruction of others, warmth and relationships with others, external supports, and the effectiveness of the supports of the community.

Parenting Stress and Health

The issues involved in raising a child with intellectual disabilities create multiple severe stressors. In many cases, parents are case managers; the primary deliverer of educational, medical, and psychological services; and the linchpin of intersystem service delivery (Breiner, 1989). There are also other responsibilities such as parenting other children, maintaining a home, and conducting the basics of self-care. These roles represent more than full-time work. Many families with a child with intellectual disabilities usually have one adult removed from the workforce to fill the multiple roles required in the home. In single-family households, parents have difficult decisions concerning whether to be fully involved in their child's case management or to work (Neece, Green, & Baker, 2012). Frequently, parents are in a difficult situation where they attempt to do both. Parents then sacrifice sleep, health, social interaction, and even work opportunities. Some parents may work but may miss out on advancement opportunities. The result of these issues is that families of children with intellectual disabilities have lower household incomes on average than families with typically functioning children (Burke & Hodapp, 2014). Financial hardship and emotional stress on families are major factors in parent involvement in their child's intervention programming and for overall positive outcomes (Farrell & Krahn, 2014).

The Family Stress Model (Boss, Bryant, & Mancini, 2016) is especially salient for families of children with intellectual disabilities. The Family Stress Model is a process by which severe economic pressure influences parents' mental health, parenting skills and involvement, and subsequently the adjustment and behavioural issues of their child (Bluth, Roberson, Billen, & Sams, 2013). The experience of financial strain becomes so stressful for parents that there is an increased likelihood of depression, feelings of inadequacy, low self-efficacy, and pessimism about their future and the future of their children. The quality of family relationships is reduced in families under stress. Families of children with intellectual disabilities have a significantly higher incidence of divorce and much higher incidence of family conflict and disagreement over major decision-making (Crnic, Arbona, Baker, & Blacher, 2009). The emotional distress that is associated with limited financial resources and economic pressures is the primary mechanism by which harsh and uninvolved parenting and child maladjustment increase. The Family Stress Model is supported across ethnic groups and geographic regions (Landers-Potts et al., 2015). The link between financial hardship and harsh and uninvolved parenting is mediated by parent anxiety, depression, and marital conflict. There is little question that financial hardship influences parents' abilities to be important members of the service delivery team.

An additional aspect of the Family Stress Model involves adult resources (Crnic, Friedrich, & Greenberg, 1983). Households with extended family resources or having friends and neighbours who can be relied upon in times of need are not only important in reducing parental stress but also provide the resources required for families to maintain employment and improve their financial situation. The availability of other adults in the home tends to reduce maternal depression (Dykens, Fisher, Taylor, Lambert, & Miodrag, 2014). Extended family and available adults that can reduce stressors related to childcare are primary factors in overcoming financial stressors. However, sometimes adults who live in the home, but do not provide childcare supports, can create a situation in which stressors predicted by the Family Stress Model are increased (Hayes & Watson, 2012).

A final component of the Family Stress Model is neighbourhood characteristics (Michelson, Davenport, Dretzke, Barlow, & Day, 2013). Families who live in neighbourhoods that are defined by high levels of poverty, unemployment, crime, and residential overcrowding result in less nurturing, warm, and supportive parenting. Neighbourhoods that have high incidence of crime and violent behaviours are directly linked to increase in children's externalizing and internalizing problems. The level of neighbourhood violence is also associated with maternal feelings of depression and maladaptive parenting. Neighbourhood characteristics are related to financial stressors as low-income families are more likely to be situated in high-risk neighbourhoods (Neppl, Senia, & Brent, 2016). The result of factors involved in the Family Stress Model is that not only are people with intellectual disabilities at high risk for mental health issues due to poor coping, language, and social skills, they are also at risk due to parenting issues related to economic stress and financial hardships leading to harsh and uninvolved parenting; and the same factors lead to lack of involvement in intersystem team delivery of services.

Family Support Services

A relatively common belief is that parents of children with intellectual disabilities, who are of low income, are people of colour, have less than a high school education or are immigrants may not value education as much as other parents because they are not actively engaged or involved in intersystem teamwork and service delivery (Landers-Potts et al., 2015). The Family Stress Model predicts that economic stressors and lack of other adult support lead to uninvolved parents who may have depression of their own (Knight, 2013). Parents may not attend meetings because they have hourly employment and work hours that take place during the school day. Any missed work will result in lower income and possible termination. Parents are sometimes placed in the position of having to choose between attending important meetings concerning multisystem implementation of interventions for their child and making enough money to pay the rent and purchase food. Most often, when freed from economic stressors, parents are involved and are valuable members of service delivery teams. There is a clear link between parental stress and the ability to create a strong partnership among educational, medical, and family systems (Cridland, Jones, Magee, & Caputi, 2014). Working to support family systems is an important aspect of long-term partnerships and affective outcomes for people with intellectual disabilities (Raspa, Bailey, Bann, & Bishop, 2014; Riechow et al., 2014).

Family Economic Control

Providing mechanisms to ease financial stress is one of the most effective mechanisms by which to improve family involvement and direct parenting skills. The professionals most involved with this level of support are that of social workers. However, other community resources, professionals, and support staff can be used to address financial issues of families. Among the most important areas of support are negotiating and discussing appropriate insurance reimbursements, completing paperwork, accessing funding for needed materials and programs, and becoming eligible for other levels of financial supports such as Social Security Disability Insurance (Wadsworth et al., 2013). In addition, assisting parents to find appropriate and adequate employment consistent with their expertise and time commitments can also assist in reducing cognitive features described in the Family Stress Model. Training programs that support improvements in income potential and the probability of employment are also effective. Parents may require community resources with the expertise and connections to assist parents with the best possible type of employment. Considering and promoting the financial status of families lead to improvements in parenting skills and the parents' abilities to serve as valuable and important members of complex intervention plans involving multiple systems (Thompson, Schalock, Agosta, Teninty, & Fortune, 2014).

Family Mental Health

Provision of mental health services is typically poorly covered by insurance, difficult to access, and may be unavailable for short-term issues (Burke & Hodapp, 2014). Moreover, availabilities are usually prioritized for those with severe and chronic psychiatric disorders. For the case of families of people with intellectual disabilities, families experience stressors that place them at risk for mental health issues. Unless parents' mental health issues are addressed, they are unlikely to be the best possible contributors to effective intervention programming for their child (Eapen, Ec, Walter, & Tay, 2014). The effectiveness of any intervention focused on an individual with intellectual disabilities will depend on their family's ability to implement that intervention. Providing families with opportunities to discuss mental health needs, address and learn coping skills, and receive counselling as needed is an effective investment in improving outcomes for the person with intellectual disabilities (Peer & Hillman, 2014).

Formal professional counselling and psychiatric services may be necessary to improve overall functioning (Woodman, Mawdsley, & Hauser-Cram, 2015). However, these intensive services are part of the family members' medical program and are outside of the purview of the team working to provide services to the person with intellectual disabilities. One option is for members of the team, often social worker or psychologist, to advise the family member having difficulties coping on the best way to receive counselling and psychiatric services. Another option is to provide other forms of support (Emerson, 2003). An important form of support is parent groups. Parent and families of people with intellectual disabilities meet and share emotions, methods of coping, tips and tricks of parenting, and other aspects of raising a person with intellectual disabilities (Song et al., 2014). Sharing ideas with other people who have experienced the same issues and concerns is a powerful level of support. It can be easy to forget that parenting a child with intellectual disabilities can be a socially isolating existence that exacerbates stressors. Yet, a weekly support group can be difficult to attend for many busy parents. In some cases, a more experienced parent-mentor relationship can be facilitated. In this relationship, an experienced and knowledgeable parent serves as a sounding board, provides information and advice, provides treatment recommendations, and serves as a willing listener to the presenting problems and stressors that inevitably will occur, all from the perspective of somebody who has experience similar issues. Whether a formal relationship with a professional psychologist, psychiatrist, or counsellor; or an informal meeting of parents sharing similar experiences, mental health support for family members is not an afterthought but a critical investment of time that will improve the outcomes of the person with intellectual disabilities (Serketich & Dumas, 1996).

Respite Services

There are no days off in parenting. All professionals on the treatment team will have days off and times to unwind at the end of the day. Parents and many family members have no opportunity to rest (Siller, Reyes, Hotez, Hutman, & Sigman, 2013). Social events such as going out to dinner or seeing a movie are often out of the question for families. This is especially true for parents who do not have extended family as an important resource. Babysitters, friends, or neighbours rarely have the skill or comfort level to supervise a child with intellectual disabilities. Communities may offer respite care through babysitters with specialized skills or a dedicated centre for providing respite care. Most of these services require payment, which is a resource that may not be available to many families. Some communities provide such respite services free of charge, but there is often a waiting list. Planning for respite services is a critical part of any intervention plan. Often parents use their respite time to garden, clean the house, or take a long bath. Providing parents with an opportunity to rest and recharge is an extraordinarily valuable support service that can assist in re-energizing and renewing tired and stressed families.

Sibling Supports

Siblings of people with intellectual disabilities experience their own levels of heightened stress (Shivers & Dykens, 2017). They are often called upon to be caregivers with responsibilities beyond those typically expected of children. Siblings often mature emotionally at a faster rate as they have had to take on some co-parenting duties. There are additional pressures such as social embarrassment, lack of parental attention to unaffected sibling, lack of financial resources, guilt, and concerns about the future of the entire family. There is no current evidence that siblings of people with intellectual disabilities have a higher than average rate of mental health issues (Shivers & Dykens, 2017). There are even a variety of studies that indicate that siblings have increased social maturity, academic achievement and improved empathy when compared to their peers (Smith, Romski, & Sevcik, 2013). Nonetheless, there are siblings who require support. Commonly, sibling support groups allow children and adolescents who share similar concerns to share resources, vent, create friendships, and discuss common features of being the sibling of a person with intellectual disabilities. A formalized plan can be made stronger by increasing support for siblings as part of the family support approach.

Marital Supports

Marriages and partnerships involving people with intellectual disabilities are under extreme stress (Eapen et al., 2014). Some of the stress is due to economic hardship, lack of rest and support, guilt, and pressures for sharing workload of parenting and household activities. Supporting marriages and partnerships creates an environment in which positive parenting skills can be implemented. A child with intellectual disabilities creates a disruptive experience in family systems and partnerships that are well beyond that of having a typically developing child (Bolourian & Blacher, 2016). There are significant strains placed on relationships. Often parents do not wish to discuss their marital stressors in a professional setting. However, acknowledging the idea that a child with intellectual disabilities can have a negative effect on a marriage or partnership can be a relief to parents. Knowing that they are not alone or unusual in having their partnership strained is often reassuring. Providing guidance and reassurance through support groups or marriage and family counsellors can provide benefit to parents.

Control

A major factor in addressing stress is to encourage parents to have as much control over the programming and treatment of the person with intellectual disabilities in the family. Often parents feel as if the role of parenting has been taken over by a team of professionals who only seek the input of the parents intermittently. Although this is discussed in the chapter on team functioning (see Chap. 6), parents should be at least equal members of all decision-making and implementing teams. Negotiating the role of the parent based on their energy, resources, confidence, skills, and willingness to take on large amounts of responsibility is an important aspect of parent control (Ault, Collins, & Carter, 2013). The goal is to have parents assert as much control over the treatment of the child as is possible. The more the parents feel in control, the more anxiety will be reduced.

Parent Skills Training

There is a well-established link between parenting and child behaviour. Inconsistent discipline, inadequate supervision, punitive or negative parenting, and poor attachment between parent and child lead to disruptive behaviours, poor academic outcomes, poor adjustment, and a lower quality of life than for children receiving positive and skilled parenting (Azad, Blacher, & Marcoulides, 2014; McIntyre, 2008). Given the additional stressors placed on parents by having children with intellectual disabilities, there is a need to create systematic parent training programs to teach generalizable skills and create a cycle of positive parenting that leads to effective outcomes. There are a host of parent skills training programs that are available. Some of those studies have received research evaluation support (Baker, 1989). Yet, the quality of studies evaluating parent training programs is typically lacking (Weisz & Kazdin, 2017). In high-quality research studies, the outcome variables focus more on parent satisfaction with the training than on whether the training led to improved child outcomes or generalizable parenting skills. Therefore, parent skills training may be an important component of educational planning

(Lundahl, Risser, & Lovejoy, 2006). Although a strong idea that is intuitively appealing, to this point supportive data are mixed.

Parent management training (PMT) is one of the best-studied psychosocial interventions for child disruptive behaviour; however, there is a substantial gap between abundant academic research and scarce availability of PMT in clinical training and practice (Forgatch & Patterson, 2010). The primary application of PMT is to provide parent training to assist in altering the child's behaviour at home. The program was originally developed to address oppositional defiant behaviours and prevent those behaviours from developing into conduct disorder (Kazdin, 1997). Most applications of PMT are to address preschool and early childhood children who have exhibited behaviour such as temper tantrums, aggression, and excessive noncompliance. The program has not been well evaluated for children with intellectual disabilities yet is a strong candidate for application to this population (Michelson et al., 2013).

Therapists work with parents to assist in developing prosocial skills in children that are incompatible with defiant or other externalizing and problematic behaviours. Parents receive instruction in social learning principles that underlie the parenting techniques taught (Aman et al., 2009). A major component is for parents to model prosocial behaviours (Chacko et al., 2016). However, there are specific behavioural techniques such as defining problem behaviours, approaches to monitoring, and tracking child behaviours; positive reinforcement procedures, token economy, and point systems to be used in the home; giving clear instructions and commands; and problem-solving difficult situations (Kazdin, 1997). Extinction and mild punishment procedures such as ignoring, response costs, and timeout are taught as replacements to corporal punishment. The focus is on a positive parenting approach using behavioural principles. Some of the instructional approaches involve role-playing, behavioural rehearsal, modelling, didactic instruction, and structured homework exercises. Attempts to evaluate the outcomes for PMT have had significant challenges. One of the primary challenges is that the average rate of attrition for parents involved in the program is 28% (Kaminski, Valle, Filene, & Boyle, 2008). This is largely due to parents involved in this research who were at high risk for negative parenting procedures. The focus of much research involves families of low socioeconomic status, multiple children with severe behaviour problems, maternal adjustment issues, parental mental health issues, and other major risk factors. However, there are positive immediate treatment outcomes such as changing parental behaviours to become more positive, less controlling, and less critical. In addition, there are some studies showing that self-reported incidents of corporal punishment have been reduced after PMT (Ollendick et al., 2016). There is statistically significant evidence that child behaviour also improves on variables of physical and verbal aggression, compliance, and destructiveness (Colalillo & Johnston, 2016). One study shows that parent perceptions of their child and parent reports of the relationship with their child also improve after PMT (Akin, Yan, McDonald, & Moon, 2017). There are mixed results on long-term outcomes of PMT. In some studies, the positive outcome initially reported lessened over time (Hagen & Ogden, 2017). There is still significant research to be done on the process of family engagement and creating behaviour change in parents, examining methods of enhancing the outcomes and generalization of the effects, the robustness of the intervention to variations and effects of time, whether PMT is an effective preventative tool, and whether the PMT can be used for multiple different populations other than young children with behaviour disorders (Fazeli, Alilou, & Beyrami, 2016). Yet, the methodology used in PMT is promising for serving as a method of developing prosocial skills in children with intellectual disabilities.

Parent-Child Interaction Therapy (PCIT) is designed for young children with emotional and behavioural disorders rather than children with intellectual disabilities (Gurwitch, Messer, & Funderburk, 2017). Yet, the focus on coaching parents to improve parent-child relationships and to change parent-child interaction patterns has a potential to be a valuable technique for parents of children with intellectual disabilities. Most commonly parents are coached by a therapist as they play with their child. The coach uses a microphone to communicate to parents, who have a small receiver in their ear. In this fashion, therapists support parents and provide real-time feedback and suggestions as they solve problems and play with their children. Although there are also some didactic and role-playing activities involved in PCIT, the real-time commentary, suggestions, and feedback represent unique components of this program. PCIT is more of an approach to improving parent-child interaction rather than a prescribed curriculum (Kennedy, Kim, Tripodi, Brown, & Gowdy, 2016). Therapists often work together to decide which skills to be focused on during each session. PCIT strongly supports parent autonomy in the development and improvement of interactions with their children. There are some studies indicating that the interactional style of both fathers and mothers in play situations with their children is positively affected by this program (Bussing, Nelson, & Kurtz, 2016). In addition, there is some evidence that children's behaviour is also affected. PCIT is based on both attachment and social learning principles to teach a parenting style that involves nurturance, good communication, and firm control. The focus is on developing and promoting an authoritative style of parenting, which has been associated with positive behavioural and mental health outcomes. A major focus of PCIT is to encourage and teach warmth and responsiveness to approve the attachment and development of a secured parent-child relationship. Like other forms of parent training, the research methodology evaluating the effectiveness of PCIT has some weaknesses (Niec, Barnett, Prewett, & Shanley Chatham, 2016). However, the interactive approach that supports both social learning theory and attachment theory has potential to be a positive method for training parents of children with intellectual disabilities.

Stepping Stone Positive Parenting Program (Triple P) is a behaviour management parent training program designed to help caregivers successfully manage disruptive and externalizing behaviours (Turner & Sanders, 2006). Triple P is the parenting program of choice in many countries, and the program's popularity is growing in the United States. Research on Triple P has been available since the 1980s. Results suggest that parental participation decreased disruptive behaviours in children, reduced parental stress, and decreased the use of coercive parenting (Prinz, Sanders, Shapiro, Whitaker, & Lutzker, 2009). In a meta-analytic study, de Graaf, Speetjens,

Smit, de Wolff, and Tavecchio (2008) found that Triple P interventions reduced dysfunctional parenting styles and increased parental competency for parents identified as having problematic parenting skills (Turner & Sanders, 2006). This program has been implemented to parents of children who have been diagnosed with autism spectrum disorder. In a small-scale evaluative study, there was a significant improvement for caregivers in the intervention group on the Parenting Scale Verbosity subscale from pretest to delayed posttest (VanVoorhis, Miller, Miller, & Stull, 2015). This program has not been widely implemented or evaluated for children with intellectual disabilities, but has many characteristics that can prove effective for this population (Marryat, Thompson, & Wilson, 2017).

Most typically the Triple P program is a 9-week small group instruction format that promotes behavioural approaches to parenting. Parents are first taught how to identify antecedents and consequences, establish goals, and monitor behaviour. Caregivers are taught positive strategies on how to teach their children new behaviours and how to use diversion from problem behaviours. Behaviour charts with rewards are commonly used. Parents are taught how to teach new behaviours and to address the function of problematic behaviours to effectively manage child behaviours in a positive way (Prinz et al., 2009). Parents are taught how to implement routines but also how to prepare and plan for environmental situations that placed the child at risk for problematic behaviours. Parents are asked to be reflective on their parenting style and to report successes and failures. Quite often the Triple P program has team leaders or instructors following up with parents via telephone to extend the effectiveness of the treatment and to encourage generalization of skills across environments (de Graaf et al., 2008).

Incredible Years Parent Training Program is a parent training program that is designed to work for children with behaviour disorder such as oppositional defiant disorder, attention deficit hyperactivity disorder, and conduct disorder (Webster-Stratton, 2001). Positive parenting practices, including contingent praise, sensitivity, scaffolding, and consistent limit setting, in contrast to negative coercive parenting behaviours and is associated with the development of children's social competence and self-regulation. The Incredible Years Parent Training Program consists of 12 weekly 2 ½ hour small group sessions. Some of the topics include rewards, limit setting, play, praise, managing challenging behaviours, addressing high-risk situations, and focusing on parent-child interaction. This program has a group focus. Groups view a videotaped vignette of parent-child interactions and hold discussions on strengths and weaknesses of what was observed. In addition to observing videotaped, parents engage in role-playing, didactic instruction, and weekly homework assignments (Webster-Stratton, 2001). When implemented with a small sample of parents of children with intellectual disabilities, the program proved successful in reducing negative parent-child interactions and child behaviour problems in comparison to a control group. The effect sizes are not especially large, yet there is reason to believe that the Incredible Years Parent Training Program has potential to be an effective parenting intervention to improve parent-child interactions and reduce negative parenting practices (Webster-Stratton & Reid, 2010).

Advocacy

Parents of children with intellectual disabilities are frequently frustrated by the systemic barriers faced to acquiring quality services, equal opportunities, adequate resources, and a host of other policy issues (Burke, Arnold, & Owen, 2015; Meppelder et al., 2014). Supporting parent advocacy is an important activity that professionals can use to strengthen and improve parents' ability to be effective deliverers of important services to the child with intellectual disabilities. For parents with the motivation and interests, teaching parents the appropriate procedures for the most effective advocating for their child can be an important part of family treatment and planning. Teams can provide personal and social supports, encourage involvements in neighbourhood or advocacy groups supporting children with intellectual disabilities, and teach the specifics about advocacy for their child and for all children with intellectual disabilities.

Involvement in a parenting group, whether a formal organization or informal meeting of parents, can provide an opportunity to share problems, emotions, and challenges to be overcome. Parents can learn from each other (Wright & Taylor, 2014). In addition, groups of parents can be far more effective in advocating for improvements in service delivery and creating policy change. By empowering parents to make policy changes and to improve the quality of services for their children, there is increased hope for improving the quality of life of their entire family. Parents involved in advocacy groups often experience increase of self-esteem, personal strengths, knowledge about disabilities, knowledge about the rights of their child and family, and a larger voice to address discrimination and influence policy decisions. Encouraging parents to network creates a powerful and informed parent to improve the quality of education and services to their children.

Advocacy can initially seem like a daunting task for a person with a disability, family, groups, or organizations (Petner-Arrey, Howell-Moneta, & Lysaght, 2016). There is generally a six-step process to effective advocacy: (1) identify the problem area and changes needed to address the problem; (2) determine which person, office, or policy is to be the target of advocacy; (3) develop a coalition of individuals and groups who will support change; (4) determine exactly when to act; (5) understand exactly what specific action is required to achieve solution of the problem areas (e.g. new funds, new legislation or regulation, new procedures); and (6) gather information and determine the incentives that will best influence decision-makers. Each form of advocacy has its own challenges (Ford, Acosta, & Sutcliffe, 2013). Whether the advocacy is for reducing opportunities for bullying in the cafeteria lines or creating an entirely new funding mechanism at the upper reaches of government, change can be made. Advocacy not only helps to create change in improved results and programs, policy, and legislation that supports children with intellectual disabilities but improves the self-efficacy of parents and their ability to suggest, develop, and implement effective treatment strategies.

Conclusions

Developing comprehensive plans for people with intellectual disabilities involves a fundamental challenge: most effective plans involve and require parent leadership and participation, yet families of children with intellectual disabilities are at risk for turmoil and disruption. Family stress, disruptions in income, guilt, marital discord, issues with siblings, and other problems often undermine the involvement of parents in programming. Effective interventions require systematically supporting and strengthening parents and families. Nearly all families experience temporary problems and require short-term support. Other families will require long-term support ranging from mental health services to job training. Involving communities as part of programming is an important aspect of a fully realized intervention plan, but the support of families by communities is one method to ensure implementation, success, and generalizability of all educational programming for people with intellectual disabilities (McConnell, Llewellyn, & Bye, 1997; Samadi, McConkey, & Kelly, 2013).

References

Akin, B. A., Yan, Y., McDonald, T., & Moon, J. (2017). Changes in parenting practices during Parent Management Training Oregon model with parents of children in foster care. *Children and Youth Services Review, 76*, 181–191. https://doi.org/10.1016/j.childyouth.2017.03.010

Aman, M. G., McDougle, C. J., Scahill, L., Handen, B., Aronold, L. E., Johnson, C., et al. (2009). Medication and parent training in children with pervasive developmental disorders and serious behavior problems: Results from a randomized clinical trial. *Journal of the American Academy of Child and Adolescent Psychiatry, 48*, 1143–1154. https://doi.org/10.1097/CHI.0b013e3181bfd669

Anderson, L., & Lakin, K. C. (1998). Parents with cognitive limitations: What do we know about providing support? *Impact, 11*(1), 6–7.

Ault, M. J., Collins, B. C., & Carter, E. W. (2013). Congregational participation and supports for children and adults with disabilities: Parent perceptions. *Intellectual and Developmental Disabilities, 51*(1), 48–61. https://doi.org/10.1352/1934-9556-51.01.048

Azad, G., Blacher, J., & Marcoulides, G. (2014). Longitudinal models of socio-economic statusImpact on positive parenting behaviors. *International Journal of Behavioral Development, 38*(6), 509–517. https://doi.org/10.1177/0165025414532172

Baker, B. L. (1989). *Parent training and developmental disabilities*. Washington, DC: American Association on Mental Retardation.

Baker, B. L., McIntyre, L. L., Blacher, J., Crnic, K., Edelbrock, C., & Low, C. (2003). Preschool children with and without developmental delay: Behavior problems and parenting stress over time. *Journal of Intellectual Disability Research, 47*, 217–230. https://doi.org/10.1046/j.1365-2788.2003.00484.x

Bluth, K., Roberson, P. N. E., Billen, R. M., & Sams, J. M. (2013). A stress model for couples parenting children with autism spectrum disorders and the introduction of a mindfulness intervention. *Journal of Family Theory & Review, 5*(3), 194–213. https://doi.org/10.1111/jftr.12015

Bolourian, Y., & Blacher, J. (2016). Impact of youth with intellectual and developmental disabilities on families: Balancing perspectives. *Current Developmental Disorders Reports, 3*(2), 116–123. https://doi.org/10.1007/s40474-016-0087-5

Boss, P., Bryant, C. M., & Mancini, J. A. (2016). *Family stress management: A contextual approach*. Thousand Oaks, CA: SAGE.

Breiner, J. (1989). Training parents as change agents for their developmentally delayed children. In C. E. Schaefer & J. M. Briesmeister (Eds.), *Handbook of parent training: Parents as co-therapists for children's behavior problems* (pp. 269–304). New York, NY: Wiley.

Burke, M. M., Arnold, C. K., & Owen, A. L. (2015). Sibling advocacy: Perspectives about advocacy from siblings of individuals with intellectual and developmental disabilities. *Inclusion, 3*(3), 162–175. https://doi.org/10.1352/2326-6988-3.3.162

Burke, M. M., & Hodapp, R. M. (2014). Relating stress of mothers of children with developmental disabilities to family–school partnerships. *Intellectual and Developmental Disabilities, 52*(1), 13–23. https://doi.org/10.1352/1934-9556-52.1.13

Bussing, R., Nelson, M. M., & Kurtz, S. (2016). Parent–Child Interaction Therapy: Treatment components and evidence-base. *Journal of the American Academy of Child & Adolescent Psychiatry, 55*(10), S351. https://doi.org/10.1016/j.jaac.2016.07.092

Carter, E. W. (2013). Supporting inclusion and flourishing in the religious and spiritual lives of people with intellectual and developmental disabilities. *Inclusion, 1*(1), 64–75. https://doi.org/10.1352/2326-6988-1.1.064

Carter, E. W., Lane, K. L., Cooney, M., Weir, K., Moss, C. K., & Machalicek, W. (2013). Parent assessments of self-determination importance and performance for students with autism or intellectual disability. *American Journal on Intellectual and Developmental Disabilities, 118*(1), 16–31. https://doi.org/10.1352/1944-7558-118.1.16

Chacko, A., Jensen, S. A., Lowry, L. S., Cornwell, M., Chimklis, A., Chan, E., … Pulgarin, B. (2016). Engagement in behavioral parent training: Review of the literature and implications for practice. *Clinical Child and Family Psychology Review, 19*(3), 204–215. https://doi.org/10.1007/s10567-016-0205-2

Chadwick, D., Wesson, C., & Fullwood, C. (2013). Internet access by people with intellectual disabilities: Inequalities and opportunities. *Future Internet, 5*(3), 376–397. https://doi.org/10.3390/fi5030376

Colalillo, S., & Johnston, C. (2016). Parenting cognition and affective outcomes following parent management training: A systematic review. *Clinical Child and Family Psychology Review, 19*(3), 216–235. https://doi.org/10.1007/s10567-016-0208-z

Cridland, E. K., Jones, S. C., Magee, C. A., & Caputi, P. (2014). Family-focused autism spectrum disorder research: A review of the utility of family systems approaches. *Autism, 18*(3), 213–222. https://doi.org/10.1177/1362361312472261

Crnic, K. A., Arbona, A. P., Baker, B. L., & Blacher, J. (2009). Mothers and fathers together: Contrasts in parenting across preschool to early school age in children with developmental delays. *International Review of Research in Mental Retardation, 37*, 3–30. https://doi.org/10.1016/S0074-7750(09)37001-9

Crnic, K. A., Friedrich, W. N., & Greenberg, M. T. (1983). Adaptation of families with mentally retarded children: A model of stress, coping, and family ecology. *American Journal of Mental Deficiency, 88*(2), 125–138.

Crnic, K. A., Neece, C. L., McIntyre, L. L., Blacher, J., & Baker, B. L. (2017). Intellectual disability and developmental risk: Promoting intervention to improve child and family well-being. *Child Development, 88*(2), 436–445. https://doi.org/10.1111/cdev.12740

de Graaf, I., Speetjens, P., Smit, F., de Wolff, M., & Tavecchio, L. (2008). Effectiveness of the Triple P Positive Parenting Program on behavioral problems in children: A meta-analysis. *Behavior Modification, 32*(5), 714–735. https://doi.org/10.1177/0145445508317134

De Ruiter, K. P., Dekker, M. C., Verhulst, F. C., & Koot, H. M. (2007). Developmental course of psychopathology in youths with and without intellectual disabilities. *Journal of Child Psychology and Psychiatry, 48*, 498–507. https://doi.org/10.1111/j.1469-7610.2006.01712.x

Dunlap, G., & Fox, L. (2007). Parent-professional partnerships: A valuable context for addressing challenging behaviours. *International Journal of Disability, Development and Education, 54*, 273–285.

Dykens, E. M., Fisher, M. H., Taylor, J. L., Lambert, W., & Miodrag, N. (2014). Reducing distress in mothers of children with autism and other disabilities: A randomized trial. *Pediatrics, 134*, e454–e463. https://doi.org/10.1542/peds.2013-3164

Eapen, V., Ec, R., Walter, A., & Tay, K. P. (2014). Conceptualisation and development of a quality of life measure for parents of children with autism spectrum disorder. *Autism Research and Treatment, 11*, e160783. https://doi.org/10.1155/2014/160783

Emerson, E. (2003). Mothers of children and adolescents with intellectual disability: Social and economic situation, mental health status, and the self-assessed social and psychological impact of the child's difficulties. *Journal of Intellectual Disability Research, 47*(4–5), 385–399. https://doi.org/10.1046/j.1365-2788.2003.00498.x

Farrell, A. F., & Krahn, G. L. (2014). Family life goes on: Disability in contemporary families. *Family Relations, 63*(1), 1–6. https://doi.org/10.1111/fare.12053

Fazeli, A., Alilou, M. M., & Beyrami, M. (2016). The effectiveness of parent management training in improving parental stress of children with attention deficit hyperactivity disorder. *Academic Journal of Psychological Studies, 5*(1), 91–101.

Floyd, F. J., Harter, K. S. M., Costigan, C. L., & MacLean, W. E., Jr. (2004). Family problem-solving with children who have mental retardation. *American Journal on Mental Retardation, 109*, 507–524. https://doi.org/10.1352/0895-8017(2004)109<507:FPWCWH>2.0.CO;2

Ford, M., Acosta, A., & Sutcliffe, T. J. (2013). Beyond terminology: The policy impact of a grassroots movement. *Intellectual and Developmental Disabilities, 51*(2), 108–112. https://doi.org/10.1352/1934-9556-51.2.108

Forgatch, M. S., & Patterson, G. R. (2010). Parent Management Training—Oregon model: An intervention for antisocial behavior in children and adolescents. In J. R. Weisz & A. E. Kazdin (Eds.), *Evidence-based psychotherapies for children and adolescents* (2nd ed., pp. 159–178). New York, NY: Guilford Press.

Guralnick, M. J. (2011). Why early intervention works: A systems perspective. *Infants & Young Children, 24*, 6–28. https://doi.org/10.1097/IYC.0b013e3182002cfe

Gurwitch, R. H., Messer, E. P., & Funderburk, B. W. (2017). Parent-child interaction therapy. In M. A. Landolt, M. Cloitre, & U. Schnyder (Eds.), *Evidence-based treatments for trauma related disorders in children and adolescents* (pp. 341–361). Cham, Switzerland: Springer. https://doi.org/10.1007/978-3-319-46138-0_16

Hagen, K. A., & Ogden, T. (2017). Predictors of changes in child behaviour following parent management training: Child, context, and therapy factors. *International Journal of Psychology, 52*(2), 106–115. https://doi.org/10.1002/ijop.12365

Harnett, A., Bettendorf, E., Tierney, E., Guerin, S., O'Rourke, M., & Hourihane, J. O. (2013). Evidence-based training of health professionals to inform families about disability. *Archives of Disease in Childhood, 98*(6), 413–418. https://doi.org/10.1136/archdischild-2012-303037

Haven, E. L., Manangan, C. N., Sparrow, J. K., & Wilson, B. J. (2013). The relation of parent–child interaction qualities to social skills in children with and without autism spectrum disorders. *Autism, 18*(3), 292–300. https://doi.org/10.1177/1362361312470036

Hayes, S. A., & Watson, S. L. (2012). The impact of parenting stress: A meta-analysis of studies comparing the experience of parenting stress in parents of children with and without autism spectrum disorder. *Journal of Autism and Developmental Disorders, 43*(3), 629–642. https://doi.org/10.1007/s10803-012-1604-y

Hewitt, A., Agosta, J., Heller, T., Williams, A. C., & Reinke, J. (2013). Families of individuals with intellectual and developmental disabilities: Policy, funding, services, and experiences. *Intellectual and Developmental Disabilities, 51*(5), 349–359. https://doi.org/10.1352/1934-9556-51.5.349

Kaminski, J. W., Valle, L. A., Filene, J. H., & Boyle, C. L. (2008). A meta-analytic review of components associated with parent training program effectiveness. *Journal of Abnormal Child Psychology, 36*(4), 567–589.

Kazdin, A. E. (1997). Parent management training: Evidence, outcomes, and issues. *Journal of the American Academy of Child & Adolescent Psychiatry., 36*(10), 1349–1356. https://doi.org/10.1097/00004583-199710000-00016 PMID 9334547.

Kennedy, S. C., Kim, J. S., Tripodi, S. J., Brown, S. M., & Gowdy, G. (2016). Does Parent–Child Interaction Therapy reduce future physical abuse? A meta-analysis. *Research on Social Work Practice, 26*(2), 147–156. https://doi.org/10.1177/1049731514543024

Knight, K. (2013). The changing face of the "good mother": Trends in research into families with a child with intellectual disability, and some concerns. *Disability & Society, 28*(5), 660–673. https://doi.org/10.1080/09687599.2012.732540

Kuo, D. Z., Houtrow, A. J., Arango, P., Kuhlthau, K. A., Simmons, J. M., & Neff, J. M. (2011). Family-centered care: Current applications and future directions in pediatric health care. *Maternal and Child Health Journal, 16*(2), 297–305. https://doi.org/10.1007/s10995-011-0751-7

Landers-Potts, M. A., Wickrama, K. A. S., Simons, L. G., Cutrona, C., Gibbons, F. X., Simons, R. L., & Conger, R. (2015). An extension and moderational analysis of the family stress model focusing on African American adolescents. *Family Relations, 64*(2), 233–248. https://doi.org/10.1111/fare.12117

Lundahl, B., Risser, H. J., & Lovejoy, M. C. (2006). A meta-analysis of parent training: Moderators and follow-up effects. *Clinical Psychology Review, 26*(1), 86–104.

Marryat, L., Thompson, L., & Wilson, P. (2017). No evidence of whole population mental health impact of the Triple P parenting programme: Findings from a routine dataset. *BMC Pediatrics, 17*, 40. https://doi.org/10.1186/s12887-017-0800-5

McConnell, D., Llewellyn, G., & Bye, R. (1997). Providing services to parents with intellectual disability: Parent needs and service constraints. *Journal of Intellectual and Developmental Disability, 22*(1), 5–17.

McIntyre, L. L. (2008). Parent training in young children with developmental disabilities: A randomized controlled trial. *American Journal on Mental Retardation, 113*, 356–368. https://doi.org/10.1352/2008.113:356-368

McIntyre, L. L., Blacher, J., & Baker, B. L. (2006). The transition to school: Adaptation in young children with and without developmental delays. *Journal of Intellectual Disability Research, 50*, 349–361.

Meppelder, M., Hodes, M., Kef, S., & Schuengel, C. (2014). Parents with intellectual disabilities seeking professional parenting support: The role of working alliance, stress and informal support. *Child Abuse & Neglect, 38*(9), 1478–1486. https://doi.org/10.1016/j.chiabu.2014.04.006

Michelson, D., Davenport, C., Dretzke, J., Barlow, J., & Day, C. (2013). Do evidence-based interventions work when tested in the "real world?" a systematic review and meta-analysis of parent management training for the treatment of child disruptive behavior. *Clinic Child and Family Psychology Review, 16*, 18–34.

Neece, C. L., Green, S. A., & Baker, B. L. (2012). Parenting stress and child behavior problems: A transactional relationship across time. *American Journal on Intellectual and Developmental Disabilities, 117*, 48–66. https://doi.org/10.1352/1944-7558-117.1.48

Neppl, T. K., Senia, J. M., & Brent, M. (2016). Effects of economic hardship: Testing the family stress model over time. *Journal of Family Psychology, 30*(1), 12–21. https://doi.org/10.1037/fam0000168

Niec, L. N., Barnett, M. L., Prewett, M. S., & Shanley Chatham, J. R. (2016). Group parent–child interaction therapy: A randomized control trial for the treatment of conduct problems in young children. *Journal of Consulting and Clinical Psychology, 84*(8), 682–698. https://doi.org/10.1037/a0040218

Ollendick, T. H., Greene, R. W., Austin, K. E., Fraire, M. G., Halldorsdottir, T., Allen, K. B., … Wolff, J. C. (2016). Parent Management Training and Collaborative & Proactive Solutions: A randomized control trial for oppositional youth. *Journal of Clinical Child & Adolescent Psychology, 45*(5), 591–604. https://doi.org/10.1080/15374416.2015.1004681

Peer, J. W., & Hillman, S. B. (2014). Stress and resilience for parents of children with intellectual and developmental disabilities: A review of key factors and recommendations for practitioners.

Journal of Policy and Practice in Intellectual Disabilities, 11(2), 92–98. https://doi.org/10.1111/jppi.12072
Petner-Arrey, J., Howell-Moneta, A., & Lysaght, R. (2016). Facilitating employment opportunities for adults with intellectual and developmental disability through parents and social networks. *Disability and Rehabilitation, 38*(8), 789–795. https://doi.org/10.3109/09638288.2015.1061605
Prinz, R. J., Sanders, M. R., Shapiro, C. J., Whitaker, D. J., & Lutzker, J. R. (2009). Population-based prevention of child maltreatment: The U.S. Triple P system population trial. *Prevention Science: The Official Journal of the Society for Prevention Research, 10*(1), 1–12. https://doi.org/10.1007/s11121-009-0123-3
Raspa, M., Bailey, D. B., Bann, C., & Bishop, E. (2014). Modeling family adaptation to Fragile X Syndrome. *American Journal on Intellectual and Developmental Disabilities, 119*(1), 33–48. https://doi.org/10.1352/1944-7558-119.1.33
Riechow, B., Kogan, C., Barbul, C., Smith, I., Yasamy, M. T., & Servili, C. (2014). Parent skills training for parents of children or adults with developmental disorders: Systematic review and meta-analysis protocol. *BMJ Open, 4*(8), e005799. https://doi.org/10.1136/bmjopen-2014-005799
Samadi, S. A., McConkey, R., & Kelly, G. (2013). Enhancing parental well-being and coping through a family-centred short course for Iranian parents of children with an autism spectrum disorder. *Autism, 17*(1), 27–43. https://doi.org/10.1177/1362361311435156
Samuel, P. S., Hobden, K. L., LeRoy, B. W., & Lacey, K. K. (2012). Analysing family service needs of typically underserved families in the USA. *Journal of Intellectual Disability Research, 56*(1), 111–128. https://doi.org/10.1111/j.1365-2788.2011.01481.x
Schein, E. H. (2016). *Humble consulting*. Oakland, CA: Berrett-Koehler.
Serketich, W. J., & Dumas, J. E. (1996). The effectiveness of behavioral parent training to modify antisocial behavior in children: A meta-analysis. *Behavior Therapy, 27*, 171–186.
Shivers, C. M., & Dykens, E. M. (2017). Adolescent siblings of individuals with and without intellectual and developmental disabilities: Self-reported empathy and feelings about their brothers and sisters. *American Journal on Intellectual and Developmental Disabilities, 122*(1), 62–77. https://doi.org/10.1352/1944-7558-122.1.62
Siller, M., Reyes, N., Hotez, E., Hutman, T., & Sigman, M. (2013). Longitudinal change in the use of services in autism spectrum disorder: Understanding the role of child characteristics, family demographics, and parent cognitions. *Autism, 18*(4), 433–446. https://doi.org/10.1177/1362361313476766
Smith, A. L., Romski, M., & Sevcik, R. A. (2013). Examining the role of communication on sibling relationship quality and interaction for sibling pairs with and without developmental disability. *American Journal on Intellectual and Developmental Disabilities, 118*(5), 394–409. https://doi.org/10.1352/1944-7558-118.5.394
Song, J., Mailick, M. R., Ryff, C. D., Coe, C. L., Greenberg, J. S., & Hong, J. (2014). Allostatic load in parents of children with developmental disorders: Moderating influence of positive affect. *Journal of Health Psychology, 19*(2), 262–272. https://doi.org/10.1177/1359105312468193
Thompson, J. R., Schalock, R. L., Agosta, J., Teninty, L., & Fortune, J. (2014). How the supports paradigm is transforming the developmental disabilities service system. *Inclusion, 2*(2), 86–99. https://doi.org/10.1352/2326-6988-2.2.86
Tuffrey-Wijne, I. (2013). A new model for breaking bad news to people with intellectual disabilities. *Palliative Medicine, 27*(1), 5–12. https://doi.org/10.1177/0269216311433476
Turner, K. M. T., & Sanders, M. R. (2006). Dissemination of evidence-based parenting and family support strategies: Learning from the Triple P – Positive Parenting Program system approach. *Aggression and Violent Behavior, 11*(2), 176–193.
VanVoorhis, R. W., Miller, K. L., Miller, S. M., & Stull, J. C. (2015). Impact of Stepping Stones Triple P on parents with a child diagnosed With autism spectrum disorder: Implications for school psychologists. *School Psychology Forum, 9*(2), 121–142.

Vohra, R., Madhavan, S., Sambamoorthi, U., & Peter, C. S. (2014). Access to services, quality of care, and family impact for children with autism, other developmental disabilities, and other mental health conditions. *Autism, 18*(7), 815–826. https://doi.org/10.1177/1362361313512902

Wadsworth, M. E., Rindlaub, L., Hurwich-Reiss, E., Rienks, S., Bianco, H., & Markman, H. J. (2013). A longitudinal examination of the adaptation to poverty-related stress model: Predicting child and adolescent adjustment over time. *Journal of Clinical Child & Adolescent Psychology, 42*(5), 713–725. https://doi.org/10.1080/15374416.2012.755926

Webster-Stratton, C. (2001). *The Incredible Years: Parents, teachers, and children training series, leader's guide*. Seattle, WA: Author.

Webster-Stratton, C., & Reid, J. M. (2010). The Incredible Years parents, teachers, and children training series: A multifaceted treatment approach for young children with conduct disorders. In J. R. Weisz & A. E. Kazdin (Eds.), *Evidence-based psychotherapies for children and adolescents* (2nd ed., pp. 194–210). New York, NY: Guilford Press.

Weisz, J. R., & Kazdin, A. E. (2017). *Evidence-based psychotherapies for children and adolescents* (3rd ed.). New York, NY: Guilford Publications.

Woodman, A. C., Mawdsley, H. P., & Hauser-Cram, P. (2015). Parenting stress and child behavior problems within families of children with developmental disabilities: Transactional relations across 15 years. *Research in Developmental Disabilities, 36*, 264–276. https://doi.org/10.1016/j.ridd.2014.10.011

Wright, A. C., & Taylor, S. (2014). Advocacy by parents of young children with special needs: Activities, processes, and perceived effectiveness. *Journal of Social Service Research, 40*(5), 591–605. https://doi.org/10.1080/01488376.2014.896850

Chapter 6
Case Management and Team Functioning

Abstract This chapter clarifies the roles, responsibilities, and limitations of school psychologists, educators, and other professionals concerning the identification, management, and coordination of services for students with intellectual disabilities. Given the complexities of assessment and treatment, multiple professionals and systems are involved in a comprehensive effort to improve the functioning of people with intellectual disabilities. Quite often, appropriate resources are available, yet they are not coordinated in a manner that provides effective and efficient services. Sometimes, therapists may work at cross purposes and even undermine the work of different professions. There is strong evidence that knowing which interventions are most effective is insufficient for effective service delivery; there must also be mindful communication and coordination among family, professionals, individuals with intellectual disabilities, and all the coordinating systems involved. There is quality research that supports specific forms of collaboration and coordination that improve service delivery through the most efficient form of case management.

Case Study

Alexandria is a 17-month-old female who has been diagnosed with Edwards syndrome (trisomy-18). Alexandria presents with Mosaic trisomy, which means that not all her cells are affected by the trisomy. Usually persons with Mosaic trisomies have fewer and less severe symptoms than people with all cells affected by the trisomy. Alexandria presents with several common concurrent medical issues, such as small size, cleft palate and micrognathia (i.e. small jaw), atrial septal defect, and omphalocele (i.e. intestines outside of the body). Most children diagnosed with Edwards syndrome do not survive past their first birthday. Alexandria already had 12 surgeries to correct cardiac defects, intestinal abnormalities, and cleft palate. She faces additional surgeries related to clenched hands and congenital vertical talus (i.e. rocker bottom foot). In addition to her physical issues, Alexandria presents with significant developmental delays. Although it is not yet possible to provide a definitive diagnosis of intellectual disabilities, all persons with Edwards syndrome have severe developmental delays that are usually characterized as severe to profound.

S. R. Shaw, A. M. Jankowska, *Pediatric Intellectual Disabilities at School*, Pediatric School Psychology, https://doi.org/10.1007/978-3-030-02992-0_6

With the complexity of Alexandria's medical and developmental needs, she has a large team of professionals providing medical and habilitative services and therapy. She has so many appointments and treatments that her mother has had to quit her job to coordinate meeting times and transport Alexandria to her appointments on time. Most days are spent driving Alexandria from one appointment to another. Alexandria's mother has a mobile file cabinet of all medical and rehabilitation reports and progress notes that are over 2000 pages and are stored in the back of the car. Alexandria's mother struggles with coordinating medical appointment timing, ensuring the treatment regimens are working towards the same goals, and frequently checking medications to ensure no interactions or adverse effects are noted. It is also clear that it Alexandria's mother is as much or more of an expert on Edwards syndrome than any of her medical or habilitative professionals. Although she has proved to be the most important member of the treatment team, financial pressures due to having to quit her job are creating significant family hardship. Alexandria's mother would like to have a professional case coordinator to relieve some of the burden on the family. Nurses and other therapists have provided some support for Alexandria's mother, yet they do not function as case managers. Currently, all professionals are involved in the silos of their specialty and subspecialty professional functions. Where Alexandria lives, there are no mechanisms or programs available for case management services.

Introduction

Intellectual disabilities are pervasive and multidomain conditions that require coordination of professionals to provide effective and efficient services (Bigby, Frawley, & Ramcharan, 2014). As illustrated in the case study, parents are frequently the case managers and coordinator of all professional services. The amount of time required to schedule, transport, and completely understand all the services is far too much for most parents to manage. Few parents have the resources, education, skills, or experience to coordinate services to develop and achieve developmental goals for the child with intellectual disabilities (Gross, Wallace, Blue-Banning, Summers, & Turnbull, 2013). As the person with intellectual disabilities ages, parents likely continue to serve as the case managers often into their middle and old age. Case management requires high energy, expertise, resources, and time and is difficult for the most energetic young parent (Minnes, Perry, & Weiss, 2015). Pressures and challenges mount over time.

Although case management is a critical component of the interaction between professional teams and families, having professionals working as a coordinated team is another important factor. Without effective coordination, treatment becomes piecemeal and lacks maximum effectiveness (DeVoss & Surmitis, 2016). There have been advances in models of team functioning and case management that maximize the quality, efficiency, and comprehensiveness of treatment and rehabilitation and that span several professions (Hughes & Wearing, 2016).

The purpose of this chapter is to describe effective case management and team functioning approaches to addressing the multidisciplinary needs of people with intellectual disabilities. In addition, specific situations requiring teamwork such as creating the components of an assessment team, educating peers concerning the needs of a child with intellectual disabilities, providing educational services in an inclusive environment within a school system, creating a medical team, and developing a team for transition from school to community are described.

Systemic Teams and Organization

Team Decision-Making Models

Providing multidomain services to people with intellectual disabilities requires mindful organization that promotes efficiency, effectiveness, case management, and synergy among systems and professionals. In effective systems, team organization is prescribed, practised, and used as a template for effective relationships and coordination of information (McLaughlin, Barr, McIlfatrick, & McConkey, 2014). However, most systems have a rather haphazard approach to team organization. Professional communication depends on personal relationships among professionals that lack consistency and quality of coordinated service delivery. For effective case management and service delivery, systems require thoughtful consideration of not only what the most effective practices are, but how those practices will be implemented across domains, among professionals, and coordinated for the most effective case management. The creation and prescription of a specific form of team organization are only part of the solution, and negotiating and effectively managing multiple individual personalities as well as multiple professional cultures is an ongoing challenge that requires investment of time and energy (Owen, Bowers, Heller, Hsieh, & Gould, 2016).

Siloed Service Delivery

Although the siloed service delivery approach to organization is not necessarily a team approach, individual professionals working without coordination with other professionals is a common situation. There are some advantages to this model (Rosenberg, Weissman, & Wong, 2014). Individual professionals are free to explore their own specialty domain in detail and efficiency because they do not need to coordinate or consider other professionals in their work. In this form of service delivery, professionals can drill deeply and provide a great deal of domain or profession-specific information. There are some professionals who prefer to work alone and may not function effectively in the context and constraints of a team system. Training for most physicians, therapists, educators, and psychologists for working within a team is nearly universal, yet there are still preferences among some subspecialists for working alone. Reimbursement mechanisms in many systems, especially private health insurance in the United States, are designed for maximum efficiency in reimbursing a single professional (Rzhetsky et al., 2014). There are rarely reimbursement mechanisms for time invested in developing teamwork. For those professionals who are in private practice or have other significant financial pressures, siloed service delivery may be necessary under some reimbursement systems. In many professional cultures, especially education, team processes are the default method as mandated by law to deliver services. In creating the culture of a team, there is a need to understanding that some professionals do not value team processes to the same degree (Rosenberg et al., 2014). There are legitimate reasons for some professionals preferring the siloed professional approach to service delivery.

Multidisciplinary Team

The most common form of professional teamwork is a multidisciplinary team. The multidisciplinary team consists of professionals representing different disciplines who coordinate the contributions of each profession, which are considered to not overlap in role and function, in order to improve patient care (Ritzema, Sladeczek, Ghosh, Karagiannakis, & Manay-Quian, 2014). The most typical form of multidisciplinary team is that all professions involved in the case meet to develop assessment and intervention strategies. After the meeting, each member of the team carries out their agreed-upon role and function separately. After each member of the team has completed their assignment, the team meets again to develop the next phase of the project. Therefore, most of the work is carried out as individuals, yet the work is coordinated via a team approach and communicated to the team after completion or to provide status updates. The primary strength of the multidisciplinary team is the fundamental agreement of shared goals among professionals. There are still important inefficiencies as, each individual profession has individually prepared reports or notes, provides services individually, and may involve duplication of services (Hardman, Drew, & Egan, 2015). Despite these inefficiencies, the multidisciplinary team allows for coordination of goals and communication of results with all members of the team. In addition, except for the time invested in the multidisciplinary team meeting, reimbursement issues are easily addressed because service can be billed via the work of each individual profession.

The composition of the multidisciplinary team is an important contributor to its overall success in providing effective service delivery (Graybill et al., 2016). When the target of service delivery is a person with intellectual disabilities, frequent members of the multidisciplinary team are teacher, speech and language pathologist, occupational therapist, psychologist, pediatrician, social worker, and nurse. Membership of the team may expand or contract based on the needs of the individual client, patient, or student. Some will involve multiple medical subspecialties, and others will require a small team (Danforth & Naraian, 2015). For teams to function effectively, there needs to be freedom to communicate and suggest innovative solutions. The composition of the team can mediate the form of communication provided during team meetings. One example is that medical directors, administrators, or school principals are sometimes members of the multidisciplinary team. The advantage of the inclusion of these professionals is that there is increased understanding of the specific issues brought up in the case and that resources may need to be allocated to provide the best possible services and outcomes. The disadvantages are that some members of the team may be reluctant to speak out or offer innovative solutions knowing that their direct supervisor is a member of the team, and their words are being evaluated. Other members of the multidisciplinary team that may be controversial are the inclusion of the person with intellectual disabilities and their family or caregiver (Heller, Gibbons, & Fisher, 2015). There is an essential advantage to having the person with intellectual disabilities and their parent or caregiver involved in all aspects of the multidisciplinary team to allow for input and control over the assessment and intervention process. In school-based multidisciplinary team meetings in the United States, parent inclusion and involvement in the multidisciplinary team is required by law (Heller et al., 2015). Again, there may be some limitations on exactly what is said during the team meeting among professionals. However, the benefit of self-advocacy and correctly identifying the needs of the client and the client's family outweigh any limitation caused by their presence (Mccallion & Janicki, 2014). Productive participation in a multidisciplinary team requires some level of practice and experience. Clients and their families are unlikely to have this practice and experience. As such, the environment of multidisciplinary team must be shaped so that clients and their families have the skills, comfort level, and opportunities to make their needs fully known to the professional elements of the team. Clients and families have veto power or at least greater weight in decision-making than other members of the team. Without a strong voice for clients and families, goals, methods, and results arising from the multidisciplinary team will be incomplete and have limited credibility, which means results and ideas for interventions are unlikely to be implemented fully with fidelity (Carney, 2014). Ensuring that all members of the multidisciplinary team have opportunities to contribute and have their ideas considered is a critical component to the success of such a team.

Interdisciplinary Team

Although multidisciplinary teams are an important method of coordinating assessment and intervention planning, all work is conducted independently. Assessment reports, case notes, and intervention plans remain specific to each profession but are coordinated to reach an agreed-upon goal. Interdisciplinary teams not only coordinate activities related to service delivery but also conduct these activities as a team (Ganz, 2014). Interdisciplinary teams blur some of the traditional boundaries among professions. An illustration of the difference between a multidisciplinary and interdisciplinary team is that in an interdisciplinary team, one report will be created that integrates information and expertise from each member of the team. Arena assessments are an example of an activity conducted by an interdisciplinary team. In arena assessments, each profession conducts a brief assessment that is observed by other members of the team (Ganz, 2014). For example, a speech and language pathologist may conduct a brief language assessment, while other members of the team observe the activity and take notes from their own professional perspective. Although the expertise of the speech language pathologist will focus entirely on language, physicians, psychologist, teachers, nurses, social workers, parents/caregivers, and others will observe the task and assimilate their information into their own expertise. As professionals are rotated through the arena assessment, a full picture of the client's overall functioning is created. The interdisciplinary team approach involves significant planning and inter-professional trust (Ganz, 2014). The benefit of an interdisciplinary team is full and complete coordination among professionals with consensus being the primary decision-making mechanism based on shared information.

Transdisciplinary Team

Interdisciplinary teams involve sharing of information across disciplines, and transdisciplinary teams move to erase completely the boundaries between professions (McLaughlin et al., 2014). In many cases, a single professional, usually the case manager, conducts many of the forms of assessment and develops interventions in consultation with other professionals. There are many forms of transdisciplinary teams in practice (Waitoller & Artiles, 2013). For example, if a psychologist is the primary case manager, then they may conduct language assessments and functional motor assessment, take family histories, take medical histories, and collect other data in close collaboration with other professionals. Typically, the advantage of a transdisciplinary team approach is that there is a single point of contact for clients and their families. With one professional responsible for most of the work, a transdisciplinary team can be part of an efficient system that can accommodate a larger number of clients than interdisciplinary or multidisciplinary teams (Parellada et al., 2013). Another advantage is that the single point of contact also serves as the case manager to assist parents and families in coordinating the number of therapies and services. Whereas the interdisciplinary team approach creates some blurriness between professional roles and functions, the transdisciplinary approach comes much closer to completely erasing these lines. Professionals from different disciplines teach, learn, and work together to accomplish an agreed-upon set of intervention goals for a client and family. The role differentiation between disciplines is defined by the needs of the situation rather than by discipline-specific characteristics. This mindset is extremely helpful in that problems are not identified as solely medical, psychological, or educational; all problems are multidomain in nature and require a coordinated approach to assessing an intervening period. The disadvantages of the transdisciplinary team are significant (Gargiulo & Metcalf, 2015). All professionals need to have a strong understanding of multiple roles and functions. There is significant sharing of expertise and teaching of fellow members of the transdisciplinary team. In addition, most states and provinces have strict professional licensing laws that prescribe exactly what activities in which each professional can engage. The result is that a psychologist engaging in activities that are identified solely for occupational therapists or physicians is likely to be illegal under the licensing laws of the state or province. Although there are some extraordinarily positive contributions to service delivery from some elements of transdisciplinary teams, in practice a pure transdisciplinary team is unwieldy and may be in contradiction of practice regulations (Rzhetsky et al., 2014).

Summary

There is a much research on different types of teams for service delivery (Brock & Carter, 2013). Sometimes evaluating the research on which form of team is most effective is difficult. The research literature can be narrowed down to the simple idea that sharing and teamwork is good. However, the outcome on which form of team creates the best and most efficient types of service delivery for people with intellectual disabilities is not as clear as many recommendations might seem. In some literature, the transdisciplinary team is considered a best practice for all decision-making (Clare et al., 2017). However, there are real challenges to making a transdisciplinary team function effectively: the team process requires a great deal of practice and expertise, and there are legal issues concerning the role and function of each professional under the state or provinces credentialing laws and regulations. The recommendation is for all systems to be mindful of their system and client needs, time required to maintain an effective team process, and formal laws and regulations (Rzhetsky et al., 2014). There is nothing wrong with siloed professional service delivery as it can be quite detailed and efficient; yet, there are significant limitations in generalizing these findings across professions. Every system must weigh the options and needs for the most effective provision of service delivery, adopt and practise the best form of systemic teamwork and organization, and not blindly follow an approach often labelled "best practices" without evidence-based consensus support in the research literature.

Specific Function Teams

Systemic teams and their organization reflect a philosophy of service delivery that each specific system (e.g. school district, hospital, mental health clinic, rehabilitation centre, vocational centre, specialized medical care) uses to meet the needs of the clients and their families. There are a variety of team organizations that assemble for specific purposes. Not all clients and families require the specific teams, but they are an important aspect of organization and management of cases.

Intraprofessional Team

Intraprofessional teams usually involve consultation of several members of the profession to assist in decision-making for either assessment or intervention planning (Perry et al., 2014). This is a team of professionals who are all from the same profession, such as a team of physical therapists or a group of psychologists collaborating on the same case. Intraprofessional teams are often used in conjunction with other forms of team problem-solving approaches. For example, a psychologist may have specific expertise in certain forms of an intervention but may seek consultation on assessment processes from a team of peer psychologists. Intraprofessional teams usually involve a specific issue to be resolved within a single profession before this information is provided to the entire service delivery team. Another common form of intraprofessional teams are teams of physicians representing specific pediatric subspecialties. In the case of people with intellectual disabilities, there are often multiple system involvements requiring coordination of medical services. The intraprofessional team may consist of a cardiologist, nephrologist, endocrinologist, neurologist, and developmental pediatrician to coordinate services to provide the specific medical treatment plan (Campbell, Robertson, & Jahoda, 2014).

Assessment Team

The assessment team typically functions in a multidisciplinary fashion, and the primary purpose is to ask the highest priority questions necessary to conduct a productive assessment. Usually the most important member of the assessment team is the client and their caregiver or parent (Moeschler, Shevell, & Genetics, 2014). They are the members of the team who can often communicate the most pressing needs that require further identification and analysis. Another important contributor to a team may be the primary care pediatrician or classroom teacher. These professionals require important answers to complete their task and understand that the assessment of these issues may require specialized expertise. The goal of the assessment team is to lay out a blueprint of all assessment procedures necessary to answer the questions presented by the referring parties, clients, and caregiver or parent.

Rehabilitation and Intervention Team

In systems that use an assessment team, there is often a complementary rehabilitation and intervention team. This team translates the information developed through the assessment team process and converts that information into a comprehensive treatment plan (Ciccarelli, Brown, Gladstone, Woodward, & Swigonski, 2014). Usually this approach is multidisciplinary in nature; however, an increasing number of systems are moving to interdisciplinary and transdisciplinary methods. The rehabilitation and intervention team is required to plan and implement evidence-based practices for the benefit of the clients and their families. Developing evidence-based interventions based on the best available research, goals of the client and caregiver or parent, and considering the results of the assessment is a complex process. In addition to these factors, this team also must consider the resources available to implement interventions. Resources can be money, time, professional expertise, training, transportation, materials, and other critical factors. All interventions developed by the team must not only meet these criteria but must also be credible, robust, and have perceived utility by the client and caregiver or parent. The rehabilitation and intervention team is a valuable method of establishing a plan and goals for the achievement of a client's potential (Moseley, Kleinert, Sheppard-Jones, & Hall, 2013). The composition of the team will vary depending on the nature of the patient's problem, yet the client and caregiver or parent is always included as a member of the rehabilitation team.

Liaison Team

The liaison team consists of a few individuals to support clients whose services cross multiple systems. Liaison teams are typically ad hoc teams to support transition processes (Scott & Havercamp, 2016). An example is a client who is being released from a juvenile detention centre and is returning to a school setting. The liaison team consists of a member of the sending system (i.e. juvenile detention centre), a member of the receiving system (i.e. school system), a liaison with understanding of both systems (often a social worker or school psychologist), and the client and caregiver or parent. The goals of the liaison team are to transition from the current system in which the client is receiving services to the receiving system. These changes can be due to development, such as moving from an elementary school to high school or from a high school situation to employment preparation; change of status, such as from a foster care setting to semi-independent living or from inpatient care to home; or legal situation, such as from incarceration to a supervised living arrangement or from living with biological family to a foster care setting. Transitions always bring challenges and are often traumatic for the person with intellectual disabilities. Failure to navigate the transition process correctly can be traumatic for people with intellectual disabilities. An example is a child who was currently in a foster care setting and was being considered for adoption. In this case, there was no transition plan in place. The potential adopting parents read the reports about the child and the child's behaviour and met the child on several occasions (when he was demonstrating his best behaviour) but were unprepared for the severity of the child's aggressive behaviours immediately after he was adopted. The potential adopting parents indicated that they wish to withdraw from the adoption process. Although this is an extreme case with much blame to go around, a systematic liaison team and a formalized transition process would have been helpful. In fairness, nearly all potential adoptive parents are actively engaged in a formal transition process (Williamson & Perkins, 2014). The case presented is unusual but illustrates a worst-case scenario for a transition that is poorly addressed. A typical transition has nine components that do not need to take place in order but need to be navigated (Shaw & Brown, 2011).

- To taper services and activities in the sending setting with the purpose of terminating medical, psychological, educational, or other therapies.
- To have professionals from the sending setting communicate to the receiving setting details about the client. Some of these details can include current functioning, examples of successful therapeutic approaches, client preferences, medical concerns and precautions, and the status of current therapeutic programming. The transfer of records is a legal matter as well and will require appropriate consents and permission before this stage can take place.
- To communicate to the client exactly what changes will be made. For everyone, change and transition are stressful. Allowing the client time to prepare mentally and emotionally is challenging. Ideally, the person with intellectual disabilities will have input into the transition process and can make as many choices for self-determination as is possible. Yet, in many cases, the transition process is not voluntary.
- Have staff members from the receiving system meet with the person with intellectual disabilities at the site of the sending system. This will give the client an opportunity to meet members of the new team in a comfortable environment.
- Have staff members from the sending system meet with staff members from the receiving system at the site of the receiving system. The physical site can be examined with any potential systemic problems or triggering stimuli identified and managed before the transition can take place.
- Staff members from the sending system report this information back to the client.
- The client visits the receiving system to explore and understand the physical environment in which they will be living or receiving therapy.
- When the transition takes place, there is continued contact with members of the therapy team from the sending system so that the client will continue to feel safe and still have access to familiar faces.
- Availability of consultation between the sending and receiving staffs can take place as needed to smooth transition and share expertise for the benefit of the client.

The purpose of the liaison team is to navigate these steps to minimize the challenges of transition. The liaison team consists of members of the sending and receiving teams. In addition to the basics of transitioning from one site of service delivery providers to another, there are frequently legal, financial, insurance, and compliance with regulations that need to be navigated. The liaison team needs to have experience in these formal processes in addition to direct services to the client.

Urgency Team

Planning for crises is a key component of any system (Poland, 1994). Although strong teamwork can help prevent many challenging situations, there remain a variety of events that are difficult to foresee and require immediate, coordinated, and concerted action. All systems require a crisis plan to address immediate issues such as fire, natural disaster, medical crises, intruders, and other issues. All hospital settings conduct drills for missing children, abducted infants, evacuation, bomb threats, aggressive patients, and other events. This form of crisis planning is a fundamental part of systems that provide services for people with intellectual disabilities. There are many situations in which the needs of a specific client may require special attention as they are at high risk for issues that would be considered urgent. The urgency team is a quick response set of professionals that are prepared, have the skills, and have practised providing services when a client-specific urgent issue arises. Examples of people with intellectual disabilities who may require an urgency team are medically fragile, uncontrolled seizures, severe allergies, severe self-injurious behaviour, aggression towards others, fire setting, running away ("eloping" or "bolting"), risk of abduction, adverse response to medications, and other issues (Owen, 2012). If any of these high-risk situations occur, then the urgency team is prepared to immediately respond and address the issue. In addition, if external supports are required, such as ambulance or police, there is a plan to contact these professionals immediately. Communication with police, medical, and ambulance services to develop a relationship concerning caregivers of the person with intellectual disabilities is helpful. There have been recent events in which people with intellectual disabilities or their caregivers have been mistaken for violent persons and have been arrested or shot by police officers. Having the urgency team communicate with these professionals in advance can reduce these unfortunate incidences. Urgency teams and crises teams are often placed as low priority in planning for services for people with intellectual disabilities. There is a high likelihood that such teams will never be required. However, having a plan, a set of individuals with expertise and experience, marshalling community resources, and educating all staff and peers about what to do in the likelihood of an urgent situation can assist in preventing disastrous consequences. Moreover, there is the peace of mind that staff, family, and clients possess through knowing that as many urgent contingencies have been considered as possible when creating a treatment plan.

Summary

The variety of activities and situations related to the provision of quality and safety living arrangements, therapies, and medical management require expertise in multiple domains. As such, specific function teams are required to generate and integrate solutions involving the best of all possible knowledge from a variety of professionals and caregivers. Planned efforts to organize and create smoothly running team processes are critical factors. Simply placing a group of diverse professionals from different professional cultures and goals and training them in the same room and calling them a team is not adequate. Regular meetings to develop an effective interpersonal team process are essential for efficient and productive action (Shaw, Glaser, & Ouimet, 2011). The investment of time to develop and practise working together will pay off when these teams are needed to provide their specific functions.

Case Management

Systemic Teams and Organization and Specific Function Teams serve valuable purposes in the development and execution of assessment, treatment, and provision of other services; there is still a requirement that the day-to-day activities of the person with intellectual disabilities are coordinated (Summers, 2015). There are several components of case management to be carried out. Among these roles are scheduling appointments; integrating information from multiple professionals into a coherent and directed intervention plan; communicating among multiple professionals (or multiple professional teams); maintaining and managing paperwork and professional reports, transportation, advocacy, financial issues such as access to funding mechanisms and insurance, appeals and legal issues; and serving as a liaison among professional systems and the person with intellectual disabilities. Case management is the most complex component of service delivery for people with intellectual disabilities. There must be expertise in multiple professional areas, strong communication skills including translation of professional jargon, awareness of community resources, and integration of the needs of the client with professional services offered (Lunsky, Hastings, Hensel, Arenovich, & Dewa, 2014). The ubiquity of technology allows for keeping scheduling calendars, contacts, and electronic copies of medical records in a single handheld device. Although there are helpful tools to assist with some aspects, case management requires a sophisticated set of multifaceted knowledge and skills. Case management is not frequently a formal professional role. Most often case management is a skill set that is developed by parents with support from a variety of professionals.

Parents

For most people with intellectual disabilities, parents are the primary case managers (Lunsky, Tint, Robinson, Gordeyko, & Ouellette-Kuntz, 2014). Parents are often self-educated as to the skills of case management. Many parents, out of necessity, become extraordinarily skilled, educated, and organized to ensure that their child receives coordinated and high-quality care.

Although parents of children with intellectual disabilities provide many benefits and advantages to high-quality case management, there are significant drawbacks to having parents in this role. Case management can be a nearly full-time job (Parellada et al., 2013). Most parents give up their careers to dedicate themselves to providing case management services. The result is that families of children with intellectual disabilities have less income than families of typically developing peers. Low income can lead to additional stressors and generally reduce the number of resources available to support the person with intellectual disabilities. High-quality health insurance is tied to plans offered by employers, yet people with intellectual disabilities receive Medicaid-based health insurance. Nonetheless, many healthcare providers have chosen not to accept clients on Medicaid, and therefore a number of medical options are reduced. Most parents as case managers are self-taught, and this leads to an uneven quality as case management. Some parents have case management peer or professional mentors, emotional and practical support, access to experts (often from published websites), and relevant expertise from previous training. However, sometimes parents are isolated and do not have a skill set that effectively generalizes to case management. Another major issue is that parents do not make objective decisions for their child. This can be both a strength and weakness. Objective decisions based on research information often yield decisions that are most likely to be effective for most people with intellectual disabilities. Yet, the parent has insight into the everyday world of the child with intellectual disabilities and has expertise into the specific issues of the child more than any other professional. A strength of having the parent as the case manager is that no one knows more about the needs of the person with intellectual disabilities as the parent (Summers, 2015). An additional problem is that frequently parents are the case managers for the person with intellectual disabilities throughout their lives. As parents become elderly, they may have their own medical, retirement, or energy concerns that make continuation as case manager a difficult proposition. Having transition plans for managing some of the case management responsibility as parents age is an important goal. As parents create their wills, identifying who will take the place of the parents as case managers after their death is important.

Nurses

For people with intellectual disability who have multiple medical concerns, often nurses serve as medical case managers. Nurses are extremely helpful for managing medical records and the variety of therapies and physician visits required. Nurses as case managers are more common in large hospitals where multiple outpatient therapies are available in one location (Singer, 2013). In some areas, home nurses serve a vital role of providing some medical care and coordination of services in the home. This form of nursing usually provides information and support for parents who are acting as case managers. Having nurses serve as case managers is becoming a less frequent role for this profession. Case managers, who are nurses, also have limitations in their knowledge of the education system and community opportunities.

Special Education Teachers

Often a special education teacher in a school system spends more hours with a student with intellectual disabilities than any other person, including parents (DeVoss & Surmitis, 2016). This detailed knowledge of the student allows them to coordinate services provided in a school setting (Ritzema et al., 2014). Much like the role of a nurse as case manager is limited to medical interactions, and the special education teacher is limited to activities to take place in school setting. Special education teachers are extraordinarily helpful in assisting parents and students with intellectual disabilities in navigating the complex special education bureaucracy that is quite common in schools.

Person with Intellectual Disabilities

An important goal for education and therapy of people with intellectual disabilities is to develop skills for self-advocacy and control of their own lives (Carter et al., 2013). Coordinating schedules, making appointments, managing financial situations, transportation, and managing records are skills that are well within the means of many people with intellectual disabilities. Case management expertise is an important daily living skill that can be taught along with other forms of adaptive behaviour. Having a person with intellectual disability engage in all the case management activities is relatively rare. Yet more of the management and decision-making activities than many professionals and family members would think can be conducted by the person with intellectual disabilities.

Professional Case Managers

Many communities have professional case managers. Hospitals, rehabilitation centres, and parenting support groups often have professional case managers with expertise spanning systems and communities (Rosenberg et al., 2014). A professional case manager can contribute to the quality of life of the people with intellectual disabilities and their families by finding resources, creating organized records, and assisting with transportation (Summers, 2015). As the importance of case management is realized, more and more agencies and support groups are developing professional case managers that may assist multiple people with intellectual disabilities as a part of their caseload. The availability of these professionals varies depending on community.

Social Workers

Social work is a diverse profession that serves many roles and functions for the lives of people with intellectual disabilities and their families (Hughes & Wearing, 2016). Social workers can serve as therapists, liaison to community agencies, support for families in finding eligible financial supports, navigation of complex governmental and nongovernmental agencies, knowledge of community resources, and a host of other incredibly useful activities. Social workers have the skills to be professional case managers, and in some cases, they serve in this role (Hughes & Wearing, 2016). More often, social workers serve to educate and support parents about the role of case manager.

Members of Parent Support Groups

There are also many communities that have resources to support the parents as case managers. For example, parent support groups provide community support where experiences are shared among parents with similar needs (Parkes, Sweeting, & Wight, 2015). There are many communities in which informational workshops take place on important case management topics such as record-keeping or types of funding available to offset costs related to the care of the person with intellectual disabilities (Gross et al., 2013). Parent support groups are highly recommended because not only do peers have a great deal of expertise and experience navigating systems in the community but also have credibility to the parent as case manager (Huff, 2015). Information in addition to understanding of the shared experience of parenting an individual with intellectual disabilities can provide valuable supports to the parent as case manager.

Other Case Managers

The case manager role is multifaceted and is often delegated among several people. It is not uncommon to have parents serve as the chief decision-maker, but specific skills are managed by a team of professionals that include several professions previously discussed. Having multiple family members involved in the case management team approach is a common situation. Family friends, attorneys, and even accountants have been used by some families as case managers (Summers, 2015).

Models of Case Management

The Clinical Case Management Model

In a clinical case management model, a clinical care professional serves as the case manager. The case manager may be a social worker, counsellor, or therapist. The case manager in a clinical case management model provides direct services for a client's individual concerns. That might include mental health services, community and employment support, or treatment for health issues. When the case manager is also providing clinical services, they may have valuable insight into the needs of the person with intellectual disabilities (Rosenberg et al., 2014). The increased level of understanding improves the case manager's ability to identify services and serve as a liaison to formal resources through community service providers.

More importantly, clinical care providers support the client to connect with informal resources such as family, friends, community, and peers. The collaboration increases the client's willingness and ability to follow through with needed services. The clinical case manager also helps the client address social, emotional, and mental barriers to services. The model is also particularly useful for people with intellectual disabilities, who need support over the course of years.

The Brokerage Case Management Model

The brokerage model is a brief approach to case management in which case workers help clients identify their needs and broker supportive services with one or two receiving agencies or service delivery locations. This model is informational in that it assumes that a person with intellectual disabilities or their family will voluntarily use needed services once they know that the services are available and they learn how to access them (Bruns, Pullmann, Sather, Brinson, & Ramey, 2015). This model works best when a client's most salient challenge is access to services, rather than availability of services. In a brokerage case management model, the case manager provides little direct service to the client. Instead, they serve as a liaison between the person with intellectual disabilities and community resources. The focus is on assessing needs, planning a service strategy, and connecting people with intellectual disabilities to services. A brokerage model places little emphasis on monitoring and measuring outcomes. The organization providing case management services in a brokerage case manager model coordinates data collection and assessment across service providers. When service providers and case managers use integrated systems for assessing needs, tracking services, and measuring outcomes, they can easily assess the effectiveness of their coordinated efforts.

The Strengths-Based Clinical Case Management Model

The strengths-based clinical case management model focuses on empowering clients and their families (Gelkopf et al., 2016). Case management focuses on creating client opportunities for growth, education, and skill development. Like a clinical case management model, the strengths-based case management model values community services, family, and intersystem partnerships. This model encourages the person with intellectual disabilities to build and nurture informal support networks and identify and access formal community services and institutional resources. However, the strengths-based case management model focuses on the development of self-advocacy for the person with intellectual disabilities, rather than assume that the case manager is expert on the client's needs (Gelkopf et al., 2016). The strengths-based model encourages and responds to the person with intellectual disability so that they may identify their own needs, take control over the search for resources and services to address those needs, and view the community as a resource instead of a barrier to success instead. Strengths-based clinical case management models involve outreach, clinical services, advocacy, and robust coordination between case managers and clients. Implementing a program based on this model requires that organizations and agencies support case managers with a robust case management system that can track highly individualized services and capture complex data and metrics.

Summary

The role of case manager may have more to do with the quality of life of the person with intellectual disabilities as any other role. Not only does this person coordinate and organize information from multiple different sources in multiple different teams but also serves as scheduler, transportation captain, negotiator, and archivist of multiple records from multiple sources and is the primary point of contact for all professionals. This multifaceted role is sometimes managed by a team of advisors and professionals. In most cases, the parent serves as the case manager (Bruns et al., 2015). This role creates demands and pressures to the important role of parenting a person with intellectual disabilities.

Educating Staff

The inclusive education movement has dramatically expanded opportunities for students with intellectual disabilities to have access the same educational opportunities as their typically developing peers. Although access to educational opportunities is a strength of inclusive education, a challenge is that the instructor of a heterogeneous and inclusive classroom may not have all the expertise that a special education teacher with extensive training on topics related to intellectual disabilities would have. Ideally, the teacher in the inclusive classroom receives support to address the diverse needs of the modern heterogeneous classroom (Danforth & Naraian, 2015). Teachers with special education skills spend a portion of the school day in small group or individual instruction for the student with intellectual disabilities. However, much of the instruction may be delivered by a teacher charged with meeting the educational and behavioural needs of a large and diverse group of students with minimal training of the needs of children with intellectual disabilities (Kurniawati, de Boer, Minnaert, & Mangunsong, 2017).

Even within a traditional model of special education in which students with intellectual disabilities are educated in relatively ability homogeneous settings that are apart from typically developing peers for most of the day, general education teachers will still encounter and be responsible for delivering some educational interventions (Danforth & Naraian, 2015). There is strong evidence that general education teachers do not find the education of students with intellectual disabilities to be rewarding and usually prefer providing most of the services to average to high cognitive ability students (Gómez-Zepeda, Petreñas, Sabando, & Puigdellívol, 2017). No matter if the educational philosophy of the school board involves inclusive education or a traditional model of special education, teachers often need to receive professional development skills and pedagogical support for academic, adaptive behaviour, and behavioural education features that are specific to students with intellectual disabilities.

General Professional Development

When professional development information is provided to teachers, physicians, and other general practitioners who may be working with people with intellectual disabilities, there is a fine line to be walked (Hatzenbuehler, Phelan, & Link, 2013). Discussions of large heterogeneous populations can often be helpful but can easily become the stuff of stereotypes and reinforce prejudices. Innocuous or true statements such as people with intellectual disabilities are at higher risk for behavioural and mental health problems than typically developing peers can be problematic (Dart, Collins, Klingbeil, & McKinley, 2014). Although this information is true, it can create a mindset, expectations, and prejudice concerning mental health of people with intellectual disabilities. General information is valuable, but perhaps the most important general information is that people with intellectual disabilities have diverse needs, skills, goals, and expectations. One of the primary goals of the general professional development session is to demystify people with intellectual disabilities. People with intellectual disabilities can learn and socialize. Although this does not appear to be a controversial statement, it may be news to general practitioners without significant experience with people with intellectual disabilities.

Although a detailed discussion of common limitations in learning, behaviour, and socialization is a useful discussion, at least as much discussion needs to be spent on common strengths (Shaw, 2016). General professional development provides information and primes teachers and pediatricians to provide the best possible services for people with intellectual disabilities.

Individualized Information

The most important document to communicate to teachers is the individualized educational plan (IEP). It is surprising how many teachers, especially in general education, have not read the IEP when a student with intellectual disabilities becomes a member of the classroom (Shaw, Gomes, Polotskaia, & Jankowska, 2015). However, the IEP may be the most efficient document from which to transmit information concerning current functioning, short-term goals, long-term goals, school-based services received, and effective methods of instruction in academics, social skills, and behavioural issues. The IEP has far more useful and productive information for educators than most psychoeducational reports (Anderson et al., 2013). There are frequently misunderstandings concerning intelligence test scores, adaptive behaviour test scores, descriptions of behaviour and background information, and even interventions in a psychoeducational report can be overwhelming and misleading to teachers in an inclusive classroom. The most common error is over interpretation of intelligence test scores. Quite often, teachers will note that an intelligence test score is extremely low and based on that data point develop expectations, fears, and concerns that may not be entirely accurate for classroom performance or constructive for educational planning (Braden & Shaw, 2009). Far more productive is the information contained in an IEP. This document is the first stage towards helping a teacher develop a plan and a mindset that leads to productive inclusive education for the student with intellectual disabilities.

An important consideration is to ensure that the teacher of the inclusive classroom is able and willing to meet the student individually. Although having teachers with strong experience teaching students with intellectual disabilities is ideal, many teachers in inclusive settings have no experience providing direct educational services to this population. The result is that there is a surprising amount of prejudice, concerns for the dynamics of the classroom environment, and low expectations. Knowing the student by name, being introduced to the parents, and being introduced to the support team can go a long way in allaying fears and concerns that many teachers have. Becoming familiar with the specific needs and goals of the student are an important part of inclusive education (Braun et al., 2015). It may seem odd that teachers need to be informed that they are providing instruction to an individual rather than a label, but in many schools and classrooms, there is minimal experience educating students with intellectual disabilities in an inclusive setting. Listening carefully to questions or concerns that the teacher may have can be helpful in targeting what information is required for there to be a successful inclusion process. For teachers not especially experienced in this area, it is important for them to know that there is a team with expertise available to support him or her in the implementation of the goals and methods described in the IEP (Shaw, 2014). In addition, teachers will likely need support in managing the balancing act between implementing the IEP and meeting the needs of the many other students, all of which have diverse individual needs. Respectful discussion and sharing information about the tension that is concerning the specialized needs of a student with intellectual disabilities and the needs of other students is productive (Shaw, Varona Prevez, & Shah, 2014). Listening, respect, and meeting the needs of all parties are required to make the education of a student with intellectual disabilities maximally effective in an inclusive environment.

Educating Peers

Contributing to the effectiveness of an inclusive classroom is peer involvement in providing education to students with intellectual disabilities (Dart et al., 2014). The evidence is strong that when a child with intellectual disabilities is introduced to an inclusive classroom, there are benefits to all class members. Improved social skills, empathy, and mastery of the academic material when the students assist in the instruction of the student with intellectual disabilities often results (Huff, 2015). The idea of preparing a classroom for the introduction of a student with intellectual disabilities can be problematic in an inclusive environment. Teaching students about specialized needs of an individual with intellectual disabilities brings the possibility of singling out the individual student. Issues such as refraining from bullying, understanding individual differences in learning, and specific accommodations to maximize the functioning of students are issues that apply to every student in the classroom and are not specific to students with intellectual disabilities. Bullying and teasing in the classroom are important issues, yet equally as important are well-meaning relationships where the student with intellectual disabilities becomes something of the class mascot (Huff, 2015). That is, students may be kind, yet do not treat the student as an equal member of the class. This can create low expectations and defeat much of the purpose of an inclusive classroom situation. Differentiating instruction and having high expectations are common and accepted practices for all students. Formal education of peers is most effective when strengths are discussed and additional information is limited to specific safety needs and concerns that go beyond those expected of all other students in the classroom. Some examples of this would include food limitations and allergies and specific safety issues. The concept of educating and preparing peers for the arrival of a student with intellectual disabilities has little research support for improving overall outcomes (Dart et al., 2014). Identifying the student with intellectual disabilities as different and requiring specialized treatment may lead to lowered expectations and reduction of the value of inclusive education.

Community Transmission

The expectation of classrooms is that there is an understanding of individual differences in learning ability at that differentiated instruction to meet the needs of all is a common assumption (Clare et al., 2017). This is not the case in the business community (Hardman et al., 2015). When people with intellectual disabilities have opportunities to work and transition from a school setting to the community setting, oftentimes employers, police, medical services, and retail establishments require increased understanding of people with intellectual disabilities. There are many examples of people with intellectual disabilities being deprived of services or treated poorly, often illegally by members of the community. Potential employers benefit from understanding the general strengths and potential of people with intellectual disabilities as well as the specific strengths of individuals being considered for employment. Much like peer education, the lack of knowledge concerning individuals with intellectual disabilities relates to failure to understand their strengths, rather than cataloguing their weaknesses (Tebes, Thai, & Matlin, 2014).

Conclusions

The movement towards delivering evidence-based interventions and applying science to the education is an important step in improving the quality of life for people with intellectual disabilities. An equally important component is how information is communicated, decisions made, resources coordinated and managed, and ideas implemented. Without mindful development of a decision-making process, outstanding science and innovative practices will not be realized. Moreover, the complexity of information that spans multiple professional domains cannot possibly be understood and employed by one person. As such, teams need to be developed, nurtured, and maintained by educational, medical, community, rehabilitation, and mental health systems to integrate and implement a variety of educational services. Team development, processes, implementation, and effectiveness are topics worthy of research and scientific study. The process of decision-making and implementation is just as important as the content of affective medical, mental health, and educational interventions.

References

Anderson, L. L., Humphries, K., McDermott, S., Marks, B., Sisirak, J., & Larson, S. (2013). The state of the science of health and wellness for adults with intellectual and developmental disabilities. *Intellectual and Developmental Disabilities, 51*(5), 385–398. https://doi.org/10.1352/1934-9556-51.5.385

Bigby, C., Frawley, P., & Ramcharan, P. (2014). Conceptualizing inclusive research with people with intellectual disability. *Journal of Applied Research in Intellectual Disabilities, 27*(1), 3–12. https://doi.org/10.1111/jar.12083

Braden, J. P., & Shaw, S. R. (2009). Intervention validity of cognitive assessment: Knowns, unknowns, and unknowables. *Assessment for Effective Intervention, 34*, 106–115.

Braun, K. V. N., Christensen, D., Doernberg, N., Schieve, L., Rice, C., Wiggins, L., … Yeargin-Allsopp, M. (2015). Trends in the prevalence of autism spectrum disorder, cerebral palsy, hearing loss, intellectual disability, and vision impairment, metropolitan Atlanta, 1991–2010. *PLoS One, 10*(4), e0124120. https://doi.org/10.1371/journal.pone.0124120

Brock, M. E., & Carter, E. W. (2013). A systematic review of paraprofessional-delivered educational practices to improve outcomes for students with intellectual and developmental disabilities. *Research and Practice for Persons with Severe Disabilities, 38*(4), 211–221. https://doi.org/10.1177/154079691303800401

Bruns, E. J., Pullmann, M. D., Sather, A., Brinson, R. D., & Ramey, M. (2015). Effectiveness of wraparound versus case management for children and adolescents: Results of a randomized study. *Administration and Policy in Mental Health and Mental Health Services Research, 42*(3), 309–322. https://doi.org/10.1007/s10488-014-0571-3

Campbell, M., Robertson, A., & Jahoda, A. (2014). Psychological therapies for people with intellectual disabilities: Comments on a Matrix of evidence for interventions in challenging behaviour. *Journal of Intellectual Disability Research, 58*(2), 172–188. https://doi.org/10.1111/j.1365-2788.2012.01646.x

Carney, T. (2014). Clarifying, operationalising, and evaluating supported decision making models. *Research and Practice in Intellectual and Developmental Disabilities, 1*(1), 46–50. https://doi.org/10.1080/23297018.2014.902727

Carter, E. W., Lane, K. L., Cooney, M., Weir, K., Moss, C. K., & Machalicek, W. (2013). Parent assessments of self-determination importance and performance for students with autism or intellectual disability. *American Journal on Intellectual and Developmental Disabilities, 118*(1), 16–31. https://doi.org/10.1352/1944-7558-118.1.16

Ciccarelli, M. R., Brown, M. W., Gladstone, E. B., Woodward, J. F., & Swigonski, N. L. (2014). Implementation and sustainability of statewide transition support services for youth with intellectual and physical disabilities. *Journal of Pediatric Rehabilitation Medicine, 7*(1), 93–104. https://doi.org/10.3233/PRM-140274

Clare, I. C. H., Madden, E. M., Holland, A. J., Farrington, C. J. T., Whitson, S., Broughton, S., … Wagner, A. P. (2017). "What vision?": Experiences of team members in a community service for adults with intellectual disabilities. *Journal of Intellectual Disability Research, 61*(3), 197–209. https://doi.org/10.1111/jir.12312

Danforth, S., & Naraian, S. (2015). This new field of inclusive education: Beginning a dialogue on conceptual foundations. *Intellectual and Developmental Disabilities, 53*(1), 70–85. https://doi.org/10.1352/1934-9556-53.1.70

Dart, E. H., Collins, T. A., Klingbeil, D. A., & McKinley, L. E. (2014). Peer management interventions: A meta-analytic review of single-case research. *School Psychology Review, 43*(4), 367–384. https://doi.org/10.17105/SPR-14-0009.1

DeVoss, J. A., & Surmitis, K. A. (2016). Partners in justice: School counselors and teachers creating classrooms for social justice. In R. Papa, D. M. Eadens, & D. W. Eadens (Eds.), *Social justice instruction* (pp. 89–102). Cham, Switzerland: Springer. Retrieved from http://link.springer.com/chapter/10.1007/978-3-319-12349-3_9

Ganz, J. B. (2014). Interdisciplinary issues and collaboration in assessment and treatment. In *Aided augmentative communication for individuals with autism spectrum disorders* (pp. 43–51). New York, NY: Springer. https://doi.org/10.1007/978-1-4939-0814-1_4

Gargiulo, R. M., & Metcalf, D. (2015). *Teaching in today's inclusive classrooms: A universal design for learning approach*. Toronto, ON: Nelson Education.

Gelkopf, M., Lapid, L., Werbeloff, N., Levine, S. Z., Telem, A., Zisman-Ilani, Y., & Roe, D. (2016). A strengths-based case management service for people with serious mental illness in Israel:

A randomized controlled trial. *Psychiatry Research, 241*, 182–189. https://doi.org/10.1016/j.psychres.2016.04.106

Gómez-Zepeda, G., Petreñas, C., Sabando, D., & Puigdellívol, I. (2017). The role of the Support and Attention to Diversity Teacher (SADT) from a community-based perspective: Promoting educational success and educational inclusion for all. *Teaching and Teacher Education, 64*, 127–138. https://doi.org/10.1016/j.tate.2017.02.002

Graybill, E., Esch, R. C., Vinoski, E., Truscott, S., Torres, A., Daniel, K., ... Crimmins, D. (2016). Including the family member in interdisciplinary team meetings: Communication trend analysis. *Small Group Research, 47*(1), 3–27. https://doi.org/10.1177/1046496415604028

Gross, J. M. S., Wallace, L., Blue-Banning, M., Summers, J. A., & Turnbull, A. (2013). Examining the experiences and decisions of parents/guardians: Participant directing the supports and services of adults with significant intellectual and developmental disabilities. *Journal of Disability Policy Studies, 24*(2), 88–101. https://doi.org/10.1177/1044207312439102

Hardman, M. L., Drew, C. J., & Egan, M. W. (2015). *Human exceptionality: School, community, and family*. Toronto, ON: Nelson Education.

Hatzenbuehler, M. L., Phelan, J. C., & Link, B. G. (2013). Stigma as a fundamental cause of population health inequalities. *American Journal of Public Health, 103*(5), 813–821. https://doi.org/10.2105/AJPH.2012.301069

Heller, T., Gibbons, H. M., & Fisher, D. (2015). Caregiving and family support interventions: Crossing networks of aging and developmental disabilities. *Intellectual and Developmental Disabilities, 53*(5), 329–345. https://doi.org/10.1352/1934-9556-53.5.329

Huff, J. (2015, August 13). *Parent to parent, peer to peer: an investigation of mutual social support groups as a resource for genetic counselors* (Thesis). Retrieved from http://bir.brandeis.edu/handle/10192/31071

Hughes, M., & Wearing, M. (2016). *Organisations and management in social work: Everyday action for change*. London, England: SAGE.

Kurniawati, F., de Boer, A. A., Minnaert, A. E. M. G., & Mangunsong, F. (2017). Evaluating the effect of a teacher training programme on the primary teachers' attitudes, knowledge and teaching strategies regarding special educational needs. *Educational Psychology, 37*(3), 287–297. https://doi.org/10.1080/01443410.2016.1176125

Lunsky, Y., Hastings, R. P., Hensel, J., Arenovich, T., & Dewa, C. S. (2014). Perceptions of positive contributions and burnout in community developmental disability workers. *Intellectual and Developmental Disabilities, 52*(4), 249–257. https://doi.org/10.1352/1934-9556-52.4.249

Lunsky, Y., Tint, A., Robinson, S., Gordeyko, M., & Ouellette-Kuntz, H. (2014). System-wide information about family carers of adults with intellectual/developmental disabilities—A scoping review of the literature. *Journal of Policy and Practice in Intellectual Disabilities, 11*(1), 8–18. https://doi.org/10.1111/jppi.12068

Mccallion, P., & Janicki, M. (2014). *Grandparents as carers of children with disabilities: Facing the challenges*. London, England: Routledge.

McLaughlin, D., Barr, O., McIlfatrick, S., & McConkey, R. (2014). Developing a best practice model for partnership practice between specialist palliative care and intellectual disability services: A mixed methods study. *Palliative Medicine, 28*(10), 1213–1221. https://doi.org/10.1177/0269216314550373

Minnes, P., Perry, A., & Weiss, J. A. (2015). Predictors of distress and well-being in parents of young children with developmental delays and disabilities: The importance of parent perceptions. *Journal of Intellectual Disability Research, 59*(6), 551–560. https://doi.org/10.1111/jir.12160

Moeschler, J. B., Shevell, M., & Genetics, C. O. (2014). Comprehensive evaluation of the child with intellectual disability or global developmental delays. *Pediatrics, 134*(3), e903–e918. https://doi.org/10.1542/peds.2014-1839

Moseley, C., Kleinert, H., Sheppard-Jones, K., & Hall, S. (2013). Using research evidence to inform public policy decisions. *Intellectual and Developmental Disabilities, 51*(5), 412–422. https://doi.org/10.1352/1934-9556-51.5.412

Owen, M. J. (2012). Intellectual disability and major psychiatric disorders: A continuum of neurodevelopmental causality. *The British Journal of Psychiatry, 200*(4), 268–269. https://doi.org/10.1192/bjp.bp.111.105551

Owen, R., Bowers, A., Heller, T., Hsieh, K., & Gould, R. (2016). The impact of support services teams: Community-based behavioral health support interventions. *Journal of Policy and Practice in Intellectual Disabilities, 14*(3), 205–213. https://doi.org/10.1111/jppi.12186

Parellada, M., Boada, L., Moreno, C., Llorente, C., Romo, J., Muela, C., & Arango, C. (2013). Specialty Care Programme for autism spectrum disorders in an urban population: A case-management model for health care delivery in an ASD population. *European Psychiatry, 28*(2), 102–109. https://doi.org/10.1016/j.eurpsy.2011.06.004

Parkes, A., Sweeting, H., & Wight, D. (2015). Parenting stress and parent support among mothers with high and low education. *Journal of Family Psychology, 29*(6), 907–918. https://doi.org/10.1037/fam0000129

Perry, J., Felce, D., Kerr, M., Bartley, S., Tomlinson, J., & Felce, J. (2014). Contact with primary care: The experience of people with intellectual disabilities. *Journal of Applied Research in Intellectual Disabilities, 27*(3), 200–211. https://doi.org/10.1111/jar.12072

Poland, S. (1994). The role of school crisis intervention teams to prevent and reduce school violence and trauma. *School Psychology Review, 23*(2), 175–189.

Ritzema, A. M., Sladeczek, I. E., Ghosh, S., Karagiannakis, A., & Manay-Quian, N. (2014). Improving outcomes for children with developmental disabilities through enhanced communication and collaboration between school psychologists and physicians. *Canadian Journal of School Psychology, 29*(4), 317–337. https://doi.org/10.1177/0829573514536529

Rosenberg, G., Weissman, A., & Wong, D. F. K. (2014). *Clinical case management for people with mental illness: A biopsychosocial vulnerability-stress model*. London, England: Routledge.

Rzhetsky, A., Bagley, S. C., Wang, K., Lyttle, C. S., Cook, E. H., Jr., Altman, R. B., & Gibbons, R. D. (2014). Environmental and state-level regulatory factors affect the incidence of autism and intellectual disability. *PLoS Computational Biology, 10*(3), e1003518. https://doi.org/10.1371/journal.pcbi.1003518

Scott, H. M., & Havercamp, S. M. (2016). Systematic review of health promotion programs focused on behavioral changes for people with intellectual disability. *Intellectual and Developmental Disabilities, 54*(1), 63–76. https://doi.org/10.1352/1934-9556-54.1.63

Shaw, S. R. (2014). Academically at-risk students and mental health issues: Information for educators. *NASP Communiqué, 43*, 23.

Shaw, S. R. (2016). Research-to-practice for school psychologists: Advances in evidence-based practice, clinical research, and implementation. *School Psychology Forum, 10*, 340–348.

Shaw, S. R., & Brown, M. B. (2011). Keeping pace with changes in health care: Expanding educational and medical collaboration. *Journal of Educational and Psychological Consultation, 21*, 79–87. https://doi.org/10.1080/10474412.2011.571549

Shaw, S. R., Glaser, S., & Ouimet, T. (2011). Developing the medical liaison role in school settings. *Journal of Educational and Psychological Consultation, 21*, 106–117. https://doi.org/10.1080/10474412.2011.571479

Shaw, S. R., Gomes, P., Polotskaia, A., & Jankowska, A. M. (2015). The relationship between student health and academic performance: Implications for school psychologists. *School Psychology International, 36*, 115–134.

Shaw, S. R., Varona Prevez, L., & Shah, S. (2014). Evidence-based interventions: Necessary, but not sufficient for a profession of scientist-practitioners. *NASP Communique, 43*(1), 17–18.

Singer, B. (2013). Perceptions of school nurses in the care of students with disabilities. *The Journal of School Nursing, 29*(5), 329–336. https://doi.org/10.1177/1059840512462402

Summers, N. (2015). *Fundamentals of case management practice: Skills for the human services*. Toronto, ON: Nelson Education.

Tebes, J. K., Thai, N. D., & Matlin, S. L. (2014). Twenty-first century science as a relational process: From eureka! To team science and a place for community psychology. *American Journal of Community Psychology, 53*(3–4), 475–490. https://doi.org/10.1007/s10464-014-9625-7

Thompson, J. R., Schalock, R. L., Agosta, J., Teninty, L., & Fortune, J. (2014). How the supports paradigm is transforming the developmental disabilities service system. *Inclusion, 2*(2), 86–99. https://doi.org/10.1352/2326-6988-2.2.86

Waitoller, F. R., & Artiles, A. J. (2013). A decade of professional development research for inclusive education a critical review and notes for a research program. *Review of Educational Research, 83*(3), 319–356. https://doi.org/10.3102/0034654313483905

Wang, M., & Singer, G. H. S. (2016). *Supporting families of children with developmental disabilities: Evidence-based and emerging practices*. New York, NY: Oxford University Press.

Williamson, H. J., & Perkins, E. A. (2014). Family caregivers of adults with intellectual and developmental disabilities: Outcomes associated with US services and supports. *Intellectual and Developmental Disabilities, 52*(2), 147–159. https://doi.org/10.1352/1934-9556-52.2.147

Chapter 7
Issues and Advances in Diagnostic Assessment

Abstract This chapter reviews assessment strategies for medical, psychological, and educational functioning for persons with intellectual disabilities. This includes a review of background information important to diagnostic assessment including (a) medical history, (b) family and home life, (c) educational history, (d) developmental history, (e) behavioural/mental health, and (f) employment/community. A review of indirect (i.e. rating scales and interviews) and direct assessment (i.e. behavioural observations) techniques is discussed. Finally, psychoeducational assessment is discussed to assist individualized educational plan teams in determining if a child requires and is eligible for special education assistance. Specific psychoeducational assessment practices are reviewed including (a) behavioural and assessment techniques, (b) cognitive assessment strategies, and (c) the evaluation of adaptive behaviour, language, basic psychological processes, academic achievement, and social/emotional functioning.

Case Study

Paul is a 5-year-old male who is about to enter formal school for the first time. He was placed in foster care at age 2 due to parental neglect. He has had five different foster homes over this period. All the foster care families reported that Paul appeared to be developmentally lagging compared to other children of his age, yet there had never been a psychological assessment or formal intervention plan put in place. For Paul, there were multiple attempts to provide early education services, but at the time that assessment was scheduled, he would move to a different foster care placement in a different location. However, now that he was entering school, a need for a complete diagnostic assessment and plan development would take place. Medical records were not remarkable, except that his birth weight was low for gestational age at 4 pounds, 14 ounces. This may be indicative of poor maternal health or environmental toxins (i.e. smoking, poor diet, drug use), but no specifics were indicated. Family history showed that both biological parents had received special education services when they were in school. His current foster care family reports that he rarely uses sentences more than three words, does not seem to understand multistep

S. R. Shaw, A. M. Jankowska, *Pediatric Intellectual Disabilities at School*, Pediatric School Psychology, https://doi.org/10.1007/978-3-030-02992-0_7

directions, does not play well with other children, and is frequently socially rejected, and he prefers spending most of his time watching television.

During school entry screening, Paul's vision and hearing were within normal limits. However, his vocabulary and language skills were significantly delayed. Some of his readiness skills such as reciting the alphabet, counting aloud, recognizing letters, and knowing the names of common objects (e.g. bottle, motorcycle, bird) were well below the expectations for a child about to enter kindergarten. The school entry screening team referred Paul for a psychoeducational assessment to determine whether special education services were appropriate.

The school psychologist interviewed Paul's current foster care parents, with whom he had lived for 14 months, and his case manager who has all documentation and reports from Paul's previous foster care settings. The purpose of the interview was to determine how he functions in the foster care setting and whether he meets the demands of home and community life. A formal measure of adaptive behaviour (i.e. AAIDD Diagnostic Adaptive Behaviour Scale) was also administered in an interview format. In addition, Paul participated in taking an intelligence test. For Paul, the Wechsler Preschool and Primary Scales of Intelligence—Fourth Edition was administered.

The results indicated that Paul has a full-scale score on the WPPSI-IV of 59. This score is in the first percentile and is consistent with an educational placement of intellectual disabilities. Based on the AAIDD Diagnostic Adaptive Behaviour Scale, four areas of adaptive behaviour were significantly impaired (i.e. more than two standard deviations below the mean for his age). For this school board in this state, Paul's reported functioning in assessment results made him eligible for a special education placement for the program entitled, "mild intellectual disabilities". However, to develop an effective individualized education plan, additional assessment information would be needed. Although the school psychologist provided diagnostic assessment information to determine eligibility for a program, additional and ongoing assessment would be required for intervention planning and effective education for Paul.

Introduction

Assessment of individuals with intellectual disabilities is a complex undertaking involving medical, psychological, educational, language, fine and gross motor, and mental health components (Virués-Ortega et al., 2014). As such, many complete assessments of persons with intellectual disabilities are multidisciplinary or interdisciplinary in nature. In addition, the purpose of assessment also varies depending on the needs of a system (e.g. screening, program eligibility, medical diagnoses, developmental assessment, cognitive, adaptive behaviour, academic achievement, mental health issues, language, progress monitoring). A common approach is to simply administer a measure of general mental ability and a measure of adaptive behaviour. If both scores fall two standard deviations below the mean or less, then the individual is considered to have a diagnosis of intellectual disabilities under most diagnostic systems. This approach may meet the bureaucratic needs of some systems (e.g., medical, legal, school) but sheds little light or useful information that can be used to develop improved functioning across environmental settings. For maximum usefulness, all assessment data are interpreted in the context of background information such as medical history, family history, developmental milestones, and the ability to function effectively and meet the needs of the environment. To meet these needs, there are a variety of techniques and available measures of varying quality. The challenge of assessment is to integrate the best possible measurement techniques to determine the current functioning of persons with intellectual disabilities to make the best possible medical, psychological, educational, and other life decisions.

Assessment techniques will vary depending on the question being answered. Some of the questions that arise when considering an assessment for a person who has or is suspected of having the diagnosis of intellectual disabilities are (Boyle et al., 2011):

- Does the individual meet eligibility criteria under IDEA for special education services as a child with intellectual disabilities?
- Does the individual meet ICD-11 criteria for intellectual disabilities/mental retardation to receive funding to offset the family cost of medical, respite, rehabilitation, and other supportive expenses?
- Does the individual meet DSM-5 eligibility criteria to receive community rehabilitative services?
- Are there additional diagnoses that are comorbid with intellectual disabilities that need to be considered and treated for most improved outcomes?
- How much progress has the individual made as result of treatment, educational programming, medications, or habilitative therapies?
- What level of supports will the individual require to be maximally functional in an employment, educational, or community environment?
- Is the individual competent to contribute to their own defence in a criminal trial?
- Does a preschool age child with language delay and demonstrating functional impairment have concurrent cognitive impairment?

The major professional challenge to any form of assessment is the case conceptualization (Greenspan, Harris, & Woods, 2015). Determining the purpose and the important questions to be answered in the assessment are the first and often forgotten stages. A one-size-fits-all assessment plan is not particularly effective in the assessment of individuals with a heterogeneous presentation of the presenting behaviours and multiple possible underlying problems. The most effective forms of assessment address the needs of the system (e.g. school, medical, rehabilitation, legal, community) and the needs of the individual and family. The most effective form of case conceptualization is to consult with representatives of the system and the individual to begin to develop questions that can be answered through the assessment process. Although it is quite common to simply administer a standardized and norm-referenced test of general intelligence, this answer is only some of the possible questions that can be answered in a comprehensive assessment. Therefore, any effective assessment must effectively meet the needs of the system and the individual and their family.

Nearly all forms of assessment are designed to answer specific questions. The formal aspect of an assessment (i.e. testing, observing, interviewing the person participating in the assessment) all work in service of answering the specific questions. As is widely known in all forms of problem-solving, the most important aspect of solving a problem is identifying the correct problem. Therefore, significant time and energy need to be invested in communicating with the referring parties and other knowledgeable people involved in the case. Effort is required to interview referring parties, caregivers, medical professionals, therapists, teachers, employers, family members, peers, and others who can effectively describe the primary issues that need to be addressed in a full assessment.

Background

A full and complete assessment requires extensive understanding of the individual's background. The most common purpose of background investigation is to create a context for the behaviour of the individual being assessed are medical, family, developmental, behavioural and emotional, school, employment, and community. Information for these backgrounds is gathered through a combination of medical record review, school record review, interview with the individual being assessed, and interviews with other people knowledgeable of the situation.

Medical History

The key to creating a useful medical history is relevance. There is no need to create an exhaustive record of typical medical information unless it is directly relevant to the case information. Medical history for individuals suspected of having intellectual disabilities is most typically divided into three sections: prenatal, perinatal, and postnatal. Any notable identifiable events or processes that are unusual and may contribute to the presenting problems are to be described in the medical history. Injuries, illness, and other events that contribute to functioning are described in detail. An example of a common sentence in psychoeducational reports concerning medical history is, "There were no remarkable or contributory events or processes in the perinatal period noted in the medical records." Obviously, the purpose of such a catch-all sentence is to communicate to the reader of a psychoeducational report that this aspect of the medical history was investigated. A subset of the medical history section is quite common in the assessment of a child with or suspected of having a diagnosis of intellectual disabilities and that is for clinical genetics. As noted in Chap. 2, many persons will have an extensive clinical and laboratory genetics record. For purposes of the assessment, information concerning genetic findings relevant to the case conceptualization is important to have collected and disseminated in a psychoeducational report.

Family/Home Life

The primary purpose of a quality family and home life history is to understand the context of supports and demands concerning the individual's daily living and independence (Luckasson & Schalock, 2013). Persons with intellectual disabilities are more likely than typical individuals to have low socioeconomic status, food and shelter insecurity, unstable foster care living arrangements, single-parent households, and other family and home life factors that make learning and performing functional behaviours difficult. Current living arrangements, who lives with the individual, who provides care, and how much care is required, are critical aspects of this information. Information such as socioeconomic status can assist in determining the level of resources that are available and can be brought to bear to promote improved functioning. For children, family constellation can help to identify the functional and emotional supports available. For adults, identifying who is providing care and what degree of independence and support are available is important. Because the primary goal of assessment is to determine the level of functioning, many times asking a family member, peer, caregiver, or guardian can provide more accurate information about functioning than any standardized and norm-referenced test. A good clinical trick is to always ask anyone you are interviewing what information they would like to have about the individual being assessed that would help to improve the everyday functioning of the individual being assessed. There is insight to be gained from family members, peers, house supervisors, roommates, and others who work daily with the individual being assessed.

Educational History

Educational history refers to formal schooling and academic training. In addition to basic information such as schools attended, attendance, grades, specialized placement, and individualized educational plans, there are also helpful teacher notes in school records that describe behaviours, communication between teachers and parents, behaviour management strategies, and additional information. Given that children spend as much time in school with a classroom teacher as they do under the supervision of their parents, teachers often provide extraordinarily valuable information that can be useful for a psychoeducational assessment (Fujiura, 2013). In many ways, teachers provide superior information because they have observed the individual being assessed under structured and cognitively and emotionally demanding situations, and teachers have a different social desirability filter when discussing functioning when compared to parents.

Developmental History

Learning the timing and completion of developmental milestones can provide an important information in the assessment process (Brown, Hatton, & Emerson, 2013). Simple information such as when the first words were spoken, two words used in combination, sitting up, standing, first steps taken, parallel play, eye contact, and so on can be helpful. Many parents, especially those with multiple children, are not especially accurate in their recall of the meeting of developmental milestones. In these situations, asking parents if they have noticed that the child being assessed reached developmental milestones at a different time line from their siblings or if failure to reach developmental milestones caused concerns at the time. Often, the timing of meeting developmental milestones is also available in medical records.

Behavioural and Mental Health

Often behavioural or mental health concerns are not effectively addressed in medical or school histories (e.g. Blasingame, 2016). The history of these concerns also may be difficult to identify in cases where the individual being assessed has gone through multiple foster care settings or communal living arrangements. Frequently, behavioural and mental health concerns are overlooked because there is an assumption that the problematic behaviours are solely a function of the intellectual disability rather than comorbid mental health problems. This overshadowing of mental health problems is a primary reason why receiving appropriate mental health services is often delayed for persons with intellectual disabilities. Moreover, behavioural problems may not be reported or recorded because of fears that professionals or caregivers may have concerning stigmatizing the individual with intellectual disabilities. Identifying the behavioural and mental health history can require a bit of detective work. Persons with intellectual disabilities are at higher risk for mental health problems; however, the presentation of symptoms may make diagnosis difficult (Hemmings & Bouras, 2016). For example, it is not uncommon for aggressive behaviours to occur and be attributed to frustration or other factors that are a function of intellectual disabilities; when in fact, the aggressive behaviours may be a symptom of major depressive disorder or anxiety disorder. Often the most productive method to interview caregivers and professionals concerning behavioural and mental health history is simply to ask whether there are any problematic behaviours that required some form of intervention, how resistant the behaviours were to intervention, and how much those behaviours affected efforts to improve overall functioning and other domains. Most people being interviewed will not be able to identify the behaviour as a possible indicator of a mental health concern but often remember problematic or maladaptive behaviours. In the case where there is a well-documented history of mental health concerns, careful description of the treatments including psychological and pharmacological treatment regimens needs to be described.

Employment and Community

An oft-ignored component of assessment is considering the needs required by home, school, employment, and community (Luckasson & Schalock, 2013). Most typically psychoeducational assessment focuses on characteristics of the individual. However, full and complete assessment provides information to facilitate the fit between the skills of the individual and the demands of their environment. Even in the cases of school-aged children, there is a need to consider eventual transition to employment and community care. Whether an immediate- or long-term part of the problem-solving process for the individual being assessed, information concerning the functional needs by employers and by the local community setting can provide valuable information leading to the development of goals for detailed intervention plans. Information from potential employers and from community transition specialists can provide valuable information that guides assessment.

Formal Assessment

Assessment is far more than an administration and interpretation of several norm-referenced and standardized tests. Psychoeducational assessment is an important part of multidisciplinary team assessment and must be flexible to meet the needs of the stakeholders in the process. The stakeholders are not only the individual being assessed and their family, but also systems such as school, medical, community, and others. To achieve useful psychoeducational assessment information, an understanding of the presenting problem is required. This often means significant information about individual's history, and the functional demands of the environment must also be assessed (Luckasson & Schalock, 2015).

Screening

A near-universal assumption about maximizing functional outcomes for persons with intellectual disabilities is that the earliest possible identification and implementation of interventions will lead to the most positive outcomes (Tassé, Luckasson, & Nygren, 2013). As such, there are numerous forms of medical screening for common causes of intellectual disabilities that occur during the prenatal, perinatal, and postnatal periods. In addition to collecting family data to determine any possible genetic risk factors for common causes of intellectual disabilities, pregnant women often undergo multiple blood tests, multiple ultrasound examinations of the foetus, and possibly amniocentesis. At birth, nearly all children receive phenylketonuria screening. During the first well-baby visits with pediatricians, the nine newborn reflexes (rooting, suck, Moro or startle, walking or stepping, grasp, tonic neck, righting, tongue thrust, withdrawal) are assessed as well as muscle tone to determine any neurological risk factors (American Academy of Pediatrics Policy Statement, 2006). Infants are examined for any dysmorphic features, unusual dimples, birthmarks, and physical asymmetries that may indicate a heightened risk for neurological or developmental issues. Parents are asked a host of questions concerning feeding, elimination, crying, sleep, attachment, evidence of intact vision and hearing, and other factors that may indicate a risk for developmental disabilities.

Pediatricians use a variety of screening measures to assess cognitive and behavioural function in young children. The most widely used is the Denver Developmental Screening Test II (DDST-2; Frankenburg, Dodds, & Archer, 1990). The DDST-2 is a 1990 revision and update of the popular Denver Developmental Screening Test. The DDST-2 is administered by pediatricians during the well-child visit. The measure typically takes 20–30 min to perform and consists of 125 total questions. Most typically, 10–50 questions are administered at any one visit. The DDST-2 is a series of important developmental milestones with the typical age range for completion of each milestone. The measure is administered via interview with parent, and frequently the pediatrician will ask a child to engage in the task so that they can see the functioning for themselves. As a screening measure, the DDST-2 does not have much specificity. However, it provides a general impression of development in fine motor, language, gross motor, and personal/social milestones. Children not achieving milestones in the expected timeframe, consistency, and quality may be referred to a subspecialist for further evaluation. The Ages and Stages Questionnaire (ASQ; Squires, Twombly, Bricker, & Potter, 2009) is a similar measure used by early childhood specialists and pediatricians and is now in its third edition. Although somewhat similar in content to the DDST-2, the ASQ is typically completed as a questionnaire to be completed by parents. Both instruments are brief and are used for children aged birth through 5 years. The advantage of these formal screening instruments is that they focus on developmental milestones and may reassure concerned parents as well as identify delays or potential long-term developmental problems.

Although some cases of intellectual disability are identified first in pediatricians' offices using formal or informal screening, the most common source of early identification for intellectual disabilities is parent report. Parents typically report concerns about lags in development that are qualitatively different behaviours than their expectations. This is especially common when parents have other children to provide a comparison. When parents note significant developmental problems, then more detailed screening tests to assist in identifying developmental delays may be administered. Examples of these more sophisticated and detailed measures include the Child Developmental Inventory (Ireton, 1992) for children 15 months through

16 years of age. The CDI can take more than 30–50 min for administration and focuses on cognition and language skills. The Parents' Evaluation of Developmental Status (Glascoe, 1997) is a detailed parent report that provides screening information for development delays.

School-Based Screening

In addition to screening that takes place in pediatricians' offices, school districts are responsible for identifying children who are at risk for developmental disabilities. All schools engage in some form of screening as a child enters kindergarten at approximately age 5. Screenings typically consist of vision, hearing, cognitive, academic readiness, and social, emotional, and motor skills. There are tests that are commonly used for school-based screening including the Brigance Screens, Developmental Profile-3 (Alpern, 2007), Developmental Indicators for the Assessment of Learning-3 (Mardell & Goldenberg, 2011), Temperament and Atypical Behaviour Scale (Neisworth, Bagnato, Salvia, & Hunt, 1999), Achenbach System of Empirically Based Assessment-Preschool Module (Achenbach, 2009), and Vineland Social-Emotional Early Childhood Scales (Sparrow, Cicchetti, & Balla, 1998). In addition to kindergarten readiness screening, most school boards have a systematic approach for screening children from ages 3 through 5. Although few, there are some school districts with a formal systematic approach to screening infants from birth through 3 years of age. The techniques used in the screening are similar to those used in a pediatrician's office.

Early Childhood Assessment

Whether through a pediatrician's office, parent referral, or through school district implemented screening; when children are identified as having a possible intellectual disability, the next stage is having a full psychoeducational assessment conducted to make an effective diagnosis or determination of eligibility for specialized programs. The major challenge for assessment is that early identification is assumed to result in more effective treatment for children with intellectual disabilities, yet the accuracy of assessment at very young ages is not especially strong, which makes firm diagnosis challenging. There are many behaviours and other developmental issues that can influence the score of a developmental or cognitive test. Children with language impairments, motor impairments, attention deficit hyperactivity disorder, prematurity, autism spectrum disorder, and those who develop at a different pace all have the risk of being identified as a child with intellectual disabilities. The assumption is that intellectual disabilities are lifelong impairments that affect multiple areas of function. Because of the emotional and social impact of a diagnosis of intellectual disabilities on individuals and families, there is a relatively high burden of proof before the diagnosis can be made.

Global developmental delay is a term that is widely used to describe lower than average intellectual functioning along with significant limitations in at least two other areas of development (e.g. social skills, motor, language; Schalock, Luckasson, & Shogren, 2007). In some cases, global developmental delay is used as a substitute or more socially acceptable term for intellectual disabilities. Other times, global developmental delay is used for children who show many of the characteristics of intellectual disabilities, but there is not compelling evidence that this is a long-term disability. In other words, there is a possibility that the child may catch up to peers. Catching up to peers can happen, especially in the areas of language and motor delays. To use global developmental delay as a synonym for intellectual disabilities is misleading. The word delay has the connotation that the child will eventually catch up to typically developing peers; children with intellectual disabilities typically do not gain ground on typically developing peers and do not typically catch up.

The other major challenge with global developmental delay is that it is extremely difficult to differentiate which specific domains may be impaired or delayed. For example, infants with motor or sensory problems may present as having cognitive impairment due to their limited ability to explore their environment. Often this is not a permanent cognitive impairment and frequently improves dramatically if the motor or sensory problems are successfully managed. In these cases, the diagnoses of global developmental delay may be more appropriate than intellectual disabilities.

Formal cognitive assessment of children aged birth through 5 assumes skills and behaviours that many children do not have. The assessment process involving working individually with a stranger, which may be completely foreign to many young children, and their lack of comfort in responding in a timely manner to requests may yield scores that underestimate the child's true cognitive ability. Likewise, young children with strong motor skills or with a great deal of experience in social interactions with adults may result in an overestimation of true cognitive ability. Cognitive assessment is typically a robust construct for school age to adult populations, but it is not especially robust for young children (Weiss, Saklofske, Holdnack, & Prifitera, 2015). This is not a matter of technical or psychometric quality of the assessment instruments, but the nature of uneven development of cognitive functions in very young children.

The most commonly used instrument for assessing development is the Bayley Scales of Infant and Toddler Development, Third Edition (Bayley, 2006). The Bayley Scales are not specifically a measure of cognitive functioning but are an overall measure of development that involves cognitive, language, motor, social, emotional, and adaptive behaviour measures. The Bayley Scales have a strong floor and ceiling, which makes it a sensitive norm-referenced measure of development. Another advantage of the Bayley is that it lends itself to multidisciplinary assessment as physical and occupational therapist is often responsible for the motor scale, speech and language pathologist for the language scale, psychologist for the social and emotional and cognitive scales, and parent/caregiver responses for adaptive behaviour.

Overall, early childhood assessment of intellectual disabilities is a difficult diagnostic task. Although there is significant pressure to make a diagnosis as early as possible to begin interventions with the highest likelihood of improving overall functioning, caution and humility are critical. Clearly, individuals who are more severely involved and have identified genetic anomalies are the easiest to identify and diagnose. Mild intellectual disabilities are more of a challenge. Quite likely, a more effective approach for infants, toddler, and preschoolers with equivocal cognitive status and a diagnosis of global developmental delay is to focus on interventions related to weak areas such as language, motor, social-emotional, and daily living skills. For early childhood, the focus on improving functionality and specific domains may be more productive than focusing on issues related to a possible diagnosis of intellectual disabilities.

Psychoeducational Assessment

For school age to adult persons, the psychoeducational assessment for purposes of diagnosis remains a challenging proposition. There are a host of complications and challenges involved in the assessment of persons with intellectual disabilities. For psychoeducational assessment, there are five primary domains. General principles in the assessment of each domain will be described followed by specific suggested instruments and techniques.

Cognitive

Most formal criteria for the diagnosis of intellectual disabilities require three parts: a standardized and norm-referenced measure of general mental ability that is more than two standard deviations below the mean, a measure of adaptive behaviour functioning that indicates significant impairment in some real-life functions, and pervasive and clear impairments that require support for nominal functioning in the person's environment. All three components are challenging, but the measure of cognitive ability brings a host of unique problems to be overcome in the assessment process.

Intelligence tests, commonly known as IQ tests, are among the most reliable and well-validated measures in clinical science (Ritchie, 2015). Yet, for historical and sociological reasons, the public has grave doubts about the utility of intelligence tests. Although there is no evidence supporting the claim, intelligence tests are widely held to be biased against some ethnic groups, unreliable and inappropriate for clinical use. Much of these concerns with little foundation stem from the history of over-interpretation and overgeneralization of intelligence test results (Jensen & McGurk, 1987; Weiss et al., 2015). The surplus meanings given to intelligence test results such as intelligence test results indicate an individual's potential, intelligence test results are a measure of one's genotype, intelligence test results are measure of one's worth and usefulness to society, and so on are completely incorrect and without any foundation (Sattler, 2008). Intelligence tests are samples of behaviour from which useful diagnostic information can be inferred. Quite likely, intelligence tests are overused in school settings. For example, there is increasing evidence that intelligence tests are not at all useful for the assessment and diagnosis of learning disabilities (Weiss et al., 2015). However, intelligence tests may be most useful in the assessment and diagnosis of intellectual disabilities. Nonetheless, there are important challenges and caveats to the use of intelligence tests for persons who are referred for a possible diagnosis of intellectual disabilities.

The administration and interpretation of intelligence tests require extensive training that typically includes multiple graduate level classes, supervised field work, and supervised internship experiences. Intelligence tests are robust and stable and are not largely influenced by fatigue or "having a bad day" (Sattler, 2008). There are important assumptions for the administration of most intelligence tests, and these assumptions are typically described in the test administration and interpretation manual. Some examples of assumptions of intelligence tests are intact visual and auditory acuity, ability to understand oral directions, English as first language, strong fine motor skills, sufficient motivation to attempt items, ability to develop rapport with the examiner, emotional regulation to address inevitable frustration when items become too difficult, and the ability to sit and attend for a significant length of time (usually 30–120 min; Flanagan & Harrison, 2012). For individuals suspected of having intellectual disabilities, many of these assumptions may not be met. Although robust and stable even when some of the assumptions are not met, validity of test scores can rightly be called into question for the assessment of many children suspected of having intellectual disabilities. Examiners must use their judgement to determine whether the test is valid or not. This decision must be made prior to scoring test items to avoid creating a likely biased post hoc explanation for unanticipated test results (Weiss et al., 2015). Some methods for addressing violations of the assumptions of standardized intelligence tests are addressed in the section below entitled, specialized situations.

Most tests of intelligence involve a variety of cognitive task ranging from vocabulary to drawing inferences from pictorial stimuli to measures of working memory. Results from this battery of tests are placed in a composite to develop an overall measure of general mental ability (aka IQ; Richards, Brady, & Taylor, 2014). Individuals with intellectual disabilities score in the lowest 2% of individuals taking the exact same test. An important note is that individuals with intellectual disabilities will have variation on the specific cognitive tasks and quite likely persons being assessed will score at or near the average range on at least some of the tests. This "subtest scatter" of high and low scores does not preclude a diagnosis of intellectual disabilities (Schalock & Luckasson, 2015). The criteria for diagnosis is overall general mental ability that is significantly below average, which is based on a composite of specific cognitive skills. Strengths on specific cognitive tasks may serve as useful information for planning interventions. Although profile analysis of the strengths and weaknesses demonstrated on intelligence tests is a common practice, the full scale or composite measure is by far the most reliable and useful metric

(Ritchie, 2015). For purposes of diagnosis of intellectual disabilities, the full scale or composite score is the primary score that should be used in making diagnostic decisions unless there are unusual circumstances. There are several norm-referenced and standardized tests of cognitive ability that are widely used.

Wechsler Scales

The Wechsler intelligence scales are the most commonly used for the diagnosis of intellectual disabilities. The three different scales are the Wechsler Adult Intelligence Scale-IV (ages 16 and over; Wechsler, 2013), the Wechsler Intelligence Scale for Children-V (ages 6–16; Wechsler, 2015), and the Wechsler Preschool and Primary Scale of Intelligence-IV (ages 4 to 6 1/2; Wechsler, 2012). These scales all have a mean (average) of 100 and standard deviation of 15. Scores approximately 70 and below are consistent with intellectual disabilities. The most common interpretation is that full-scale scores between 69 and 50 are consistent with mild intellectual disabilities and 35–49 consistent with moderate intellectual disabilities. The Wechsler scales typically have a floor of 4 standard deviations below the mean, meaning that full scale scores lower than 40 are not possible (Simeonsson, Granlund, & Bjorck-Akesson, 2003). An important assumption of the Wechsler scales is that intelligence is a function of performance, and not capacity. Wechsler originally defined intelligence as an individual's ability to adapt and constructively solve problems in the environment. Noncognitive factors such as expressive language delays, receptive language issues, motor issues, sensory impairment, inattentiveness, or motivation to perform can all play major factors in a full-scale score. As such, the Wechsler is not an appropriate measure for all persons being considered for the diagnosis of intellectual disabilities. An important, yet subtle and often ignored factor is that Wechsler assumes that intelligence cannot be seen or its existence clearly verified and therefore cannot be reliably measured directly (Weiss et al., 2015). But performance and function can be reliably measured and overall mental ability inferred from performance. Certainly, over the 75 years that Wechsler scales have been assessing intelligence, this is a reasonable approach that has proved effective in the typical population. However, for persons with intellectual disabilities and often multiple other impairments that influence function, significant caution and humility must be exercised when inferring general intelligence from performance (Kaufman, Reynolds, Liu, Kaufman, & McGrew, 2012). The Wechsler scales are outstanding and well-developed norm-referenced measures of general mental ability.

Stanford-Binet

The lineage of the Stanford-Binet goes back to 1905. The Stanford-Binet Intelligence Scale, Fifth Edition, was published in 2003 (Roid & Barram, 2004). The Stanford-Binet is an individually administered intelligence test and closely resembles the strengths and weaknesses of the Wechsler scales. The Stanford-Binet is for persons aged 2–85. The Stanford-Binet provides assessment of five factors of cognitive ability that include fluid reasoning, knowledge, quantitative reasoning, visual spatial processing, and working memory. Theoretically, there is little difference between the Stanford-Binet and Wechsler scales in the assessment of general mental ability. The Stanford-Binet may have some improvements in that there are several items that require no or minimal oral responses from the examinee and there are many manipulatives in the assessment. Although this may be effective and appropriate for persons with limited expressive language, there are significant problems with a child who has motoric impairments. There is a brief battery called the Stanford-Binet Intelligence Scales for Early Childhood (Roid, 2005), which is a subset of the larger Stanford-Binet and is targeted for children aged 2–5 years and 11 months. Although many of the items and design are taken directly from the broader Stanford-Binet, there is an emphasis on nonverbal tasks. Like the Wechsler scales, the Stanford-Binet has a mean of 100 and standard deviation of 15 and a range of scores between 40 and 160. Limitations of the Stanford-Binet for assessment of persons with intellectual disabilities are similar to that of the Wechsler scales.

The Kaufman Assessment Battery for Children-II (Kaufman & Kaufman, 2004) is a widely used measure of general intelligence that purports to be a culturally fair measure of cognitive ability for children aged 3–18. Rather than dividing intelligence into verbal and nonverbal, which has been the traditional approach in assessment of intelligence, the K-ABC-II divides information into simultaneous and successive processing. An advantage of the K-ABC-II over the Wechsler and Stanford-Binet is that many of the tasks are less culturally loaded (i.e. symbolic, abstract, and language reduced). Moreover, the activities are engaging and much like play tasks. Although the engaging activities can help with some aspects of motivation, it is not clear whether the K-ABC-II and its claims of cultural fairness are entirely consistent with research evidence.

The Woodcock Johnson Tests of Cognitive Abilities—Fourth Edition (Shrank, McGrew, Mather, & Woodcock, 2014) shares much with the previously reported measures of cognitive functioning. This individually administered test of intelligence is designed to be an effective measure for people aged 2 through the mid-1990s. This is a wide-ranging measure of assessment that covers many performance factors. The primary difference between the Woodcock-Johnson and the other measures is that the Woodcock-Johnson has few manipulatives and only a couple of the tests are timed. This makes the Woodcock-Johnson a much stronger test for individuals who may have motor difficulties and unable to physically manipulate blocks and beads, which are common tasks among the other important measures.

In terms of technical sophistication, all the above tasks are professionally designed, well developed, normed on a representative sample, and have adequate reliability, validity, and freedom of evidence of bias. In terms of a measure of overall general mental ability using the composite index, there is little to choose between these measures. The primary differences are quite specific in terms of the types of tasks that are being measured. Another important factor is the year in which a test was normed and published. Because of the Flynn effect (the reliable observation that intelligence test scores are increasing at a rate of about 0.3 IQ points per year), test using older normative samples will yield higher composite IQ scores than those using recently developed measures (Ritchie, 2015). Because the criterion for composite intelligence test scores for diagnosis of intellectual disabilities is typically 70, a newer test is more likely to yield lower scores due to the artefact of the Flynn effect and result in more frequent scores below 70. Interpretation of intelligence test scores for an individual having multiple tests over time needs to consider which tests were administered and when they were published. Professional decisions need to be made in terms of which types of task will allow an individual to perform in a manner consistent with their overall mental abilities.

Measures of intelligence have not changed a great deal over the last 50 years. Most measures do not represent significant changes in how intelligence is assessed. Many intelligence measures are more theoretically based than they have been in the past. The primary issue is that much of society, including the great number of psychologists and educators, have dismissed or called into question the value of cognitive assessment. The positive component of this criticism is that the results of intelligence tests should be interpreted with humility and caution when concerning the predictive value and scope of the meaning of intelligence test scores, which are valuable and important yet limited. However, standardized and norm-referenced intelligence test scores are the most reliable and valid for the diagnosis of intellectual disabilities of any measure in psychology with no evidence of bias concerning ethnic groups or socioeconomic status (Ritchie, 2015). Cognitive assessment is the foundation from which a diagnosis of intellectual disabilities is made. Nonetheless, professional judgement of an experienced and well-trained clinician remains that foundation of quality cognitive assessment and the test scores serve to provide information to assist in diagnosis and future planning.

Adaptive Behaviour

Adaptive behaviour is the other major factor involved in diagnosing intellectual disabilities. Consistent with Wechsler's conceptualization of intelligence, adaptive behaviour is an approach to assessing one's ability to adapt and constructively solve problems. Yet, tests of cognitive ability do so in a standardized and one-on-one situation in which adaptation and constructively solving problems are inferred from performance on a test; adaptive behaviour represents observations and reports of how the individual functions in their environment. Among the skills that comprise adaptive behaviour are literacy; self-direction; concepts of money, number, and time; interpersonal skills; social responsibility; self-esteem; gullibility; social problem-solving; following rules such as obeying laws, workplace rules, and social interaction; personal care; job skills; use of money; safety; healthcare; travel and transportation; and use of communication devices such as email, texting, telephone, and the Internet (Stadler, Becker, Gödker, Leutner, & Greiff, 2015). The advantages of this approach are that the artificial and performance-driven assumptions of cognitive assessment are eliminated from consideration. Whereas cognitive assessments are based on constructs that must be inferred from performance, adaptive behaviour represents a collection of specific skills that can be the basis from which to develop interventions to improve functioning. The disadvantages are that adaptive behaviour measures rely on reports from caregivers, teachers, and interviews with the individual being assessed. There can be a significant amount of error concerning accurate recall, the psychological filter used by each respondent, and potential bias. Diagnostic criteria vary as to how to interpret adaptive behaviour measures for purposes of meeting the criteria as a person with an intellectual disability. ICD and DSM require that a composite measure of adaptive behaviour be approximately two standard deviations below the mean (Wei, Oakland, & Algina, 2008). For these two definitions, a composite score is the metric of interest for diagnosis. For the American Association on Intellectual and Developmental Disabilities (Schalock et al., 2007) definition of intellectual disabilities, at least two of ten subdomains of adaptive behaviour must be impaired to meet this component of the diagnostic criteria for eligibility. In cases where the issue of performance on standardized measures of cognitive ability confounds inferences about intellectual functioning, adaptive behaviour may be the best indicator of general functional ability. As is typical of all the criteria for a diagnosis of intellectual disabilities, one of the most important aspects of any diagnosable psychiatric issue is impairment of real-world functioning. Adaptive behaviour reflects the strengths and weaknesses in real-life functioning.

There are multiple available measures of adaptive behaviour that are relatively similar in scope and detail. Most of these assessment instruments involve behaviour checklists or interviews with caregivers or teachers. The key variable is that the respondent reporting on the adaptive behaviour must have multiple opportunities to see the individual engage in these opportunities over a long period. At least 6 months of time spent with the individual is required. This makes assessment extremely difficult for persons who have been had multiple caregivers, have receive care through institutional settings, or have been raised in multiple foster care settings. Consistent observation is necessary because most of the instruments involve a continuum of how regularly the individual engages in adaptive and functional adaptive behaviour and how completely, what quality, or how effectively does the individual meet the needs of their environment. Adaptive behaviour measures are administered in a standardized fashion (i.e. interview or checklist) and are norm-referenced. Among the high-quality adaptive behaviour measurements available are Scales for Independent Behaviour-Revised (Bruininks, Woodcock, Weatherman, & Hill, 1996a), Vineland Adaptive Behaviour Scales-III (Sparrow, Cicchetti, & Salnier, 2016), Inventory for Client and Agency Planning (Bruininks, Woodcock, Weatherman, & Hill, 1996b), Adaptive Behaviour Assessment System-II (Harrison & Oakland, 2003), and AAIDD Adaptive Behaviour Scales (Tasse, Balboni, Schalock, & Zhang, 2010). There is also important overlap between general measures of adaptive behaviour and more specific measures such as social skills and maladaptive behaviour measures. In addition, some early childhood measures such as the Bayley Scales also include adaptive behaviour assessment within the scale itself (Bayley, 2006).

Academic Achievement

In the case of preschool children and adults being considered for diagnosis of intellectual disabilities, academic skills are subsumed under the category of adaptive behaviour. Basic literacy, number concepts, and written language are assessed in all the basic adaptive behaviour scales described above. School-based assessment of intellectual disabilities most often requires that functioning in the school be the primary adaptive behaviour that is affected. However, for the case of school-aged children where eligibility for specialized education is concerned, a full and complete standardized and norm-referenced measure of academic achievement is to be administered in most situations. Academic achievement test scores below two standard deviations from the mean are not necessary for a formal diagnosis of intellectual disabilities based on most definitions; however, there must be some evidence of significant impairment in academic skills for a student to be eligible for specialized educational services. This can be confusing because many measures of academic achievement have a floor that is too high for younger grades. For example, on several measures of academic achievement, if a child receives a raw score of zero correct, this may result in a standard score of 80. The reason for this is that a 5-year-old kindergarten student is not expected to have many academic skills in reading or mathematics. A child who has seriously impaired academic skills due to intellectual disabilities at age 5 will not differ dramatically from a typical 5-year-old. This makes early diagnosis difficult in younger grades because the differences between intellectually disabled and typically developing students are challenging to discriminate. However, the gap between typically developing students and students with intellectual disabilities will reliably grow over time. This phenomenon is known as a cumulative deficit (Flanagan & Harrison, 2012). A common occurrence when assessing academic achievement is that for children with intellectual disabilities, there may be a decrease in standard scores over time. This does not necessarily mean that that child is losing skills or deteriorating in function. As a norm-referenced measure, most academic achievement tests simply provide a relative rank of skills compared to a distribution of age peers. For most cases, decreasing standard scores simply indicate that the child is losing ground to age peers or not improving at the same rate as age peers. Interpretation of raw scores is necessary to determine whether a child is losing absolute skills over time. In many cases, interviewing teachers is a good method of determining whether the child is losing absolute skills or simply has a decrease in standard scores due to an artefact of a norm-referenced test.

There are multiple norm-referenced standardized tests that are widely used for the assessment of school-aged children with intellectual disabilities. All of which are professionally designed and normed and have sufficient psychometric characteristics. Although there are specific diagnostic tests for each subdomain of academic skills such as the Test of Early Math Ability-2 (Ginsburg & Baroody, 2003) or the Mather-Woodcock Group Writing Test (Mather, 1997) among dozens of domain-specific tests of academic skills, for the assessment of individuals referred for a possible diagnosis of intellectual disabilities, comprehensive academic achievement tests are usually used. Among the widely used individually administered tests of comprehensive academic achievement are Kaufman Tests of Educational Achievement (Kaufman, 2014), Peabody Individual Achievement Test (Markwardt, 1997), Wechsler Individual Achievement Test (Wechsler, 2009), Woodcock-Johnson Tests of Achievement (Shrank, Mather, McGrew, & Woodcock, 2014), Test of Academic Achievement Skills (Gardner, 1999), and several others.

Behaviour

Behavioural and mental health problems are common in persons with intellectual disabilities referred to as "dual diagnosis". In many cases, symptoms that may indicate a diagnosable mental health problem are often ignored by caregivers, educators, and clinicians because of a process known as "diagnostic overshadowing". This is when maladaptive behaviours are attributed entirely to the logical consequences of intellectual disabilities and the possible mental health conditions are overshadowed by the intellectual disability. Too often, behaviours that could be attributed to mental health issues may be identified as consistent with or evidence of autism spectrum disorder (Kendall & Owen, 2015). There are a variety of teacher, caregiver and parent, and self-report behavioural instruments that assist in making diagnosis. However, most of these measures are norm-referenced measures that compare behaviours to a typically developing normative sample. The result is that many of these checklist result in an overestimation of mental health problems in persons with intellectual disabilities primarily due to inherent communication and cognitive deficits influencing results of these psychiatric or behavioural measures (Pearl & Mayes, 2016).

The Reiss Screen for Maladaptive Behavior (Reiss & Valenti-Hein, 1990) and the Reiss Scales for Children's Dual Diagnosis (Reiss & Valenti-Hein, 1994) are excellent and brief checklists completed by teachers, caregiver and parents, and others who know the individual well enough to rate whether each of 60 symptoms of psychiatric disorders are no problem, a problem, or a major problem in the person's life that negatively affect functioning. This screening instrument is designed to determine if the individual should be referred to professionals for more advanced professional diagnosis by subspecialist such as a psychiatrist. Mental health and psychiatric diagnosis always have complicating factors. For persons with impaired coping skills, communication skills, social skills, motor skills, and community experience for chronological age, diagnoses for persons with intellectual disabilities increase the difficulty of diagnosis by an order of magnitude.

Language

Language is a central component of cognitive functioning. Without any form of semiotic medium, it is impossible for persons to develop abstract reasoning. A person without any form of communication is unlikely to mentally progress much past the cognitive capacity of a typically developing 2-year-old child. Language is also a keystone variable when it comes to behaviour and mental health issues as well. Language skills are not only required for communication with others, but also for self-talk, which is essential for self-regulation, self-calming, and mental representation of problems and overall reasoning (Fu, Lincoln, Bellugi, & Searcy, 2015). Therefore, disentangling language from cognitive, adaptive behaviour, academic achievement, and mental health is nearly impossible. Language is an extraordinarily complex construct that is difficult for many psychologists and educators to assess. Conducting a multidisciplinary assessment with a speech and language pathologists conducting the language assessment can add a great deal of expertise and nuance to the assessment results.

One measure that is widely used by educators and psychologists is the Clinical Evaluation of Language Fundamentals-5 (Wiig, Semel, & Secord, 2013). The CELF-5 is an excellent measure of receptive language, expressive language, language structure, and language content. There is also a core language score which is the composite language index. This measure is for persons aged 5–21 years and 11 months. The CELF-5 does not have an especially sensitive floor and may not be accurate would lower functioning persons. Aspects of language such as phonology, morphology, syntax, and semantics are well assessed by the CELF-5 and other measures. An important feature for persons with intellectual disabilities and autism spectrum disorder is limitations in pragmatics. Pragmatics includes all aspects of the communication process such as conversation turn-taking, reading and exhibiting body language that is appropriate to assist in the communication, personal space, inferring intent of the speaker, and using context to infer and communicate meaning. Any strong assessment of language for persons with intellectual disabilities needs to include some component of pragmatics in the assessment process.

Specialized Situations

The commonly used measures of cognitive ability, adaptive behaviour, and other components that are usually used in psychoeducational assessment are effective for most cases where diagnosis of intellectual disabilities is being considered. However, this population is heterogeneous and is at risk of sensory and medical issues, behavioural and mental health problems, attention issues, motor impairments, language problems, and a host of other issues that may make traditional assessment challenging. Moreover, there are confounding factors such as the presence of autism spectrum disorders in conjunction with intellectual disabilities, malingering in cases where an individual may benefit or be motivated to perform in a manner much lower than their true functioning, and persons with extremely low levels of functioning who may not be appropriate for typical standardized and norm-referenced measures. There are no children who are "untestable". However, the assessment and diagnosis of intellectual disabilities is a complex and professional undertaking that is not amenable to cookie-cutter procedures.

Sensory Impairments

Most domains of psychoeducational assessment assume intact visual and auditory acuity. Before a formal assessment for diagnosis of intellectual disabilities can be undertaken, formal and accurate vision and hearing screening are required. Much like responses to standardized cognitive tasks, responses to auditory and visual stimuli can also be affected by the same confounding factors affecting performance (e.g. motivation, understanding directions, fine motor skills, oral communication), thus, making inferences about vision and hearing unclear. There are screening measures that are virtually performance free such as, auditory and visually evoked potentials; yet, these are often not widely available, and inferences concerning functional vision and hearing acuity are questionable (Shannon, Félix, Krumholz, Goldstein, & Harris, 1984).

To provide information supporting a diagnosis of intellectual disabilities, the clinician is required to infer cognitive functioning via performance, but not have performance heavily influenced by sensory impairment. As such, the clinician must select instruments that minimize the effect of any possible sensory impairments. For example, a cognitive assessment that depends solely on oral instructions and oral responses is unlikely to be an effective measure of cognitive ability for a person with hearing loss. Likewise, entirely visual tasks such as block design on the Wechsler scales or response to incomplete matrices on multiple measures of cognitive ability are inappropriate for a person with visual impairments. Psychoeducational assessment of persons with sensory impairments is more than simply taking care of how information is presented to the person being assessed and method of response; there is also the probability that cognitive processing is significantly different for persons with sensory impairments. Persons with sensory impairments have a host of challenges adapting to their environment, and it is difficult to differentiate challenges and ability to adapt to the environment due to sensory impairment or due to intellectual disabilities. There are measures and techniques for cognitive assessment of persons with hearing and vision impairment.

In the case of persons with visual impairment, verbal or haptic forms of assessment are used. Most commonly, oral directions with oral responses are the most common form of assessment. However, there must be caution taken to ensure that the forms of questions and answers do not require extensive visual experience. For example, the question, "What colour are strawberries?" may be inappropriate because there is a higher probability of getting the item correct if the person being assessed has visual experience. Also note that few people with visual impairments have mastered braille reading. Moreover, even the most proficient braille readers are significantly slower than typical sighted reading. Understanding common issues directly related to the sensory impairment is a key feature of psychoeducational assessment.

For persons with auditory impairment, there are also multiple measures available that involve limited oral instructions. Measures such as the Raven's Progressive Matrices (Raven, Raven, & Court, 1998), Leiter International Performance Scale,

Third Edition (Roid, Miller, Pomplun, & Koch, 2013), and Wechsler Nonverbal Scale of Ability (Wechsler, 2015) require no oral response, and directions can be administered via gestures and modelling. The Universal Nonverbal Intelligence Test—Second Edition (Bracken & McCallum, 2015) is designed with standardized gestures that are taught to examinees and used for directions and for responses. Students with sign language skills are most effectively assessed in their preferred language within clinician who shares those language skills. Usually, cognitive assessment of persons with sensory impairments is a subspecialty area requiring specialized training and experience.

Motor Impairment

Performance from which cognitive abilities are inferred requires motor skills. Even in extreme cases where eyeblink or eye movement is used as the response communication, some degree of motor movement is required. However, motor impairments are common for persons who are being assessed for possible intellectual disabilities. Cerebral palsy, significant tremors, nystagmus, apraxia, neuromuscular control, and other disorders of fine motor movement are common for a host of genetic and idiopathic causes of impaired cognitive functioning. When there are questions about fine motor skills, it can be helpful to have an assessment conducted by an occupational therapist to determine the role that fine motor impairment plays in the ability of the person being assessed to adapt to their environment and appropriate modifications for accurate assessment. Establishing an effective response mechanism is important. Altering a standardized instrument can be problematic, and all deviations from standardization procedures need to be recorded.

Malingering

Malingering is intentionally performing in such a way that a diagnosis of intellectual disabilities can be made. Malingering is not the same as a lack of motivation to respond or engage in the assessment process. The goal of malingering is to "fake bad" to receive a diagnosis. Malingering is rare in childhood. However, there are reported cases of parents coaching children on how to give incorrect responses to tests of cognitive ability and those same parents underestimating the child's functional ability on adaptive behaviour scales. The purpose of such parent-driven malingering is often to receive additional financial supports from government programs such as Social Security Disability Insurance. Again, these are rare events (Lyle & Simplican, 2015). More common incidents of malingering in the assessment of intellectual disabilities relate to legal matters for adolescents and adults. Competence to stand trial and using intellectual disabilities as a diagnosis to mitigate punishment are common. There are multiple methods to assess malingering.

There are formal measures such as the Test of Memory Malingering (Tombaugh, 1999) and the Word Memory Test (Green, 2004). Strong assessment of background, record review, and interviewing those who know the person being assessed well can assist in determining the history of presenting symptoms of intellectual disabilities.

Severe and Profound Intellectual Disabilities

Providing psychoeducational assessment to persons who are severely impaired is a clincal challenge. Under the DSM-5 and ICD-11 diagnostic criteria, these persons would be classified as severe to profound in their degree of intellectual disabilities. They typically require continuous and extensive supports for elementary functioning and may also have multiple disabilities, including medical involvement. For purposes of a psychoeducational assessment, few of the standardized and norm-referenced assessments of mental ability are appropriate. Nearly all widely used measures have a floor with a standard score of 40. People with a composite intelligence test score of less than 40 are difficult to assess. Quite often psychological reports have the phrase "untestable" for these individuals. All people are testable, yet it may be difficult to create a strong estimate of general mental ability.

Providing exact numbers representing a standardized composite score of intelligence below 40 is a meaningless exercise. A standard score of 40 is equivalent to a 0.0064 percentile rank. A standard score of 25 is equivalent to a 0.0000601 percentile rank. There may be some diagnostic or program eligibility ramifications to providing composite standard scores. However, if a person clearly has a strong evidence of intellectual disability, a formal score cannot be achieved; the DSM-5 allows for a diagnosis of intellectual disabilities, severity unspecified. Although the use of a Wechsler scales or Stanford-Binet assessment of intelligence is not recommended, even accurate standard scores at this level are unlikely to add significant functional value.

Descriptive measures can be productive and useful for educational planning. There are four simple examples of creative assessment that can provide useful information for extremely low-functioning persons. For persons with profound levels of intellectual disabilities, classical conditioning could provide valuable information. For example, using a penlight to elicit a pupillary response paired with the ringing of the bell can provide valuable information. After the pairing is successful, typically 8–15 presentations, then ring the bell alone and carefully observe for pupillary response. This form of learning is extremely simple yet clearly demonstrates a form of effective instruction. Another example is to use simple Piagetian tasks to determine whether sensorimotor tasks such as coordination of reactions, secondary, and tertiary reactions that demonstrate cause-and-effect, object permanence, and internal representational thought. A series of toys such as rattles and brightly coloured objects can provide an improvisational laboratory to determine the skills that a low-functioning individual represents. The third approach can be complex but is a potentially useful description. This is a form of the Fantz preference test (Langlois et al., 1987) that is well known in developmental psychology for assessment of infants. This idea is based on the human preference for novelty. An example would be to hold up to similar objects such as large yellow balls in the left hand and in the right hand. Repeat the presentation until the person becomes bored or satiated to looking at the objects. Then change so one of the hands holds a large blue cube. Observe carefully to see if the person's gaze shifts to the new stimulus. This would indicate that the person can discriminate between objects. One could easily vary tasks by shape, colour, utility, familiarity, or a host of variables. Shifts in gauge demonstrate the ability to discriminate. The final example would be trials required to learn a task. For example, an individual is presented with two blocks and teaches them to stack one on top of the other. Instruction methods may include modelling, hand-over-hand teaching, oral directions, and other mechanisms—all with heavy social reinforcement for success. The number of trials required for an individual to successfully complete the task independently is then counted. Once success on the task has been achieved, other activities can be pursued during the assessment process. After a period of 20 min or so, the block stacking task is reintroduced. Then the number of trials required to be successes is counted again. If the individual successfully completes the task with fewer trials or with fewer required teaching interventions, then learning of the task can be inferred. This indicates that learning is possible and can provide some information about which forms of teaching and learning techniques are more successful. These are simple assessment techniques that go well beyond standardized and norm-referenced assessment. Detailed descriptions of the methods used for this descriptive form of assessment will need to be included in the psychoeducational assessment report. To conduct any of these qualitative assessment techniques, clear understanding and evaluation of the assessment needs, theories of cognitive development, comfort levels, and skills of the individual must be determined via record review, background information, and assessment of adaptive behaviour through interviews with caregivers, teachers, or others having knowledge of the individual being assessed.

An important feature of individuals who may be resistant or unable to complete the standardized assessment process is that performance may be inconsistent and extremely context specific. For example, some persons are easily fatigues and may provide useful responses for 10 min or less. Assessing these individuals over a period of several sessions is important to determine the consistency of performance. There are also limitations as to the inferences that can be made by the performance of the individual. It is far better to say that a person "did not successfully complete a task" rather than "cannot successfully complete a task". Although typically most psychoeducational assessment is conducted without parents or caregivers present, it is often helpful to have them present during assessment. Frequent checks with the parents with phrases like, "have you ever seen her engage in this behaviour before?" and then follow up with "under what conditions did you see her engage in this behaviour?" simply because an individual does not show the behaviour in the artificial and unique situation of formal testing does not mean they are unable to complete the behaviour in another context.

Another option for individuals who are difficult to assess with standardized instruments is the Developmental Assessment for Students with Severe Disabilities—Third Edition (DASH-3) (Dykes & Mruzek, 2012). This is a criterion-referenced tool to measure specific skills for persons of all ages with severe, multiple, physical, and sensory disabilities. The DASH-3 can also be an effective instrument for persons with autism. This measure allows for identification of skills that could not be assessed due to task resistance, skills that are not performed independently, and skills that are considered priorities for interventions. The scales of the DASH-3 include sensorimotor, language, social-emotional, activities of daily living, and academics. This measure uses a combination of interviews with caregivers and teachers and direct assessment to develop the skill levels on each of the scales. This measure can also be used in repeated measures to track progress over time.

Autism

The diagnosis of autism spectrum disorder has become extraordinarily common as the incidence rates are now estimated to be 1 in 68 (Centers for Disease Control, 2014). As mentioned in previous chapters, the rise of incidence of autism is likely due to shifting definitions, societal awareness, and availability of treatments and funding that are earmarked solely for persons with a diagnosis of autism. In addition, the diagnoses of intellectual disabilities have decreased over the same period. Autism is most typically assessed via the Autism Diagnostic Observation Schedule (Lord, Rutter, DeLavore, & Risi, 2008) and the Autism Diagnostic Interview (Rutter, LeCouteur, & Lord, 2008). However, a large percentage (estimated to be between 25% and 55%) of children diagnosed with autism spectrum disorder also have intellectual disabilities. These two conditions can co-occur. Caution in diagnosis is required because many of the characteristics of autism spectrum disorder such as language delays, social deficits, and stereotyped or unusual behaviours are also common for individuals with severe and profound intellectual disabilities. Currently, there is not enough specificity in the available psychoeducational instrumentation or in the socially derived diagnostic criteria for autism and intellectual disabilities to differentiate with the above instruments described.

Summary

The psychoeducational assessment of persons with intellectual disabilities is extraordinarily complex. This is an area in which there have not been major visible changes in the field due to advances in research. However, the quality of assessment tools available, the emphasis on early screening and early identification, and the focus on function have resulted in subtle changes in the scope and purpose of psychoeducational and diagnostic assessment. Although the criteria are simple:

standardized and norm-referenced intelligence test scores below two standard deviations from the mean, significantly impaired adaptive behaviour, and the onset of symptoms occurs before the age of 18; the act of conducting psychoeducational assessment for a diagnosis that is considered lifelong requires attention to detail and strong understanding of the nature of cognitive abilities.

References

Achenbach, T. M. (2009). *The Achenbach system of empirically based assessment (ASEBA): Development, findings, theory, and applications*. Burlington, VT: University of Vermont Research Center for Children, Youth, & Families. Vineland Social Emotional Early Childhood Scales.

Alpern, G. D. (2007). *Developmental profile-3*. Los Angeles, CA: Western Psychological Services.

American Academy of Pediatrics Policy Statement. (2006). Identifying infants and young children with developmental disorders in the medical home: An algorithm for developmental surveillance and screening. *Pediatrics, 118*, 405–420.

Bayley, N. (2006). *Bayley scales of infant and toddler development-third edition: Administration manual*. San Antonio, TX: Harcourt Assessment.

Blasingame, G. D. (2016). Assessment, diagnosis, and risk management of sexual offenders with intellectual disabilities. In A. Phenix & H. M. Hoberman (Eds.), *Sexual offending* (pp. 227–246). New York, NY: Springer. Retrieved from http://link.springer.com/chapter/10.1007/978-1-4939-2416-5_11

Boyle, C. A., Boulet, S., Schieve, L. A., Cohen, R. A., Blumberg, S. J., Yeargin-Allsopp, M., … Kogan, M. D. (2011). Trends in the prevalence of developmental disabilities in us children, 1997–2008. *Pediatrics, 127*(6), 1034–1042. https://doi.org/10.1542/peds.2010-2989

Bracken, B. A., & McCallum, R. S. (2015). *Universal nonverbal intelligence test* (2nd ed.). Itasca, IL: Riverside Publishers.

Brown, I., Hatton, C., & Emerson, E. (2013). Quality of life indicators for individuals with intellectual disabilities: Extending current practice. *Intellectual and Developmental Disabilities, 51*(5), 316–332. https://doi.org/10.1352/1934-9556-51.5.316

Bruininks, R. H., Woodcock, R. W., Weatherman, R. F., & Hill, B. K. (1996a). *Scales of independent behaviour – Revised*. New York, NY: Houghton Mifflin Harcourt.

Bruininks, R. H., Woodcock, R. W., Weatherman, R. F., & Hill, B. K. (1996b). *Inventory for client and agency planning*. Rolling Meadows, IL: The Riverside Publishing Company.

Centers for Disease Control. (2014). *Prevalence of autism spectrum disorder among children aged 8 years autism and developmental disabilities monitoring network, 11 sites, United States, 2010*. (2014, April 25). Retrieved May 18, 2017, from https://web.archive.org/web/20140425185152/http://www.cdc.gov/mmwr/preview/mmwrhtml/ss6302a1.htm?s_cid=ss6302a1_w

Dykes, M. K., & Mruzek, D. W. (2012). *Developmental assessment for individuals with severe disabilities* (3rd ed.). Los Angeles, CA: Western Psychological Services.

Flanagan, D. P., & Harrison, P. L. (2012). *Contemporary intellectual assessment, third edition: Theories, tests, and issues*. New York, NY: Guilford Press.

Frankenburg, W. K., Dodds, J., & Archer, P. (1990). *The Denver II technical manual*. Denver, CO: Denver Developmental Materials.

Fu, T. J., Lincoln, A. J., Bellugi, U., & Searcy, Y. M. (2015). The association of intelligence, visual-motor functioning, and personality characteristics with adaptive behavior in individuals with Williams syndrome. *American Journal on Intellectual and Developmental Disabilities, 120*(4), 273–288. https://doi.org/10.1352/1944-7558-120.4.273

Fujiura, G. T. (2013). The demarcation of intellectual disability. *Intellectual and Developmental Disabilities, 51*(2), 83–85. https://doi.org/10.1352/1934-9556-51.2.083

Gardner, M. F. (1999). *Test of academic achievement skills*. New York, NY: ATP.

Ginsburg, H., & Baroody, A. (2003). *TEMA-3 examiners manual* (3rd ed.). Austin, TX: PRO-ED.

Glascoe, F. P. (1997). *Parents' evaluation of developmental status (PEDS)*. Nashville, TN: Ellsworth & Vandermeer Press.

Green, P. (2004). *Word memory test*. Kelowna, BC: Author.

Greenspan, S., Harris, J. C., & Woods, G. W. (2015). Intellectual disability is "a condition, not a number": Ethics of IQ cut-offs in psychiatry, human services and law. *Ethics, Medicine and Public Health, 1*(3), 312–324. https://doi.org/10.1016/j.jemep.2015.07.004

Harrison, P. L., & Oakland, T. (2003). *Adaptive behavior assessment system – Second edition*. San Antonio, TX: The Psychological CorporationIndividuals with Disabilities Education Act, 20 U.S.C. § 1400 (2004).

Hemmings, C., & Bouras, N. (2016). *Psychiatric and behavioural disorders in intellectual and developmental disabilities*. Cambridge, England: Cambridge University Press.

Ireton, H. (1992). *Child development inventory*. Minneapolis, MN: Behaviour Science Systems.

Jensen, A. R., & McGurk, F. C. J. (1987). Black-white bias in "cultural" and "noncultural" test items. *Journal of Personality and Individual Differences, 8*, 295–301.

Kaufman, A. S. (2014). *Kaufman tests of educational achievement* (3rd ed.). New York, NY: Pearson.

Kaufman, A. S., & Kaufman, N. L. (2004). *Kaufman assessment battery for children* (2nd ed.). San Antonio, TX: Pearson.

Kaufman, S. B., Reynolds, M. R., Liu, X., Kaufman, A. S., & McGrew, K. S. (2012). Are cognitive g and academic achievement g one and the same g? An exploration on the woodcock–Johnson and Kaufman tests. *Intelligence, 40*(2), 123–138. https://doi.org/10.1016/j.intell.2012.01.009

Kendall, K., & Owen, M. J. (2015). Intellectual disability and psychiatric comorbidity: Challenges and clinical issues. *Psychiatric Times, 32*(5), 60–63.

Langlois, J. H., Roggman, L. A., Casey, R. J., Ritter, J. M., Rieser-Danner, L. A., & Jenkins, V. Y. (1987). Infant preferences for attractive faces: Rudiments of a stereotype? *Developmental Psychology, 23*, 363–369.

Lord, C., Rutter, M., DeLavore, P. C., & Risi, S. (2008). *Autism diagnostic observation schedule*. Los Angeles, CA: Western Psychological Services.

Luckasson, R., & Schalock, R. L. (2013). What's at stake in the lives of people with intellectual disability? Part ii: Recommendations for naming, defining, diagnosing, classifying, and planning supports. *Intellectual and Developmental Disabilities, 51*(2), 94–101. https://doi.org/10.1352/1934-9556-51.2.094

Luckasson, R., & Schalock, R. L. (2015). Standards to guide the use of clinical judgment in the field of intellectual disability. *Intellectual and Developmental Disabilities, 53*(3), 240–251. https://doi.org/10.1352/1934-9556-53.3.240

Lyle, M. L., & Simplican, S. C. (2015). Elite repudiation of the R-word and public opinion about intellectual disability. *Intellectual and Developmental Disabilities, 53*(3), 211–227. https://doi.org/10.1352/1934-9556-53.3.211

Mardell, C., & Goldenberg, D. S. (2011). *Developmental indicators for the assessment of learning* (4th ed.). New York, NY: Pearson.

Markwardt, F. C. (1997). *Peabody individual achievement test – Revised*. New York, NY: Pearson.

Mather, N. (1997). *Mather Woodcock group writing test*. Rolling Meadows, IL: Riverside.

Neisworth, J. T., Bagnato, S. J., Salvia, J., & Hunt, F. M. (1999). *Temperament and atypical behaviour scale*. Baltimore, MD: Brookes.

Pearl, A. M., & Mayes, S. D. (2016). Methods and procedures for measuring comorbid disorders: Psychological. In J. L. Matson (Ed.), *Comorbid conditions among children with autism spectrum disorders* (pp. 45–63). New York, NY: Springer. Retrieved from http://link.springer.com/chapter/10.1007/978-3-319-19183-6_3

Raven, J., Raven, J. C., & Court, J. H. (1998). *Manual for Raven's progressive matrices and vocabulary scales. Section 1: General overview*. Oxford, England: Oxford PsychologistsPress/San Antonio, TX: The Psychological Corporation.

Reiss, S., & Valenti-Hein, D. (1990). *Reiss scales for children's dual diagnosis: Test manual.* Worthington, OH: IDS Publishing.

Reiss, S., & Valenti-Hein, D. (1994). Development of a psychopathology rating scale for children with mental retardation. *Journal of Consultation and Clinical Psychiatry, 62*, 28–33.

Richards, S. B., Brady, M. P., & Taylor, R. L. (2014). *Cognitive and intellectual disabilities: Historical perspectives, current practices, and future directions*. New York, NY: Routledge.

Ritchie, S. (2015). *Intelligence: All that matters*. London, England: Hodder & Stoughton.

Roid, G. (2005). *Stanford-Binet Intelligence Scales for Early Childhood–Fifth Edition*. Lutz, FL: Pro-Ed.

Roid, G., & Barram, R. (2004). *Essentials of Stanford–Binet intelligence scales (SB5)*. Hoboken, NJ: Wiley.

Roid, G. H., Miller, L. J., Pomplun, M., & Koch, C. (2013). *Leiter international performance scale-third edition*. Wood Dale, IL: Stoelting.

Rutter, M., LeCouteur, A., & Lord, C. (2008). *Autism diagnostic interview – Revised*. Los Angeles, CA: Western Psychological Services.

Sattler, J. M. (2008). *Assessment of children: Cognitive foundations* (5th ed.). San Diego, CA: Sattler.

Schalock, R. L., & Luckasson, R. (2015). A systematic approach to subgroup classification in intellectual disability. *Intellectual and Developmental Disabilities, 53*(5), 358–366. https://doi.org/10.1352/1934-9556-53.5.358

Schalock, R. L., Luckasson, R. A., & Shogren, K. A. (2007). The renaming of mental retardation: Understanding the change to the term intellectual disability. *Intellectual and Developmental Disabilities, 45*(2), 116–124. https://doi.org/10.1352/1934-9556(2007)45[116:TROMRU]2.0.CO;2

Shannon, D. A., Félix, J. K., Krumholz, A., Goldstein, P. J., & Harris, K. S. (1984). Hearing screening of high-risk newborns with brainstem auditory evoked potentials: A follow-up study. *Pediatrics, 73*, 22–26.

Shrank, F., Mather, N., McGrew, K., & Woodcock, R. (2014). *Woodcock Johnson tests of achievement: IV*. New York, NY: Houghton Mifflin Harcourt.

Shrank, F., McGrew, K., Mather, N., & Woodcock, R. (2014). *Woodcock Johnson tests of cognitive ability—Fourth edition*. Rolling Meadows, IL: The Riverside Publishing Company.

Simeonsson, R. J., Granlund, M., & Bjorck-Akesson, E. (2003). Classifying mental retardation: Impairment, disability, handicap limitations, or restriction? In H. N. Switzky & S. Greenspan (Eds.), *What is mental retardation?* (pp. 309–329). Washington, DC: American Association on Mental Retardation.

Sparrow, S. S., Cicchetti, D., & Balla, D. A. (1998). *Vineland social emotional early childhood scales*. New York, NY: Pearson.

Sparrow, S. S., Cicchetti, D., & Salnier, C. A. (2016). *Vineland adaptive behaviour scales-III*. New York, NY: Pearson.

Squires, J., Twombly, E., Bricker, D., & Potter, L. (2009). *The ASQ user's guide for the ages and stages questionnaire: A parent—Completed, child monitoring system* (3rd ed.). Baltimore, MD: Paul Brookes.

Stadler, M., Becker, N., Gödker, M., Leutner, D., & Greiff, S. (2015). Complex problem solving and intelligence: A meta-analysis. *Intelligence, 53*, 92–101. https://doi.org/10.1016/j.intell.2015.09.005

Tasse, M. J., Balboni, G., Schalock, R. L., & Zhang, D. (2010). AAIDD diagnostic adaptive behaviour scales. *Journal of Applied Research in Intellectual Disabilities, 23*, 436.

Tassé, M. J., Luckasson, R., & Nygren, M. (2013). AAIDD proposed recommendations for ICD–11 and the condition previously known as mental retardation. *Intellectual and Developmental Disabilities, 51*(2), 127–131. https://doi.org/10.1352/1934-9556-51.2.127

Tombaugh, T. N. (1999). *Test of memory malingering*. New York, NY: Pearson.

Virués-Ortega, J., Pritchard, K., Grant, R. L., North, S., Hurtado-Parrado, C., Lee, M. S. H., … Yu, C. T. (2014). Clinical decision making and preference assessment for individuals with intellectual and developmental disabilities. *American Journal on Intellectual and Developmental Disabilities, 119*(2), 151–170. https://doi.org/10.1352/1944-7558-119.2.151

Wechsler, D. (2009). *Wechsler individual achievement test – IV*. New York, NY: Pearson.

Wechsler, D. (2012). *Wechsler preschool and primary scale of intelligence – Fourth edition*. New York, NY: Pearson.

Wechsler, D. (2013). *Wechsler adult scale of intelligence — Fourth edition*. New York, NY: Pearson.

Wechsler, D. (2015). *Wechsler intelligence scale for children — Fifth edition*. New York, NY: Pearson.

Wei, Y., Oakland, T., & Algina, J. (2008). Multigroup confirmatory factor analysis for the adaptive behavior assessment system-ii parent form, ages 5–21. *American Journal on Mental Retardation, 113*(3), 178–186. https://doi.org/10.1352/0895-8017(2008)113[178:MCFAFT]2.0.CO;2

Weiss, L. G., Saklofske, D. H., Holdnack, J. A., & Prifitera, A. (2015). *WISC-V assessment and interpretation: Scientist-practitioner perspectives*. San Diego, CA: Academic Press.

Wiig, E. H., Semel, E., & Secord, W. A. (2013). *Clinical evaluation of language fundamentals-5*. New York, NY: Pearson.

Chapter 8
Educational Interventions and Accommodations

Abstract This chapter provides guidance on educational interventions and accommodations for the students with intellectual disabilities. It reviews the most recent findings regarding such interventions and accommodations including discussion of the integration of educational and mental health. This chapter emphasizes the role of the educators, psychologists, and school professionals working collaboratively to address the child's unique educational and mental health needs. There is a significant science of educational interventions and accommodations that can be implemented for the benefit of people with intellectual disabilities.

Case Study

The multidisciplinary team at Eastern Elementary School met to discuss the development of an individualized educational plan (IEP) for James. James has moved into the community with his family and is preparing to enter third grade. In his previous school, James received educational services as a student with intellectual disabilities. However, based on the IEP that was created in his previous school, the team could not determine exactly how to proceed with educational planning for the upcoming school year. The IEP document was one page in length with half of that page dedicated to receiving the signatures of the members of the multidisciplinary team. The goal listed was that James receives "an appropriate education for his grade and ability level." The approaches to education were described as "receive services in an inclusive grade two environment and receive supports as needed." James's mother was a member of the multidisciplinary team. She stated that the previous school assured her that this was common procedure for developing IEPs and that much of the details have been left to the discretion of the teacher and parent. The Eastern Elementary School multidisciplinary team wanted to develop a clear and functional document that can serve as the basis for educational programming. The multidisciplinary team at Eastern Elementary School includes James's mother, the school psychologist, the inclusive classroom teacher, the special education consultant, the speech and language pathologist, and the school administrator. This team set out to develop a detailed plan using psychological and

S. R. Shaw, A. M. Jankowska, *Pediatric Intellectual Disabilities at School*, Pediatric School Psychology, https://doi.org/10.1007/978-3-030-02992-0_8

educational assessment results to determine his exact level of current functioning; develop measurable goals; create specific instructional techniques to improve reading, writing, mathematics, social skills, speech and language, adaptive functioning, and behaviour management; possible barriers to achieving the goals were identified; evidence-based interventions were described with consideration of school resources, parent acceptability, and teacher training; and a progress monitoring was considered. This complex IEP required 3 weeks and several meetings to develop. James's mother was surprised and a bit frustrated that the process required such a long period to complete. However, after the completion of the nine-page IEP, she was impressed that the school multidisciplinary team developed such a detailed and well-considered program. Upon reading the IEP from his previous school, the professionals at Eastern Elementary School were not prepared to provide the best possible educational services for James. The development of a strong IEP is a cornerstone for delivery of effective educational interventions and accommodations. In some cases, IEP development is considered a paperwork exercise to achieve compliance with state regulations and federal special education law. This approach is certainly in violation of the spirit, if not the letter, of special education law, and clearly misses an opportunity to improve overall instruction and service delivery for students with intellectual disabilities.

Introduction

The most effective forms of education involve individualized instruction based on the current needs of each student. In the case of students with intellectual disabilities, the individualization is codified into individualized educational plans (IEPs; Downing, 2010). The elements of quality teaching for effective learning are somewhat beyond the scope of this book. However, when providing instruction to students with intellectual disabilities, knowing what forms of remediation and accommodations can be effective, are critical considerations.

Expectations for academic success can be problematic or supportive in reaching educational goals. In 1968, *The Pygmalion Effect* (Rosenthal & Jacobson, 1968) was published and had profound influence on the role of expectations in achieving educational goals. This book was widely influential and still carries a significant consideration in teacher education. The logic of this approach is that once teachers were told that students had low intelligence or high intelligence that students were perceived and treated in predictable ways. Those believed to have high intelligence were engaged more frequently, supported in a more positive fashion, and ultimately were higher achievers. Those believed to have low intelligence were often ignored, discouraged from exploration and classroom contribution, and ultimately were lower achievers. The study was extraordinarily poorly designed and of questionable ethical consideration (Thorndike, 1968). It is relevant to note that the research upon which *The Pygmalion Effect* was created were rejected from peer-reviewed journals due to methodological insufficiencies. The authors chose to write up their findings in a book, which was not peer-reviewed. A modern influence with stronger scientific support is the modern theory of *Mindsets* by Dweck (2006). In this approach both students and teachers who believe that general intelligence can be influenced by hard work and strong study habits result in higher achieving students than students and teachers who believe that general intelligence is innate and uninfluenced by work habits. Although there has been criticism of this research and application of findings, the idea of mindsets is influential in education and has some utility (Mercer, Ryan, & Williams, 2012).

An example of expectation setting is a common misinterpretation of intelligence test scores. For all students with intellectual disabilities, there exists a psychological report with measures of general mental ability that have results showing that the individual is in the lowest 2% of age peers. A major misinterpretation is that the results of a standardized intelligence test are referred to as a student's "potential" (Reschly & Grimes, 2002). Intelligence tests are samples of behaviour from which reliable inferences can be made about overall problem-solving ability and are not the same thing as potential. There are also many other variables that are effectively predicted with intelligence test scores (Sattler, 2008). However, potential is complex. Potential represents the highest ability at which one can function in the best of all possible environments. What the best of all possible environments is a theoretical concept and cannot be determined directly. As psychologists, therapists, physicians, and educators, our mission is to search for the most appropriate remediation and accommodation of skills so that the student can achieve at the highest possible level. Using intelligence test scores as a measure of potential creates an artificial ceiling of achievement (Reschly & Grimes, 2002). Having a student achieve academically, in adaptive behaviours, in social skills, and in other domains well above that of the lowest 2% of age peers (i.e., necessary scores for diagnosis or placement), is not only possible but it is common. There is no question that individuals with intellectual disabilities have challenges to be overcome. But intelligence test scores represent current functioning and should not be interpreted as an uppermost limit at which a student can achieve. Low expectations limit achievement.

Individualized Educational Plan Development

Although the development of an IEP for students with intellectual disabilities is codified in laws and regulations, the development of these Individualized Education Plans (IEP) is often exercised in paperwork and compliance rather than meeting their intended purpose of developing a roadmap to effective education (Sturmey & Didden, 2014). Inclusive education provides students with intellectual disabilities access to educational opportunities, but individualized techniques and procedures required for effective education are often ignored or minimized (O'Neill, Albin, Storey, Horner, & Sprague, 2014). The process of IEP development is typically conducted as a multidisciplinary team approach. There are some basic rules and IEP development that are helpful in maximizing the probability that the good ideas in this document are implemented and reflect the reality of the education of the student with intellectual disabilities (Barnett, Daly, Jones, & Lentz, 2004).

Current Functioning

Often the current functioning section of an IEP includes little more than the results of norm-referenced and standardized test that are copied from psychoeducational reports (Decker, Hale, & Flanagan, 2013). This information provides one level of understanding of current functioning. However, all norm-referenced tests provide only information concerning the relative rank of the individual compared to age peers. These tests are designed to be stable and are therefore not amenable to change (Sattler, 2008). An IEP can be most productive when current functioning data are presented in a ratio scale (i.e., equal intervals between numbers and a zero point) that are sensitive to change over time. Such data can include percentage of time on task, words read per minute, words written correctly per minute, percentage of days without a toileting accident, number of aggressive (operationally defined as hitting, kicking, spitting, scratching, and aggressively yelling at another person) incidents, and similar behaviours (Beavers, Iwata, & Lerman, 2013). An academic intervention can be extraordinarily effective in increasing the speed of learning new skills, but scores on a norm-referenced test may not change. If a child can read four words per minute prior to the implementation of the IEP and eight words per minute after the implementation of the IEP, then word reading speed improved 100%. Reporting and documenting these forms of assessment data are critical evaluating IEP-based interventions (Hosp, Hensley, Huddle, & Ford, 2014).

Details and Accountability

No matter what type of intervention is developed in an IEP, specifics matter (Courtade, Test, & Cook, 2014). One function of an IEP is for educational systems to be fully accountable for the process of educating students with specialized needs, including intellectual disabilities. All forms of intervention need to have a point person accountable for the implementation, the details of exactly what processes will be included in the intervention, a timeline for when the interventions will begin and for how long will they be implemented, the resources required for implementing interventions, and in what location will the interventions occur. Another important detail is to include exactly how long initial interventions will be implemented before data will be analysed to determine the extent to which progress towards goals has been achieved.

Assessment to Intervention

Assessment serves multiple purposes, including eligibility for special education services, diagnosis, and assessment of progress. Converting assessment data directly into interventions is a challenge. The preponderance of the evidence is clear that patterns and profiles from standardized norm-referenced measures of intelligence and academic achievement do not lead to more effective design of educational interventions than simple teacher observations (Kehoe, 2015). The same limitations apply to neuropsychological instrumentation and neurological imaging and testing (Lloyd & Kennedy, 2014). These forms of assessment information provide information upon which to design strong educational interventions. A better system is to focus on the goals required for maximum functioning given the demands of the environment in the school and in daily practice. A reasonable assumption is that the methods used for instruction are effective for all persons but may need to be slightly altered in presentation for students with intellectual disabilities.

Goals

Goals can be thought of as short-term formative goals or academic year length summative goals. At a maximum, progress towards short-term goals need to be evaluated and considered every 9 weeks—although usually short-term goals are less than 9 weeks and are formative. If there is failure to make progress towards these goals, then there remain opportunities for changing the details of the educational plan. Long-term goals refer to end of the academic year evaluation and are summative in nature. The other domains to be considered are systemic goals versus individual goals. Systemic goals are those mandated by formal authorities. They may refer to standardized academic achievement test scores, guidelines of minimum performance, or some other formal goal, which may or may not be reasonable given the current functioning of the individual student (Mitchell, 2014). Individual goals refer to goals that are specific to the individual with intellectual disabilities that are derived via discussion with the multidisciplinary team. The most valuable members of the team for establishing goals are typically the students themselves, teachers, and parents. All goals whether short term or long term, systemic or individual, are most useful when using the simple and widely adopted SMART acronym (i.e., specific, measurable, agreed-upon, reasonable, and time-based; Cook & Cook, 2013).

Impediments to Learning and Strengths

For IEP to be successful and useful, a description of strengths and impediments to achieving goals is added. Such descriptions can assist teachers, psychologists, and other therapists to modify evidence-based interventions to meet the specific needs of the student. Strengths can be divided into three primary categories: intrapersonal and interpersonal strengths, support strengths, and available resources. Intrapersonal and interpersonal strengths refer to the specific skills and talents of the student. This involves a description of the specific cognitive, social, executive processing, and motor strengths that can be used to support effective achievement of IEP goals. Interpersonal strengths refer specifically to social skills and relationships with specific individuals (Seong, Wehmeyer, Palmer, & Little, 2015). Sometimes intrapersonal strengths can be specific such as, "This student has a special fondness for Mrs. Neal, the speech and language pathologist, as he listens and follows her directions more so than with any other adult". Other times interpersonal strengths can be general such as, "This student is eager to please and responds well to oral instructions and prosocial encouragement". Support strengths involve resources outside of the school setting that promote effective learning and generalization of tasks achieved in an IEP. Some support strengths include a family heavily involved and expert in the education of their child, involvement of an independent behaviour analysis or therapist, and effective medical support such as psychiatry or developmental pediatrics. Support strengths can be incorporated into an IEP to help support effective instruction (McDonnell, Mathot-Buckner, Thorson, & Fister, 2001). No matter how severe the involvement or how much support a student with intellectual disabilities requires, there are always strengths that support learning, social skill development, and academic achievement (Kleinert et al., 2015).

Impediments to learning involve behavioural, sensory, motor, social, or cognitive components may require accommodations for effective instruction to take place (Gilson, Carter, & Biggs, 2017). Often impediments to learning are described in the IEP and influence short-term goals to be achieved. This is because many times academic and behavioural goals cannot be achieved unless the impediments are resolved first (Gilson et al., 2017). The team developing the IEP must always make the challenging decision on whether to attempt to remediate and remove the impediments or accommodate and work around the impediments. It is critical to know under what conditions do the impediments impair learning and under what conditions are the effects of these impediments minimized (Feng & Sass, 2013).

Evidence-Based Treatments and Intervention

Evidence-based intervention does not necessarily mean that every intervention must be taken word for word from programs evaluated and published in scholarly journals (Lane, Kalberg, & Shepcaro, 2009). Evidence-based interventions require that the preponderance of research evidence support a practice being implemented. Evidence-based treatments and interventions require interpretation of the supporting research literature to help guide individual decisions on the types of interventions inserted into an IEP and implemented. The shift from authoritative decision-making, in which decisions are based on intuition, unsystematic observation, and tradition, to empirically based decision-making allows clinicians to avoid biases and poorly supported conclusions based solely on experience (Gambrill, 2016; Guyatt et al., 1992). This change first occurred in the medical world and later spread to other fields such as nursing, occupational therapy, psychology, and education (Gambrill, 2016). In psychology and education, evidence-based interventions have the potential to influence and significantly improve the quality of services provided by psychologists (Levant & Hasan, 2008).

A similar philosophy has been applied to education as well. The recently enacted American Federal law called the Every Student Succeeds Act (ESSA) (2015) defines four levels of evidence-based interventions that have been codified into law. Per ESSA, "strong" evidence refers to research showing a statistically significant effect on student outcomes from at least one experimental study. The terms "moderate" and "promising" require evidence from quasi-experimental study or correlational studies that make statistical corrections for selection bias. Federal funding streams strongly favour educational systems that apply strong, moderate, and promising evidence. In addition, there is a fourth category made up of activities that have a research-based theoretical rationale but lack direct empirical support. This fourth category is only considered acceptable if there are "ongoing efforts to examine the effects" on student outcomes.

Despite the growing expectations to use evidence-based interventions in psychology and education, a major challenge in the use of evidence-based interventions is that the construct is interpreted in multiple ways for multiple purposes (Rycroft-Malone et al., 2004). The various definitions, including the ESSA guidelines, imply the use of research to inform practice, but any single definition remains too vague to establish a standard of evidence-based interventions. As such, the label of evidence-based interventions has frequently been used as a talisman that means different things to different people.

One major problem is that the label of evidence-based intervention has become something of a Good Housekeeping seal of approval that is used to market textbooks, programs, workshops, and other for-profit educational activities (Ioannidis, 2016a). The quality of the evidence is usually low. Often research is cherry picked, and only the few studies finding positive effects are included in marketing materials and websites. A common situation is that a research study of poor methodological quality is published in a journal with relatively low standards. With this publication, salesmen or marketers can make the case that their intervention is evidence-based. This is not the intended purpose of the evidence-based movement in education (Ioannidis, 2016a). However, professionals and parents implementing interventions that are labelled as "evidence-based" must take this designation with a grain of salt and conduct their own review of research to determine if the intervention is truly evidence-based (Ioannidis, 2016b). There are formal reviewing bodies that do an excellent job of independently verifying whether an intervention is truly evidence based. The What Works Clearinghouse (https://ies.ed.gov/ncee/wwc/) reviews the educational literature on a host of interventions and develops an independent conclusion based on the four levels of evidence-based interventions from ESSA. The Cochrane Reviews (http://www.cochranelibrary.com/cochrane-database-of-systematic-reviews/) serve a similar function in medicine- and medical-related therapies.

Given that students with intellectual disabilities have rare and sometimes unique educational needs, the likelihood that interventions to address the individualized needs of students will have been thoroughly evaluated in the scientific literature is low (Odom et al., 2005). Most often, interventions would be in the promising or research-based rationale categories. Moreover, even when there is an intervention that is clearly supported in the research literature and can rightly be called an evidence-based intervention, often the intervention must be modified to a large degree to meet the available resources, strengths of the student, and impediments to learning of the student. In these cases, the evidence-based intervention may need to be changed so much that it may not be consistent with the specifics of the intervention described in the evidence base. Most research supporting evidence-based practices involve improvement of the average performance of a group of students over time. Evidence-based interventions that have been rigourously evauated still have no guarantee that the intervention will be effective for every student. As such it is important to evaluate the effectiveness of any intervention for each individual student with evaluation methods are described in the IEP.

Practice-based evidence is a related and perhaps more useful concept than evidence-based practices (Politte, Howe, Nowinski, Palumbo, & McDougle, 2015). In the education and IEP development for students with intellectual disabilities, searches for the necessary interventions to achieve stated goals cannot be effectively met by the available research literature (Test et al., 2009). In these cases, interventions that have a research, theory, or general practice rationale can be implemented. Just like evidence-based interventions, practice-based evidence requires that effective outcomes be measured carefully to determine whether they are effective for the specific individual. Even in the cases of evidence-based practices or practice-based evidence, an important consideration is to always remember what the "I" stands for in an IEP—programs cannot be a one-size-fits-all no matter what the preponderance of research would support. Individualizing instruction is an essential component to meet the unique needs of students with intellectual disabilities.

General Rules of Instruction

What are the common characteristics of students with intellectual disabilities that require a change in approach for effective schooling? In other words, what are the characteristics that are commonly observed in persons with low intelligence that are different from typically developing peers that directly influence learning and teaching. The default state is that there are no differences (Pennington & Courtade, 2015). All students can learn. The question is at what level can they learn, what are the most effective approaches, and how consistent with the expectations of school systems can teaching and learning be. The general template is that there are five major components that often, but not always, differentiate typically developing learners from students with intellectual disabilities (Lundberg & Reichenberg, 2013). If students with intellectual disabilities are to be taught in an inclusive classroom, then these components can be used to differentiate instruction. Nothing substitutes for an individualized educational approach, but this is a template to be used in searching for the highest level of achievement that can be attained.

Generalization

The learning characteristic that is critical in all of education is generalization. Students typically learn a fact, rule, algorithm, or procedure through direct instruction (Shaw, 2008). Then it is up to the students to apply that fact, rule, algorithm, or procedure to appropriate situations. For example, very young children learn that 1 + 1 = 2. There are few differences between high ability and low ability students in how quickly or completely they learn this one fact. However, rarely do teachers need to teach high ability children what 1 + 2 equals. These students understand the concept of addition quickly and generalize this concept to novel situations. Students with low general mental ability learn each fact almost as quickly and completely as do high ability students. Yet, they have significant difficulty with generalization. Thus, lower functioning students require many repetitions and numerous facts before they begin to generalize the overall concept to novel situations. Because most instruction is incomplete—that is, we only teach the facts, rules, algorithms, or procedures and do not teach how to generalize or apply this information—students with intellectual disabilities progress through the curriculum at a much slower pace.

The same issue is encountered when teaching adaptive behaviour skills such as social skills. Social skills training is extraordinarily effective for teaching a specific skill set in a classroom environment (Root, Saunders, Spooner, & Brosh, 2017). Yet, as soon as the students leave the classroom environment and move to recess, lunch room, bus line, and hallways, they often fail to generalize the social skills taught. The result is limited application and effectiveness of the social skills training. If academic or social skills instruction are to be effective, then a plan for generalization must be implemented. In the case of academic instruction, much more in the way of practice activities and then guided scaffolding to learn how to apply the rule or algorithm to a novel situation is required. In the case of social skills instruction, the targeted social skill must be practised in multiple situations and multiple events for generalization to begin to occur (Wilson, McKenzie, Quayle, & Murray, 2014).

Issues of generalization are common for all levels of intellectual ability. Currently, many states and provinces are primarily concerned with formal instruction being generalized only to the point that students can demonstrate their learning on standardized multiple-choice tests (Adibsereshki, Abkenar, Ashoori, & Mirzamani, 2015). This is an important form of generalization but hardly represents complete and effective education.

Functionally, students with low general mental ability require anywhere from 5 to 10 times the number of practice opportunities before a skill is generalizable compared to students of average to above average general mental ability (Browder, Ahlgrim-Delzell, Spooner, Mims, & Baker, 2009). Therefore, instruction of students with low general mental ability is far less efficient and more time-consuming than instruction of typically developing peers.

Concreteness

A common observation among first grade teachers is that children with intellectual disabilities tend to be at or near grade level in learning mathematics skills yet are far behind in reading skill development (Coyne, Pisha, Dalton, Zeph, & Smith, 2012). The explanation for this difference is simple: math instruction in first grade tends to involve manipulatives and be concrete. Blocks, rods, number lines, and other concrete activities are widely used as illustrations of mathematical concepts. Reading involves black squiggles on a white page that represent sounds and thoughts. Reading is an abstract activity (Flores, Hinton, Strozier, & Terry, 2014). The more that instruction and material can become concrete, the less of a gap there will be between high and low ability students (Knight, Spooner, Browder, Smith, & Wood, 2013). Intellectual ability measures assess abstract and inferential reasoning (Sattler, 2008). People with intellectual disabilities tend to have impaired abstract reasoning skills but have concrete thinking skills (such as rote memory) far closer to average (Reschly & Grimes, 2002). Consider the dimension of abstract versus concrete information presentation, examples, student output, and practice in developing instruction. The level of concreteness is an excellent dimension upon which to differentiate instruction.

The mantra for concrete instruction is to see it, hear it, touch it, and do it (Mechling, Ayres, Foster, & Bryant, 2015). There are a host of forms of active learning such as classroom without walls, experiential learning, interactive instruction, experimentation, dramatic recreation, and other methods that allow full student participation in the learning experience. Oddly, many of these forms of instruction have been specifically dedicated to the teaching of gifted or students with high intelligence. In fact, these interactive forms of instruction, although useful for many levels of student ability, are essential for constructive instruction of students with intellectual disabilities. The traditional method of instruction involves reading of texts and lectures (Neil & Jones, 2014). These traditional methods are abstract. The abstract form of instruction involving reading of text and lectures may be relatively dull for all levels of general mental ability but represents an efficient method of transmitting information to students of average to high general mental ability. This form of abstract construction is most often completely ineffective for students with intellectual disabilities.

The dimension of concreteness refers to more than just direct sensory perception of the information. Concreteness can also refer to relevance to individuals (Lee, Browder, Flowers, & Wakeman, 2016). Many of us remember taking algebra in high school and asking the instructor, "When will we ever have the opportunity to use algebra? How is this going to be useful in my life?" Too many of us, algebra was extremely abstract because we could not understand the utility of this subject to our lives. Relevance of information is a form of concreteness. For nearly every level of cognitive ability, there is a requirement that students relate to the material, and it has relevance. Effective instruction requires that no matter what subject you are teaching that you can answer the question, "Why is this useful to me?" This is not simply a matter of motivation to learn the material but also a form of abstraction. Even abstract concepts such as money, time, history, philosophy, politics, and calculus can be made more concrete if the purpose of these activities to everyday life becomes clear. By making abstract concepts more relevant, it is far more likely that the new information will be assimilated into information that is currently stored in long-term memory. For example, studying the Magna Carta can be abstract and isolated if studied as a document written in another continent in the year 1215. However, many students can understand how an historic abstraction has relevance to their lives. For example, the Magna Carta is relevant because current interactions with government and police forces are based on this historic document. The ability to take an abstract concept and make it relevant to students is an important factor for students of any ability level (Lang & Rispoli, 2015). For students with intellectual disabilities, concreteness is a major variable in determining not only motivation but ability to accommodate and assimilate new information to what is already learned.

Efficient Long-Term Storage and Recall

The issue of generalization and concreteness in instruction relates to an important variable in the acquisition of new knowledge, that is, the ability to assimilate and store information in long term and the ability to efficiently recall that information for use (Mechling et al., 2015). A simple, yet useful, model of cognitive processing of information involves a storage mechanism that includes four parts: (1) attention is directed towards incoming sensory information; (2) sensory information is stored in short-term memory, which has limited durability and capacity; (3) information is further used or processed through working memory; and finally (4) information in working memory that can be tied to previously existing information in long-term memory can be added to long-term memory, which is a practically limitless store of information (Dahlin, 2011). Information in long-term memory also provides a template that indicates how attention should be focused to gain the most useful knowledge; influences unconscious strategies that can expand the capacity and durability of short-term memory, which is context specific; influences how information in working memory can best be used; and provides a scaffold from which to build new long-term memory. The basic concept is that the more one knows, the easier it is to learn new information. Students with intellectual disabilities generally have important weaknesses at every step of this process. Attention may be impaired at a deep level involving brainstem abnormalities or simply due to lack of knowledge on how and where to direct attentional resources. Short-term memory is the cognitive process in which people with intellectual disabilities most often are minimally impaired. Rote memory is a relative strength (Bruni & Hixson, 2017). The old finding in cognitive psychology that people can remember seven bits of information plus or minus two bits is equally valid for people with borderline intelligence or mild intellectual disabilities. There may be some weaknesses because working memory has a contextual component. For example, chess experts have a large short-term memory for chess boards; gardeners have large short-term memory for soil quality and so on. If a person has limited situational expertise, then short-term memory may not have the contextual expertise that allows people to make shortcuts (i.e., the ability to chunk information into useful bits). Working memory is the blackboard or desktop of memory—it is where information is not only stored but mentally manipulated. Working memory is where new information combines with previously learned information to solve problems and think usefully (Collins, Evans, Creech-Galloway, Karl, & Miller, 2007). As new information proves to be useful in solving problems, it is also assisted in moving to long-term memory and permanent storage.

There are two categories of teaching strategies that can make use of this information for classroom issues and communication. The first strategy is to pre-organize information. Because attention, short-term memory, and working memory are largely influenced by previous knowledge, students are assisted by reminding students what previous knowledge they have that is relevant to the new incoming information (Shaw, 2008). An easy method to pre-organize information is to simply provide a preface before any new information is provided. For example, "last week we discussed a type of word that describes a noun and we call those words adjectives. Does everybody remember talking about adjectives? Now we are going to discuss a similar, but slightly different, type of word called an adverb. These are words that describe verbs." This simple prompt reminds students what information that they have stored in long-term memory is most relevant for learning the new task. By providing a cognitive prompt, the relevant information from long-term memory is primed; attention, short-term memory, and working memory are maximized. This simple prompt will help all students. However, there is likely to be a disproportionately positive affect on students with intellectual disabilities.

The second strategy is to provide supports to address limitations in short-term and working memories (Shaw, 2008). Nearly every learner takes advantage of strategies and uses artificial support to address our limitations. Most of us have calendars to keep track of appointments, to do lists to monitor and remind us of activities, notebooks to allow us to record quick thoughts before they disappear, and a host of other techniques that we use to overcome limitations in working and short-term memory. In addition, we use supports to help overcome our limitations in working memory. If any of us were requested to add a column of ten three-digit numbers, then our first response would be to get a paper and pencil to write down each of those numbers because we know that such a task would easily outstrip the capacity of short-term memory and working memory. Supports to increase speed of processing are also important. Many of us have had the situation where we are taking notes, but the speaker is going so fast that we cannot write fast enough to keep up with the words being spoken. At that point, the information not only does not get written down but it is completely lost in our cognitive processing system. The ability to take notes using shorthand or an outlining system is a mechanism that we use to support our deficiencies and speed of processing. Students with intellectual disabilities have more severe functional limitations in each of the aspects of cognitive processes, but do not have a repertoire of strategies to overcome these limitations (Shaw, 2008).

For academic skills, there are some basic tricks and skills that can be helped to improve on these limitations in storage and recall of information (Browder, Hudson, & Wood, 2013). A common problem with new readers is that decoding skills are slow and effortful. The slow and effortful decoding skills often mean that when sounding out a word that by the time the student gets to the second part of the word to sound out they have already forgotten the first half of the word and the word goes unread. Often students start out by memorizing the 250 most common words (often called the Dolch list) when learning basic reading skills (Denton & Al Otaiba, 2011). Teaching students as many as the 1000 most common words as sight words to be memorized allows students to take advantage of the relative strength in short-term memory and take stress from the relatively weak working memory. Mathematics activities place heavy emphasis on working memory. One approach to accommodate this weakness is to teach basic math skills on an abacus. An abacus allows for students to learn the process of mathematics and understand the deeper meanings of the concept (unlike a calculator) yet reduces the burden on working memory. The complexity of math is that in a simple equation such as $8 + 4 = X$, the learner must store the first number in working memory, then the operation, then the second number, apply the algorithm, and produce an answer. These processes severely tax working memory. On an abacus, the first number is entered on the abacus by sliding the appropriate beads into place. The information for the first number is stored in the abacus, and then the second number is added. The final number of beads are counted in an answer is achieved. By storing the information on the abacus through the sliding of beads, there are significant relief from working memory, but the process increases understanding of mathematical concepts. The abacus has advantages of being concrete and improving the deeper understanding of mathematics processes that can lead to improved generalization. Because mathematics is often tested with paper and pencil (an abstract task), students often need to use an abacus as a scaffold to develop paper and pencil math skills (Lee et al., 2016). Writing skills can be heavily affected by motor performance. If handwriting is slow and effortful, then there is an extra burden placed on working memory as described in the notetaking scenario above. The ability to speed the recording of written language through keyboarding skills or voice-to-text software can significantly decrease the burden on working memory and improve written language. These are some examples of methodology that can be used to maximize cognitive strengths and improve storage, organization, and recall of information. Examples can be used for students of any ability, yet in a heterogeneous or inclusive classroom, students with intellectual disabilities are likely to see the most benefit from such methods (Shaw, 2008).

Although academic skills are considered the most important goal for many persons with borderline intelligence and mild to moderate intellectual disabilities, teaching functional and daily living skills also requires careful organization to improve the storage and recall of skills. A simple example of this is to ask students to anticipate and carry out the next skill to be conducted. “It is time to brush your teeth. Please do the first step in toothbrushing. Do you know what to do next? Okay, do the next step." Linking in sequencing one activity to another in a task analysed approach to complex activities adds to the sequential organization of steps. In other words, teaching step one and step two of every activity is valuable; yet, it is even more valuable to teach that the completion of step one is a cue to begin step two (Leaf et al., 2015). The sequential linking of steps is an excellent approach to organizing information for teaching functional and daily living skills with the goal of as much independence as is possible.

Academic Engaged Time and Discipline

A critical variable for all students is the amount of time in a classroom that is dedicated to learning new material, practicing new material, reviewing information, and demonstrating information on teacher made tests (Grossman, Cohen, Ronfeldt, & Brown, 2014). Collectively, these activities are known as academic engaged time. Academic engaged time is a classroom variable that is highly predictive of academic performance and student behaviours conducive to learning (Grissom, Loeb, & Master, 2013). Typically, about 20–25% of the school day is involved in academic engaged time (Grissom et al., 2013). The remainder of the school day involves transitions, interruptions, disciplinary activities, downtime or free time, and nonacademic activities such as assemblies and lunchtime. This appears to be extraordinarily inefficient. There is a reason why students who are homeschooled often go through the exact same curriculum and are finished with the academic lessons expected of them after about 2 h of work. Managing a classroom of 20–30 students is an extraordinarily difficult task. Even increasing academic engaged time to 30% of the school day is an intensive exercise of planning, organization, and classroom discipline (Grossman et al., 2014). Yet, there is no question that all students would benefit from more opportunities to learn new information, practice, review old information, and demonstrate knowledge. In an inclusive classroom, all students would benefit from increases in academic engaged time; but students with intellectual disabilities will see even larger gains in academic and social skill development.

As mentioned above, students with intellectual disabilities have difficulty with generalization of skills. Most typically this means that to learn a new skill, students require many times more practice activities than for children who are typically developing. Extra practice requires extra time. If academic engaged time were increased only slightly, then there would be more opportunities for extra practice activities and academic improvement (Shaw, 2008). There are several methods for increasing academic engaged time; however all methods require intensive effort and preparation that is quite challenging to maintain for most teachers. The first approach is to systematically reduce transition times. Setting a stopwatch to time transitions from one topic to another or from the beginning of class to preparation to learn can become classroom goals. Students are rewarded as a class for reducing their transition time until transition times are minimized. Some teachers even practice and rehearse transition times as if transitioning were a drill to be made maximally efficient. The second approach is to increase speed in rehearsal activities. For example, if students have a worksheet of mathematics problems to complete for practice and you would typically give them 20 min to complete the worksheet, only allow students 10 min to complete the task. When given 20 min to complete a task, most students will waste upwards of 10 min before they begin work on the assignment. By reducing the time allowed, downtime is minimized, and concentrated practice is more likely. There are some students in the classroom who may experience extreme anxiety over being put under time pressures. The primary measure of success is not necessarily completion of a worksheet but concentrated time and effort in practising in rehearsal of mathematics problems. This concentrated effort is what is rewarded. In such a speeded classroom, teachers are required to have additional materials prepared for practice in rehearsal because students are working at a more intense and rapid rate. A functional side effect of the speeded classroom is that there are fewer behaviour problems and disruptions. By minimizing the downtime and maximizing academic engaged time in a classroom, there are fewer opportunities for distracted or problematic behaviours. These simple techniques sound easy to adopt but require energy and planning. In an inclusive classroom containing students with intellectual disabilities, all students will benefit; yet, students with intellectual disabilities will disproportionally see benefits in learning due to increased rehearsal time that can help to overcome limitations in generalization (Shaw, 2008).

Detailed Classroom Disciplinarian Management Plan

There are several available classroom disciplinary techniques. Most of them are quite effective. The primary issue is that teachers must be mindful in having an organized classroom with clear and explicit expectations communicated effectively to students (Medeiros, Rojahn, Moore, & van Ingen, 2014). In addition, it is a worthwhile investment of time to have to remind students of classroom rules and the consequences for violating those rules (Poppen, Sinclair, Hirano, Lindstrom, & Unruh, 2016). Also, positive and prosocial behaviours are also worthy of instruction in the classroom. Time invested in classroom discipline instruction is typically results in a net gain in academic engaged time. A short amount of time invested in instruction concerning discipline will result in significant time savings in managing disciplinary problems in the classroom that can be disruptive (Schaafsma, Kok, Stoffelen, & Curfs, 2015).

The major concern for students with intellectual disabilities is that most formal classroom disciplinary techniques involve a punitive response (e.g., losing a privilege, writing the student's name on the blackboard, receiving a strike, being sent to the principal's office) for violating a classroom rule. Punitive responses can be extremely effective if children completely understand the appropriate behaviour but choose to violate the rule (Sennott, Light, & McNaughton, 2016). In the case of students with intellectual disabilities, they may not know exactly what the appropriate behaviour would be (Sennott et al., 2016). Punitive responses are not effective if children do not understand the appropriate behaviours and feel they have no choice but to violate the rule. In these cases, the punitive response can result in emotional outbursts and anger due to frustration (Will & Hepburn, 2015). The general statement is that punitive approaches work very well when the problem is a "won't do" problem, but do not work well at all if the problem is a "can't do" problem. The assumption that all children have the requisite skills to comply with the basic classroom rules may not be met by children without significant school experience or those who have intellectual disabilities.

Meta-Academic Skills

In a long-term project involving improving academic functioning of 142 students with borderline general mental ability, academic techniques were put into place so that students' achievement improved from average standard scores on a standardized test of academic achievement (Wechsler Individual Achievement Test) from 67.2 to 89.4 during a 16-week intensive academic intervention program (Shaw, 2008). Although this seems successful, the problem was that despite improvements in skills, only 17 of the 142 students demonstrated an improvement in school grades. It became quite clear that academic skills are necessary but not sufficient for academic success. Further analysis indicated that meta-academic skills, the skills required for success at school that are not traditional academic topics such as reading, writing, and mathematics, were severely impaired for these children with borderline general mental ability.

Meta-academic skills are not taught directly in school but are assumed to be learned through the process of school-based socialization (Shaw, 2008). Students with low general mental ability tend not to indirectly learn and apply the skills to their functioning in the classroom. Rather than learn meta-academic skills that lead to further opportunities to profit from quality academic instruction, many students learn classroom survival skills that may be counterproductive to learning (Jameson, McDonnell, Johnson, Riesen, & Polychronis, 2007). For example, some students develop survival skills such as the ability to make excuses, to blame others for poor quality work or for getting assignments, copying the work of others, and so on (Jameson et al., 2007). Students have learned that these survival skills can be effective in circumventing classroom rules, performance expectations, and their own self-image as intelligent and capable people. Direct instruction of meta-academic skills has been an important feature in improving not only the ability to profit from quality instruction but also effective functioning in a classroom so that higher grades can be achieved (Hudson, Browder, & Wood, 2013).

Meta-academic skills are comprised of five major areas: executive processes, social skills, school adaptation, coping with medical issues, and coping with behavioural issues (Shaw, 2008). *Executive processes* include attentional control, cognitive inhibition, inhibitory control, working memory, and cognitive flexibility that are applied for the person to achieve a goal (Kirk, Gray, Riby, & Cornish, 2015). Direct teaching and practice in these areas have been effective interventions for children with attention deficit hyperactivity disorder and preschool children (Lee & Carlson, 2015). Recent evidence demonstrates that instruction in these skills is useful for reducing risky behaviours and increasing homework completion (Claro, Boulanger, & Shaw, 2015). *Social skills* are the basic interpersonal skills required for success in school. Often social skills are taught so that interpersonal skills such as friend making, conflict resolution, and play activities are the primary focus (Lee & Carlson, 2015). However, social skills can also be related directly to classroom functioning and include cooperative learning, teamwork for group projects, communicating with adults, communicating with peers, and effective communication through digital media (appropriate Facebook, chat, Snapchat, and other modes of peer discussion). *School adaptation* involves skills such as following classroom rules, independent learning for homework, test preparation, responding to criticism, and other meta-academic skills directly related to classroom specific behaviour. Because students with intellectual disabilities have a higher probability of *medical issues*, the ability to adhere to medical treatments, understand methods of minimizing side effects of medication, appropriate diet and sleep hygiene, communicating with medical professionals, and other behaviours to assist in coping with medical issues are taught in this section. In addition, students with intellectual disabilities have a higher probability of *mental health issues* as well. As such, learning to communicate with behavioural therapist or counsellor, adhering to and practising activities discussed in therapy or counselling, identifying key triggers for maladaptive behaviour or mental health crises, and addressing the social stigma of mental health problems combined with intellectual disabilities. There are increasing curricula available to directly teach meta-academic skills using many of the same techniques that address generalization, concreteness, and storage and recall (Shaw, 2008). For people with intellectual disabilities, time invested in instruction of meta-academic skills is likely to result in an efficient academic instruction and classroom discipline as well.

Resources

A major challenge of inclusive classrooms is that resources are limited (Campbell-Whatley, Dunaway, & Hancock, 2016). It is quite simple for a psychologist or book author to put forth ideas and innovative practices that may be effective and supported by research literature yet implementing these ideas can be nearly impossible without appropriate resources. Among the resources that are required for effective development and implementation of the activities described in an IEP are time, material, personnel, parental support, skills and knowledge, confidence, and data collection support. Without any of these categories of resources, an IEP cannot be successfully carried out. Before recommending an intervention or instructional technique to be included into an IEP, an analysis of resource requirements versus actual resources available is a critical feature (Anagnostou et al., 2014). Without appropriate resources, an IEP is simply a wish list rather than an actionable plan to promote learning for students.

Teachers as Professionals

Related to the topic of resources in developing and carrying out an IEP is the culture of innovation and teacher professionalism. IEPs are typically developed by a multidisciplinary team, where teachers serve as an equal member. Ideally, the teacher must agree to and support the elements in the IEP because the teacher will be implementing most of the ideas presented (Dillenburger et al., 2014). There are many cultures and environments in which teachers may feel pressured to implement educational interventions that may not be possible to be implemented given the resources that are available. Such an approach to educational intervention development may be perceived as coercive, and thus it is unlikely that interventions will be implemented with any sense of integrity or fidelity. Considering resources and teacher comfort level with innovation and individualized educational interventions is critical component of an effective intervention plan.

Physical/Sensory Accommodations

Implementing an IEP for students with multiple disabilities, including physical and sensory impairments, in an inclusive classroom is a resource intensive undertaking. Most large school systems have professionals (e.g., orientation and mobility experts for visually impaired, signing or manual communication for hearing impaired, mobility supports, medical support) with expertise in applying technology and other resources to meet the needs of students with multiple impairments. However, there are few of these professionals, and this resource is always stretched thin (Losinski, Sanders, & Wiseman, 2016). There is a requirement that these experts work with the primary teacher in an inclusive setting to teach many of the specific skills and exactly how to use and troubleshoot any technology for the benefit of students. This element becomes a transdisciplinary approach where specific professionals teach and provide resources to the inclusive education teacher. However, such an approach requires extensive time and energy (i.e., resources) on the part of the implementing inclusive classroom teacher. These opportunities and resources are to be included into an IEP.

Behavioural Treatment and Counselling

Programming for behavioural, emotional, and mental health concerns for students with intellectual disabilities is an important aspect of any IEP. Often, behavioural, emotional, and mental health issues are not included in a comprehensive educational program (Vlissides, Beail, Jackson, Williams, & Golding, 2017). The assumption is often that maladaptive behaviours are secondary to intellectual disabilities and are often unavoidable. Moreover, behaviour issues are treated entirely as issues to be operantly conditioned through behaviour management methods or by psychiatric care and psychotropic drugs. Although these are often entirely appropriate approaches, counselling for students with intellectual disabilities is frequently ignored as a possible option for long-term improvement of emotional and behavioural issues (Hassenfeldt, Lorenzi, & Scarpa, 2014). There is a long history of diagnostic "overshadowing", which means that mental health issues are minimized and attributed entirely to the intellectual disability (Scott & Havercamp, 2016). Many students with intellectual disabilities have no mental health or behavioural issues requiring planning and service delivery. Yet, students with intellectual disabilities are at higher risk for experiencing mental health and behavioural problems. As such, a comprehensive plan to address maladaptive behaviours, impaired social skills, emotional regulation, anxiety, depression, and other issues is a critical component of an IEP.

To a large degree, the characteristics of students with intellectual disabilities involving challenges with generalization, need for concreteness, difficulty storing and recalling information, increasing engage time, and a systematic disciplinary program are just as important for addressing behavioural, emotional, and mental health issues as they are for academic instruction. The primary approach to address issues for students with intellectual disabilities is the use of behaviour analytic techniques; that is, operant conditioning using elements of functional behaviour analysis. Functional behaviour analysis involves a structured observation of the antecedents of the target behaviour, topographical description of the behaviours, discriminate stimulus surrounding the behaviour, and the consequences of the behaviour (Mohammadzaheri, Koegel, Rezaee, & Rafiee, 2014). By altering aspects of the environment, most commonly the consequences of behaviour, the frequency, severity, and duration of problematic behaviours can be changed. This behavioural approach is well suited for students with challenges and with generalization, abstractness, storing and recalling information, need for increased academic engaged time, and a systematic disciplinary program.

Conducting an Functional Behaviour Assessment

There are several components to the creation of a successful functional behaviour analysis (Sugai et al., 2000).

- Identification and description of observable and measurable target behaviours.
  - Onset of behaviours.
  - Duration of behaviour.
  - Frequency of behaviour.
  - Severity of behaviour.
  - Description of what the behaviour looks like.
- Analysis of the events directly relating to the onset of target behaviour.
  - What happens directly before the behaviour?
  - What happens directly after the behaviour?
  - Situations in which the behaviour never occurs?
- Analysis of the environment.
  - What are the expectations for behaviour?
  - What are the peer characteristics that may influence behaviour in the environment of interest? (e.g., modelling of behaviour, peer group dynamics, bullying or teasing).
  - What are the school or classroom characteristics that may influence behaviour? (e. g., classroom rules, teacher characteristics, disciplinary system, communication with parents, issues in transportation).
  - What are the family characteristics that may influence behaviour? (e.g., socioeconomic status, disciplinary practices, relationships between parents and child, communication and trust with school, achievement expectations).
  - What are the community characteristics outside of the school that may influence behaviour? (e.g., police/community relationships, prevalence of violence and crime, relationship between school and community, school funding and resources from the community).
- Identification of the strengths of the student that can be used to develop and implement any behaviour change efforts.
  - Involves information derived from psychoeducational assessment.
  - Interview information from parents, teachers, and the student.
  - Review of behavioural history.
- Determining which consequences are most reinforcing to the student.
  - Derived from interviews with student, parent, and teacher.
  - Review the analysis of short- and long-term consequences of the behaviour of interest to determine which consequences lead to the maintenance of the behaviour.
- Development of hypothesis concerning the function of the behaviour.
  - All behaviours serve a function. Reducing behaviours that are problematic in a school setting but serve an important function for the student will be challenging, if not impossible. Behaviour change is most effective when a

problematic behaviour can be replaced by a benign or helpful behaviour that serves the same function.

The information required to address a behavioural component in an IEP is complex and often requires multiple members of a multidisciplinary team. The important aspect of functional behaviour assessment is that the document is a tentative plan that evolves based on continuously collecting new information about the behaviour of interest. A scientific approach, in which hypotheses are created based on the functional behaviour assessment and tested based on collection of information on the frequency, severity, and duration of behaviour over time, is the most effective way to use a functional behaviour analysis in the context of creating behaviour change goals in an IEP.

Behavioural Intervention Plans

Behaviour intervention plans involve the specific programming that are described in an IEP that are directly related to the results of the functional behaviour assessment (Hanley, Iwata, & McCord, 2003). There are many components to the development and implementation of an effective behaviour intervention plan (Sugai et al., 2000).

- Analysis of resources, especially time, is an important consideration in the development of a behaviour intervention plan. Any training or coaching in the specific skills required to implement the behaviour intervention program is to be carried out prior to implementation.
- The student and parent are important members of the team to develop a behaviour intervention plan. Often the student and parent have insights into techniques that have been successful. By having student and parent as a critical member of the behaviour intervention plan team, there is more likely to be support for and acceptance of the plan by all parties involved. Success of implementation depends on this.
- The specifics of the changes in the environment, antecedents, and consequences are identified with individual roles and responsibilities established, the duration of the intervention agreed upon, and the methods of evaluation developed.
- Among the forms of interventions involved may be:
  - Adjusting the environment to prevent problems and promoting positive behaviours that serve a similar function as the maladaptive behaviours.
  - Teaching specific skills that are replacement or incompatible behaviours to the problem issues.
  - Manage the consequences so that positive behaviours are reinforced, and problem behaviours are minimized in both long and short term.
- Classroom-wide interventions may be effective and appropriate for a behaviour intervention plan, yet individualized approaches are often superior. This is

especially true in that consequences that may be reinforcing for one student are not reinforcing for others.

- Resources are to be developed so that consequences of the behaviour are administered consistently and immediately. Consistent and immediate presentation of consequences minimizes the possibility that there is a long-term chaining and accidental reinforcement of problem behaviours.
- Elements of a least restrictive environment are important guidelines for behaviour intervention plans. The educational environment should be as closely aligned to typically developing peers as is possible. Always note that method using restraint or aversive consequences has the result of increasing the probability of emotional reactions that may be counterproductive to the behaviour intervention plan.
- Ensure that all decisions consider resources required. Most commonly, the greater the resources required to implement the plan, the least likely the plan will be implemented with fidelity. Using data to ensure that the implementation of the program is minimally disruptive to the teacher's typical classroom approach is helpful in ensuring behaviour intervention plan maintenance. Elements of a least restrictive environment are not only important for the legal rights and functioning of the student with intellectual disabilities but also increase the likelihood that a program will be maintained and implemented with fidelity.

There are criticisms to using strictly behavioural approaches to addressing behaviours of students with intellectual disabilities. Some of these criticisms include the following: the programming does not consider the students' goals for their own behaviour, does not typically consider self-advocacy in selection of the behaviours to be changed, generalization of the skill beyond an environment that can be strictly controlled (e.g., the classroom) is difficult, parent involvement in behavioural program is rare and could be extremely helpful, and there is an overemphasis on increasing compliant behaviours rather than increasing functional behaviours (Dessemontet, Bless, & Morin, 2012).

Counselling

One form of addressing behaviour, emotions, and mental health issues that is frequently ignored is the tool of counselling. Many students with intellectual disabilities can benefit from targeted discussion, individual or small group instruction of coping skills, and rehearsal of behaviours, verbalizations, and coping mechanisms (Prout & Nowak-Drabik, 2003). To a large degree, the high risk of people with intellectual disabilities for developing mental health problems is due to concrete problem-solving abilities for an abstract world (Prout & Nowak-Drabik, 2003). Having a relationship with a professional counsellor can teach appropriate skills via coaching and encouragement (Szymanski & King, 1999). Allowing students to control, self-advocate, and select the skills to be developed has the advantage of increasing motivation to change behaviours. Although most often implemented for students with mild intellectual disabilities, there is evidence that students with moderate intellectual disabilities can also profit from effective counselling. As is the case for most clients, students with intellectual disabilities benefit as much from the therapeutic liaison between client and counsellor as any substantive work on learning and applying new coping skills.

Even for the case of mental health counselling, many of the attributes of learners with intellectual disabilities apply to the counselling session as well (Shaw, 2008). For example, generalization must be built into all counselling sessions. Any skill developed in an individual or group counselling environment will need to be practised in multiple environments and in multiple situations. This form of guided practice beyond a therapy session to lunch room, hallway, multiple different classrooms, buses, home, church, and other environments and situations is required to maximize the probability of generalization. The degree of abstractness has long been considered an impediment to effective counselling for students with intellectual disabilities. Talking about specific coping mechanisms and skills can become quite abstract. The mantra of see it, feel it, hear it, and do it—and all with relevance to the student—applies to mental health counselling as well as academic skill development. The ability to efficiently store and recall information is also an issue. All counselling sessions are most effective when they begin with a review of the information that was discussed in the last counselling session and open discussion of any opportunities in which the student had to apply the skills they learned during the last session. Once this brief review and evaluation of the effectiveness of the previous lessons learned are addressed, then new coping skills are linked explicitly to previously learned information. In this fashion, the counsellor is assisting the student with intellectual disabilities to store new information by helping them understand how it relates to previously learned information. With minor adjustments, counselling students with intellectual disabilities can serve a long-term positive goal of improving coping skills, reducing maladaptive behaviours, and improving adaptive skills all within the framework of an interpersonal relationship (Prout & Nowak-Drabik, 2003). In addition, allowing students with intellectual disabilities to be equal contributors in a counselling process also supports self-advocacy and control of the treatment process. Although not appropriate for all persons with intellectual disabilities, counselling is an often overlooked tool to improve adaptive function.

Conclusions

Creating IEPs that are based on evidence-based interventions, are responsive to students with intellectual disabilities, and are credible and feasible in their implementation in inclusive setting are all important aspects of developing school-based interventions (Sturmey & Didden, 2014). Improved understanding of the cognitive abilities and emotional skills of students with intellectual disabilities allows multidisciplinary teams to develop such effective planning. The keys to effective evidence-based interventions in an IEP are careful matching of resource requirement of programming with available resources and continuous collection and evaluation of data to guide the process towards goals in an iterative fashion (Odom et al., 2005).

References

Adibsereshki, N., Abkenar, S. J., Ashoori, M., & Mirzamani, M. (2015). The effectiveness of using reinforcements in the classroom on the academic achievement of students with intellectual disabilities. *Journal of Intellectual Disabilities, 19*(1), 83–93. https://doi.org/10.1177/1744629514559313

Anagnostou, E., Zwaigenbaum, L., Szatmari, P., Fombonne, E., Fernandez, B. A., Woodbury-Smith, M., ... Scherer, S. W. (2014). Autism spectrum disorder: Advances in evidence-based practice. *Canadian Medical Association Journal, 186*(7), 509–519. https://doi.org/10.1503/cmaj.121756

Barnett, D. W., Daly, E. J., III, Jones, K. M., & Lentz, F. E., Jr. (2004). Response to intervention empirically based special service decisions from single-case designs of increasing and decreasing intensity. *The Journal of Special Education, 38*(2), 66–79.

Beavers, G. A., Iwata, B. A., & Lerman, D. C. (2013). Thirty years of research on the functional analysis of problem behavior. *Journal of Applied Behavior Analysis, 46*(1), 1–21. https://doi.org/10.1002/jaba.30

Browder, D. M., Ahlgrim-Delzell, L., Spooner, F., Mims, P. J., & Baker, J. N. (2009). Using time delay to teach picture and word recognition to identify evidence-based practice for students with severe developmental disabilities. *Exceptional Children, 75*, 343–364.

Browder, D. M., Hudson, M. E., & Wood, A. L. (2013). Teaching students with moderate intellectual disability who are emergent readers to comprehend passages of text. *Exceptionality, 21*(4), 191–206. https://doi.org/10.1080/09362835.2013.802236

Bruni, T. P., & Hixson, M. D. (2017). Beyond sight words: Reading programs for people with intellectual disabilities. *Behavioral Development Bulletin, 22*(1), 249–257. https://doi.org/10.1037/bdb0000062

Campbell-Whatley, G. D., Dunaway, D. M., & Hancock, D. R. (2016). *A school leader's guide to implementing the common core: Inclusive practices for all students*. London, England: Routledge.

Claro, A., Boulanger, M.-M., & Shaw, S. R. (2015). Targeting vulnerabilities to risky behavior: An intervention for promoting adaptive emotion regulation in adolescents. *Contemporary School Psychology, 19*(4), 330–339. https://doi.org/10.1007/s40688-015-0063-9

Collins, B. C., Evans, A., Creech-Galloway, C., Karl, J., & Miller, A. (2007). Comparison of the acquisition and maintenance of teaching functional and core content sight words in special and general education settings. *Focus on Autism and Other Developmental Disabilities, 22*, 220–233.

Cook, B. G., & Cook, S. C. (2013). Unraveling evidence-based practices in special education. *The Journal of Special Education, 47*(2), 71–82. https://doi.org/10.1177/0022466911420877

Courtade, G. R., Test, D. W., & Cook, B. G. (2014). Evidence-based practices for learners with severe intellectual disability. *Research and Practice for Persons with Severe Disabilities, 39*(4), 305–318. https://doi.org/10.1177/1540796914566711

Coyne, P., Pisha, B., Dalton, B., Zeph, L. A., & Smith, N. C. (2012). Literacy by design a universal design for learning approach for students with significant intellectual disabilities. *Remedial and Special Education, 33*(3), 162–172. https://doi.org/10.1177/0741932510381651

Dahlin, K. I. E. (2011). Effects of working memory training on reading in children with special needs. *Reading and Writing, 24*(4), 479–491. https://doi.org/10.1007/s11145-010-9238-y

Decker, S. L., Hale, J. B., & Flanagan, D. P. (2013). Professional practice issues in the assessment of cognitive functioning for educational applications. *Psychology in the Schools, 50*(3), 300–313. https://doi.org/10.1002/pits.21675

Denton, C. A., & Al Otaiba, S. (2011). Teaching word identification to students with reading difficulties and disabilities. *Focus on Exceptional Children, 2011*, 254345149.

Dessemontet, R. S., Bless, G., & Morin, D. (2012). Effects of inclusion on the academic achievement and adaptive behaviour of children with intellectual disabilities. *Journal of Intellectual Disability Research, 56*(6), 579–587. https://doi.org/10.1111/j.1365-2788.2011.01497.x

Dillenburger, K., Röttgers, H.-R., Dounavi, K., Sparkman, C., Keenan, M., Thyer, B., & Nikopoulos, C. (2014). Multidisciplinary teamwork in autism: Can one size fit all? *The Educational and Developmental Psychologist, 31*(02), 97–112. https://doi.org/10.1017/edp.2014.13

Downing, J. (2010). *Academic instruction for students with moderate and severe intellectual disabilities in inclusive classrooms*. Thousand Oaks, CA: Corwin.

Dweck, C. S. (2006). *Mindset: The new psychology of success*. New York, NY: Random House Publishing Group.

ESSA (2015). Every Student Succeeds Act of 2015, Pub. L. No. 114-95 § 114 Stat. 1177 (2015–2016).

Feng, L., & Sass, T. R. (2013). What makes special-education teachers special? Teacher training and achievement of students with disabilities. *Economics of Education Review, 36*, 122–134. https://doi.org/10.1016/j.econedurev.2013.06.006

Flores, M. M., Hinton, V. M., Strozier, S. D., & Terry, S. L. (2014). Using the concrete-representational-abstract sequence and the strategic instruction model to teach computation to students with autism spectrum disorders and developmental disabilities. *Education and Training in Autism and Developmental Disabilities, 49*(4), 547–554.

Gambrill, E. (2016). Evidence-based practice and policy: Choices ahead. *Research on Social Work Practice, 16*(3):338–357.

Gilson, C. B., Carter, E. W., & Biggs, E. E. (2017). Systematic review of instructional methods to teach employment skills to secondary students with intellectual and developmental disabilities. *Research and Practice for Persons with Severe Disabilities, 42*(2), 89–107. https://doi.org/10.1177/1540796917698831

Grissom, J. A., Loeb, S., & Master, B. (2013). Effective instructional time use for school leaders: Longitudinal evidence from observations of principals. *Educational Researcher, 42*(8), 433–444. https://doi.org/10.3102/0013189X13510020

Grossman, P., Cohen, J., Ronfeldt, M., & Brown, L. (2014). The test matters: The relationship between classroom observation scores and teacher value added on multiple types of assessment. *Educational Researcher, 43*(6), 293–303. https://doi.org/10.3102/0013189X14544542

Guyatt, G., Cairns, J., Churchill, D., Cook, D., Haynes, B., Hirsh, J., … Tugwell, P. (1992). Evidence-based medicine: A new approach to teaching the practice of medicine. *JAMA, 268* (17), 2420–2425.

Hanley, G. P., Iwata, B. A., & McCord, B. E. (2003). Functional analysis of problem behavior: A review. *Journal of Applied Behavior Analysis, 36*(2), 147–185. https://doi.org/10.1901/jaba.2003.36-147

Hassenfeldt, T. A., Lorenzi, J., & Scarpa, A. (2014). A review of parent training in child interventions: Applications to cognitive–behavioral therapy for children with high-functioning autism. *Review Journal of Autism and Developmental Disorders, 2*(1), 79–90. https://doi.org/10.1007/s40489-014-0038-1

Hosp, J. L., Hensley, K., Huddle, S. M., & Ford, J. W. (2014). Using curriculum-based measures with postsecondary students with intellectual and developmental disabilities. *Remedial and Special Education, 35*(4), 247–257. https://doi.org/10.1177/0741932514530572

Hudson, M. E., Browder, D. M., & Wood, L. A. (2013). Review of experimental research on academic learning by students with moderate and severe intellectual disability in general education. *Research and Practice for Persons with Severe Disabilities, 38*(1), 17–29. https://doi.org/10.2511/027494813807046926

Ioannidis, J. P. A. (2016a). Evidence-based medicine has been hijacked: A report to David Sackett. *Journal of Clinical Epidemiology, 73*, 82–86. https://doi.org/10.1016/j.jclinepi.2016.02.012

Ioannidis, J. P. A. (2016b). Why most clinical research is not useful. *PLoS Medicine, 13*(6), e1002049. https://doi.org/10.1371/journal.pmed.1002049

Jameson, J. M., McDonnell, J., Johnson, J. W., Riesen, T., & Polychronis, S. (2007). A comparison of one-to-one embedded instruction in the general education classroom and one-to-one massed practice instruction in the special education classroom. *Education & Treatment of Children, 30*, 23–44.

Kehoe, M. (2015). *The effectiveness of applied behavior analysis*. .Education Masters. Retrieved from http://fisherpub.sjfc.edu/education_ETD_masters/307

Kirk, H. E., Gray, K., Riby, D. M., & Cornish, K. M. (2015). Cognitive training as a resolution for early executive function difficulties in children with intellectual disabilities. *Research in Developmental Disabilities, 38*, 145–160. https://doi.org/10.1016/j.ridd.2014.12.026

Kleinert, H., Towles-Reeves, E., Quenemoen, R., Thurlow, M., Fluegge, L., Weseman, L., & Kerbel, A. (2015). Where students with the most significant cognitive disabilities are taught implications for general curriculum access. *Exceptional Children, 81*(3), 312–328. https://doi.org/10.1177/0014402914563697

Knight, V. F., Spooner, F., Browder, D. M., Smith, B. R., & Wood, C. L. (2013). Using systematic instruction and graphic organizers to teach science concepts to students with autism spectrum disorders and intellectual disability. *Focus on Autism and Other Developmental Disabilities, 28*(2), 115–126. https://doi.org/10.1177/1088357612475301

Lane, K. L., Kalberg, J. R., & Shepcaro, J. C. (2009). An examination of the evidence base for function-based interventions for students with emotional and/or behavioral disorders attending middle and high schools. *Exceptional Children, 75*, 321–340.

Lang, R., & Rispoli, M. (2015). Introduction to the special issue behavioral interventions to enhance academic outcomes. *Behavior Modification, 39*(1), 3–7. https://doi.org/10.1177/0145445515568928

Leaf, J. B., Leaf, R., McEachin, J., Taubman, M., Ala'i-Rosales, S., Ross, R. K., … Weiss, M. J. (2015). Applied behavior analysis is a science and, therefore, progressive. *Journal of Autism and Developmental Disorders, 46*(2), 720–731. https://doi.org/10.1007/s10803-015-2591-6

Lee, A., Browder, D. M., Flowers, C., & Wakeman, S. (2016). Teacher evaluation of resources designed for adapting mathematics for students with significant cognitive disabilities. *Research and Practice for Persons with Severe Disabilities, 41*(2), 132–137. https://doi.org/10.1177/1540796916634099

Lee, W. S. C., & Carlson, S. M. (2015). Knowing when to be "rational": Flexible economic decision making and executive function in preschool children. *Child Development, 86*(5), 1434–1448. https://doi.org/10.1111/cdev.12401

Levant, R. F., & Hasan, N. T. (2008). Evidence-based practice in psychology. *Professional Psychology: Research and Practice, 39*(6), 658–662. https://doi.org/10.1037/0735-7028.39.6.658

Lloyd, B. P., & Kennedy, C. H. (2014). Assessment and treatment of challenging behaviour for individuals with intellectual disability: A research review. *Journal of Applied Research in Intellectual Disabilities, 27*(3), 187–199. https://doi.org/10.1111/jar.12089

Losinski, M., Sanders, S. A., & Wiseman, N. M. (2016). Examining the use of deep touch pressure to improve the educational performance of students with disabilities a meta-analysis. *Research and Practice for Persons with Severe Disabilities, 41*(1), 3–18. https://doi.org/10.1177/1540796915624889

Lundberg, I., & Reichenberg, M. (2013). Developing reading comprehension among students with mild intellectual disabilities: An intervention study. *Scandinavian Journal of Educational Research, 57*(1), 89–100. https://doi.org/10.1080/00313831.2011.623179

McDonnell, J., Mathot-Buckner, C., Thorson, N., & Fister, S. (2001). Supporting the inclusion of students with moderate and severe disabilities in junior high school general education classes: The effects of classwide peer tutoring, multi-element curriculum, and accommodations. *Education & Treatment of Children, 24*, 141–160.

Mechling, L. C., Ayres, K. M., Foster, A. L., & Bryant, K. J. (2015). Evaluation of generalized performance across materials when using video technology by students with autism spectrum disorder and moderate intellectual disability. *Focus on Autism and Other Developmental Disabilities, 30*(4), 208–221. https://doi.org/10.1177/1088357614528795

Medeiros, K., Rojahn, J., Moore, L. L., & van Ingen, D. J. (2014). Functional properties of behaviour problems depending on level of intellectual disability. *Journal of Intellectual Disability Research, 58*(2), 151–161. https://doi.org/10.1111/jir.12025

Mercer, S., Ryan, S., & Williams, M. (2012). *Psychology for language learning: Insights from research, theory and practice*. Basingstoke, England: Palgrave Macmillan.

Mitchell, D. (2014). *What really works in special and inclusive education: Using evidence-based teaching strategies*. London, England: Routledge.

Mohammadzaheri, F., Koegel, L. K., Rezaee, M., & Rafiee, S. M. (2014). A randomized clinical trial comparison between pivotal response treatment (prt) and structured applied behavior analysis (aba) intervention for children with autism. *Journal of Autism and Developmental Disorders, 44*(11), 2769–2777. https://doi.org/10.1007/s10803-014-2137-3

Neil, N., & Jones, E. A. (2014). Studying treatment intensity: Lessons from two preliminary studies. *Journal of Behavioral Education, 24*(1), 51–73. https://doi.org/10.1007/s10864-014-9208-6

O'Neill, R. E., Albin, R. W., Storey, K., Horner, R. H., & Sprague, J. R. (2014). *Functional assessment and program development*. Ontario, Canada: Nelson Education.

Odom, S. L., Brantlinger, E., Gersten, R., Horner, R. H., Thompson, B., & Harris, K. R. (2005). Research in special education: Scientific methods and evidence-based practices. *Exceptional Children, 71*, 137–148.

Pennington, R. C., & Courtade, G. R. (2015). An examination of teacher and student behaviors in classrooms for students with moderate and severe intellectual disability. *Preventing School Failure: Alternative Education for Children and Youth, 59*(1), 40–47. https://doi.org/10.1080/1045988X.2014.919141

Politte, L. C., Howe, Y., Nowinski, L., Palumbo, M., & McDougle, C. J. (2015). Evidence-based treatments for autism spectrum disorder. *Current Treatment Options in Psychiatry, 2*(1), 38–56. https://doi.org/10.1007/s40501-015-0031-z

Poppen, M., Sinclair, J., Hirano, K., Lindstrom, L., & Unruh, D. (2016). Perceptions of mental health concerns for secondary students with disabilities during transition to adulthood. *Education and Treatment of Children, 39*(2), 221–246. https://doi.org/10.1353/etc.2016.0008

Prout, H. T., & Nowak-Drabik, K. M. (2003). Psychotherapy with persons who have mental retardation: An evaluation of effectiveness. *American Journal on Mental Retardation, 108*(2), 82–93. https://doi.org/10.1352/0895-8017(2003)108<0082:PWPWHM>2.0.CO;2

Reschly, D., & Grimes, J. (2002). Best practices in intellectual assessment. In A. Thomas & J. Grimes (Eds.), *Best practices in school psychology* (Vol. 4, pp. 763–773). Washington DC: National Association of School Psychologists.

Root, J., Saunders, A., Spooner, F., & Brosh, C. (2017). Teaching personal finance mathematical problem solving to individuals with moderate intellectual disability. *Career Development and Transition for Exceptional Individuals, 40*(1), 5–14. https://doi.org/10.1177/2165143416681288

Rosenthal, R., & Jacobson, L. (1968). *Pygmalion in the classroom*. New York, NY: Holt, Rinehart & Winston.

Rycroft-Malone, J., Seers, K., Titchen, A., Harvey, G., Kitson, A., & McCormack, B. (2004). What counts as evidence in evidence-based practice? *Journal of Advanced Nursing, 47*(1), 81–90. https://doi.org/10.1111/j.1365-2648.2004.03068.x

Sattler, J. M. (2008). *Assessment of children: Cognitive foundations* (5th ed.). San Diego, CA: Sattler.

Schaafsma, D., Kok, G., Stoffelen, J. M. T., & Curfs, L. M. G. (2015). Identifying effective methods for teaching sex education to individuals with intellectual disabilities: A systematic review. *The Journal of Sex Research, 52*(4), 412–432. https://doi.org/10.1080/00224499.2014.919373

Scott, H. M., & Havercamp, S. M. (2016). Systematic review of health promotion programs focused on behavioral changes for people with intellectual disability. *Intellectual and Developmental Disabilities, 54*(1), 63–76. https://doi.org/10.1352/1934-9556-54.1.63

Sennott, S. C., Light, J. C., & McNaughton, D. (2016). AAC modeling intervention research review. *Research and Practice for Persons with Severe Disabilities, 41*(2), 101–115. https://doi.org/10.1177/1540796916638822

Seong, Y., Wehmeyer, M. L., Palmer, S. B., & Little, T. D. (2015). Effects of the self-directed individualized education program on self-determination and transition of adolescents with disabilities. *Career Development and Transition for Exceptional Individuals, 38*(3), 132–141. https://doi.org/10.1177/2165143414544359

Shaw, S. R. (2008). An educational programming framework for a subset of students with diverse learning needs borderline intellectual functioning. *Intervention in School and Clinic, 43*(5), 291–299. https://doi.org/10.1177/1053451208314735

Sturmey, P., & Didden, R. (2014). *Evidence-based practice and intellectual disabilities*. Hoboken, NJ: Wiley.

Sugai, G., Horner, R. H., Dunlap, G., Hieneman, M., Lewis, T. J., Nelson, C. M., … Ruef, M. (2000). Applying positive behavior support and functional behavioral assessment in schools. *Journal of Positive Behavior Interventions, 2*(3), 131–143. https://doi.org/10.1177/109830070000200302

Szymanski, L., & King, B. H. (1999). Practice parameters for the assessment and treatment of children, adolescents, and adults with mental retardation and comorbid mental disorders. *Journal of the American Academy of Child & Adolescent Psychiatry, 38*(12), 5S–31S. https://doi.org/10.1016/S0890-8567(99)80002-1

Test, D. W., Fowler, C. H., Richter, S. M., White, J., Mazzotti, V., & Walker, A. R. (2009). Evidence-based practices in secondary transition. *Career Development for Exceptional Individuals, 32*, 115–128. https://doi.org/10.1177/0885728809336859

Thorndike, R. L. (1968). Reviewed work: Pygmalion in the classroom by Robert Rosenthal and Lenore Jacobson. *American Educational Research Journal, 5*(4), 708–711.

Vlissides, N., Beail, N., Jackson, T., Williams, K., & Golding, L. (2017). Development and psychometric properties of the Psychological Therapies Outcome Scale – Intellectual Disabilities (PTOS-ID). *Journal of Intellectual Disability Research, 61*(6), 549–559. https://doi.org/10.1111/jir.12361

Will, E., & Hepburn, S. (2015). Applied behavior analysis for children with neurogenetic disorders. In R. M. Hodapp & D. J. Fidler (Eds.), *International review of research in developmental disabilities* (Vol. 49, pp. 229–259). Orlando, FL: Academic Press.

Wilson, S., McKenzie, K., Quayle, E., & Murray, G. (2014). A systematic review of interventions to promote social support and parenting skills in parents with an intellectual disability. *Child: Care, Health and Development, 40*(1), 7–19. https://doi.org/10.1111/cch.12023

Chapter 9
Future Directions to Support People with Intellectual Disabilities

Abstract The concluding chapter discusses future trends in research and application for people with intellectual disabilities. Although predicting what might happen in the dynamic fields of research, education, and social policy development is always hazardous, there are trends in all fields that can lead to improvement in assessment, diagnosis, medical, educational, therapy, service delivery, and policy development. Given the direction of professional trends, there can be reasonable speculation about the direction of the field. This chapter also discusses some of the aspects of prevention and prophylactic treatment to reduce problematic behaviours and increase quality of life for people with intellectual disabilities, their families, and communities. Ultimately, improvement of service delivery for people with intellectual disabilities will depend on the ability of professionals, parents, individuals with intellectual disabilities, policymakers, and other stakeholders to implement the advances in research and the ability of educators and service providers to guide future directions in research.

Case Study

Eva's parents had discussed many aspects of Eva's disability, diagnosis, educational, and medical therapies and participated in genetic counselling that is common when having a child with a severe intellectual disability. Eva's parents were highly educated and provided excellent participation and support for their child's care. However, they wanted to spend time with the psychologist and developmental pediatrician who had made the original diagnosis. Upon meeting these professionals, Eva's parents had two primary questions: (1) What is it that caused this developmental disability? and (2) How can we begin to organize a search for a cure for this developmental disability so that Eva can have a life that is normal?

These are common questions that parents ask professionals. The answers to these questions are not what Eva's parents wanted to hear. The answer to question one is that we rarely know the exact cause of the disability. The answer to question two is

S. R. Shaw, A. M. Jankowska, *Pediatric Intellectual Disabilities at School*, Pediatric School Psychology, https://doi.org/10.1007/978-3-030-02992-0_9

that with few exceptions, there is little hope of a cure for intellectual disabilities. What Eva's parents were looking for is understandable and laudable. Their desire is to do anything that they can to help their child and other children who are experiencing similar issues. At this point, it is important to be humble and understanding when presenting the state of research. Searching for a specific cause and attempting to cure developmental disabilities are several steps beyond the current state of scientific literature.

The discussion with Eva's parents was not easy. Having a child with severe intellectual disabilities was an emotional challenge. The stressors of raising Eva, guilt over the possibility that they may have done something wrong, worry that God has punished them, and having a family life that deviated from their expectations and dreams have been taking a toll on both parents and their relationship. Most of the discussion concerned what Eva's parents can do to make a difference. Eva's parents were discouraged from trying to find the ultimate cause of her developmental disability. In addition, searching for a cure is something that could only reap benefits in a generation or two, if ever. The discussion turned towards two areas where parents can make an enormous difference: advocating for their child to receive the best possible evidence-based practice available and to advocate for policies and allocation of resources by governmental and nongovernmental agencies and foundations to support research into improving the lives of persons with disabilities. Eva's parents have significant resources and influence. By serving as an advocate for their child and for all children with intellectual disabilities, quite likely they will have a significant impact. Eva's parents were also encouraged to prepare Eva to develop self-advocacy skills. Parents and people with intellectual disabilities are frequently driving forces in research and innovative service delivery to people with intellectual disabilities, and research and practice benefit from having parents serve as advocates and voices committed to improving lives.

Future Directions

Describing future trends in the education and clinical service for people with intellectual disabilities is speculative in nature. However, the growth of advances in knowledge, innovation, and service delivery over the last 10 years has been greater than any other time in the study of intellectual disabilities (Richards, Brady, & Taylor, 2014). It is common to think about advances in genetics, diagnostics, and medical treatments (Wallace, 2016). Yet, there have been just as many advances in the areas of classroom instruction, methods of service delivery, coordination of professional teams, and creating effective community policies. Although there are significant challenges in changing the way that society considers people with intellectual disabilities, the future is promising for improving the quality of life for people with intellectual disabilities, their family, and their communities.

The Problems with Prediction

Searching for a Cure

Searching for a cure for intellectual disabilities will always be problematic. There is no single cause or single mechanism responsible for all intellectual disabilities (Altermark, 2014). Intellectual disabilities are heterogeneous set of developmental issues that are caused by hundreds, if not thousands, of different polygenetic, single-gene defects, environmental, prenatal, perinatal, infectious, hormonal, and postnatal factors (Clark et al., 2018). There are likely to even be multiple causes where these factors interact. Any cure will necessarily be piecemeal (Bölte, 2014). That is, there will need to be a cure for each specific causal factor and the interactions among factors. To this point the only effective cures are to treat infectious or medical processes leading to intellectual disabilities, such as meningitis, encephalitis, some metabolic disorders, reduction in childhood illnesses such as whooping cough and measles, renal transplants of failing kidneys, and similar general medical factors (Generoso et al., 2018). Likewise, prevention of intellectual disabilities has been effective in addressing perinatal factors and prenatal and postnatal environmental factors such as improved methods in obstetrics; improved nutrition; reduction of prenatal risk factors such as smoking, alcohol, and drug use; and reductions in environmental toxins such as lead and other heavy metals and air and ground pollution (Gupta, Gupta, & Shirasaka, 2016). Quite likely, addressing these factors has reduced the incidence of intellectual disabilities. Advocacy to continue and improve upon these medical, societal, and environmental policy actions is required to prevent some developmental disabilities. Although this seems intuitive, there are societal pressures to discontinue mandatory vaccines for childhood illnesses, remove government regulations concerning pollution, reduce access to prenatal and postnatal medical care, and reduce government supports for nutritional programs for pregnant mothers and infants (Johnson, Carrillo & Mehta, 2016). Maintaining these societal advances may prove to be a political challenge. Even if these advances are maintained, such factors account for a small percentage of the causes of intellectual disabilities.

Most of the causes of intellectual disabilities are genetic. The most common genetic disorders, Down syndrome and fragile X syndrome, account for about 30% percent of all persons with intellectual disabilities combined (Bailey, Raspa, Bishop, & Holiday, 2009; Potier & Reeves, 2016). Efforts to create a cure for these two major disorders are extraordinarily complex and many years away, if it is at all possible. For Down syndrome there are animal models using pharmaceuticals that can improve the size of the cerebellum and improve functioning of the hippocampus, thus leading to improved memory and learning (Clark, Fernandez, Sakhon, Spanò, & Edgin, 2017). These animal models have yet to be translated into any efforts to apply to human trials. The complexity of working with humans with an extra copy of chromosome 21 and the overexpression of each of the 300–500 genes the chromosome carries is overwhelming (Inglis, Lohn, Austin, & Hippman, 2014).

People committed to a cure for intellectual disabilities often get overly excited about animal trials or computer simulations that demonstrate the ability to repair or replace neural structures with medication, therapies, stimulation, or other mechanisms. People become optimistic about new technologies and buzzwords such as neural plasticity, epigenetics, and stem cells and the use of clustered regularly interspaced short palindromic repeats (CRISPR) technology to create DNA sequencing as a potential treatment (Wojtal et al., 2016).

A reasonable approach to integrating medical and genetic advances with educational and therapeutic service delivery is through the understanding of developmental trends. For example, in the case of Prader-Willi syndrome, it is well documented that most people with the specific genetic disorder will have significant issues with diet and foraging for food (Singh et al., 2017). As soon as the confirmatory genetic testing has established the diagnosis, behavioural, nutritional, and therapeutic interventions can be installed prior to the development of food foraging. This form of prophylactic treatment has potential to integrate science with practice and prevent significant problematic issues from occurring. There are certainly challenges to developing understandings of the development of behavioural phenotypes for specific genetic disorders. However, the high probability of specific functional deficits developing over time make the implementation of prophylactic approach is a potentially important goal of research of people with intellectual disabilities.

Prevention

Environmental Issues

The most significant advances in the prevention of intellectual disabilitics are through improvements in environmental factors, especially prenatal care (Wilkinson, Skene, Crespigny, & Savulescu, 2016). However, there have been significant advances in perinatal and postnatal care that lead to the reduction of the incidence of intellectual disabilities as well.

Prenatal exposure to teratogens is one of the major nongenetic causes of intellectual disabilities. This is especially true of foetal alcohol effects. There have been large-scale public health service announcements that have publicized the importance of avoiding ingestion of alcohol during pregnancy, especially during the first trimester. Foetal alcohol effects often occur because the mother was unaware of her pregnancy during the first trimester and continued to drink significant amounts of alcohol (Gupta et al., 2016). There is no clear level of safe alcohol ingestion, but severity of the foetal alcohol effects is a function of amount of alcohol ingestion and the timing of the alcohol ingestion to the foetal development. Other lifestyle factors expose a developing foetus to teratogens or a generally nonoptimal foetal environment. Exposure to maternal cigarette smoking, illicit drug use, some prescription drug use, and malnutrition are contributing factors to intellectual disabilities (Richards et al., 2014). There was a significant amount of public attention given to maternal use of crack cocaine during pregnancy (dos Santos et al., 2018). The initial reports were that this form of cocaine use would lead to a generation of children with significant brain damage that results in attention deficit hyperactivity disorder, oppositional defiant disorder, and intellectual disabilities. There is no question that cocaine in the bloodstream can pass through the blood-brain barrier and effect foetal development (dos Santos et al., 2018). However, most of the effects on the foetus from crack cocaine and opioid users appear to be due to other health factors (Bushman, Victor, Ryan, & Perron, 2018). Among those factors are that crack cocaine users tend to be polysubstance abusers and often use alcohol, are malnourished, and have poor prenatal care. The interaction among these factors results in impairment in the developing brain and functional loss of cognitive ability. There is often an interaction effect as parents of low general mental ability are more likely to be exposed to teratogens and an unhealthy maternal lifestyle. Therefore, the polygenetic causation of low general mental ability can interact with teratogens to dramatically impair functions (Singer, Min, Lang, & Minnes, 2016). A major focus of prevention of intellectual disabilities is to reduce alcoholism, drug addiction, and improve nutrition for women of childbearing age.

Improvement in Perinatal Care

Improvements in obstetrics have resulted in a reduction of perinatal trauma and functional impairments due to brain injury (Matsuda et al., 2018). The use of forceps and suction devices for supporting delivery of neonates occasionally resulted in brain trauma. In nearly all cases, the use of these devices was uneventful despite many neonates having bruising and skull compression during the process. A small number experience brain trauma and shearing types of injuries that lead to functional impairments. In some cases, those impairments were severe enough to lead to functional intellectual disabilities. The serious decision for obstetricians is that in difficult births, the alternative to using forceps or vacuum forms of extraction was to place a child at risk for anoxia during the birth process. The current trend is that the number of caesarean sections has increased dramatically over the last 25 years (Dan, Hochner-Celnikier, Solnica, & Loewenstein, 2017). Although an extreme intervention for the mothers, avoiding the difficult journey through the birth canal and possibility of anoxia or forceful extraction has resulted in fewer perinatal injuries with fewer long-term consequences.

Public Policy

Public policies to reduce injury and preventable illness have served to reduce incidence of intellectual disabilities (e.g., Trasande, 2017). There is a history of excellent public service campaigns to communicate the dangers of prenatal alcohol ingestion on the developing foetus. Foetal alcohol effects represent the single most common preventable cause of intellectual disabilities (Gupta et al., 2016). Other forms of prevention such as encouraging seatbelt use, warning about shaken babies, facilitating improved maternal nutrition, and other community health efforts to improve the quality of maternal and foetal health are important in reducing intellectual disabilities (dos Santos et al., 2018). Perhaps the most important public policy is the increase of vaccinations to prevent a variety of childhood diseases, many of which can negatively affect intellectual functions. There are many aspects of childhood diseases that can result in high fever, sepsis, and other effects on major organ systems such as kidney, liver, heart, lungs, and brain that can have negative cognitive consequences. Despite lack of evidence, there remains a misperception that vaccines can cause seizures, intellectual disabilities, and autism (Tomlinson et al., 2014). Negative effects from vaccines are extraordinarily rare, less than 1 in one million cases; yet thousands of lives are saved, and the negative cognitive consequences of childhood illnesses are dramatically reduced (Wilkinson et al., 2016). Vaccines serve the purpose of reducing incidents of intellectual disabilities and are an important part of public policy. Reducing pollution and environmental toxins, especially exposure to heavy metals such as lead and cadmium, can also serve as important public policy decisions to reduce incidence of intellectual disabilities (Johnson et al., 2016; Lee et al., 2017).

Societal Factors

Related to environmental issues are societal factors that can lead to conditions that, if addressed, can lead to the reduction of intellectual disabilities. Although social and political changes to address the societal factors are extraordinarily challenging, they are likely to be positive investments that will result in improved functioning and development of the next generation of schoolchildren and adults (Shogren et al., 2017).

Poverty is an important risk factor for intellectual disabilities. In many cases poverty is not causal but a co-occurrence with intellectual disabilities (Graham, 2005). Some cases have people in poverty due to low education and inability to find gainful employment that is caused by the intellectual disability. Other cases involve the extreme financial burden and inability of caregivers to hold high income jobs due to having a child with intellectual disabilities that result in poverty. Poverty also means that there are minimal resources to support the family member with intellectual disabilities and provide effective interventions (Bitler, Hoynes, & Kuka, 2017). Although poverty may be causal only in rare situations, societal efforts to reduce poverty in the overall population may reduce the incidence of intellectual disabilities and allow for more effective interventions.

Poverty is a multisystem risk factor, and one of the most important risk factors is in the domain of healthcare (Crnic, Neece, McIntyre, Blacher, & Baker, 2017). Most nations consider healthcare to be a right provided to all members of the society.

In most countries, healthcare services are not entirely equitably distributed but are reasonably close. Most healthcare in the United States is administered through employers and large numbers of people in poverty or close to poverty who do not have adequate healthcare insurance (Anjum, 2016). Lack of access to healthcare combined with poverty leads to high risk of poor maternal nutrition, untreated drug and alcohol use, likelihood of prematurity and low gestational weight, and a host of other factors that could be used to reduce the incidence of intellectual disabilities (Esmonde & Booker, 2016). Moreover, lack of comprehensive healthcare likely results in delayed identification of developmental problems and delays in application of early intervention services (Graham, 2005).

Conclusions

Despite important scientific advances, the future of service delivery to people with intellectual disabilities and their family will depend largely on public policy decisions and funding. There are many simple ideas that have been known to be effective in preventing and intervening for many years but have been incompletely implemented. In some cases, public policy has retreated from best practices (Bitler et al., 2017). Poverty is increasing, the percentage of persons in the United States with healthcare insurance is decreasing, and there are many people who are resistant to scientific information and refused to have their children vaccinated endangering themselves, their children, and the community (Bryson, 2018). Advances in science are necessary for basic information and require effective scientific communication to the public to address important political and public policy decisions that affect the lives of people with intellectual disabilities and their families.

Training and Professional Preparation

The training and professional preparation of teachers, therapists, physicians, psychologist, and other service providers to persons with intellectual disabilities is always a challenge as the multicomponent aspect of these tasks makes preservice and in-service training complex (Alexander, Ayres, & Smith, 2015). Service providers are expected to implement evidence-based practices, engage in documentation and compliance with state regulations and federal laws, understand the complexity of increasing functionality of the clientele, integrating issues in cultural and linguistic diversity, and supporting the human and civil rights of the clientele. Providing preservice training in these domains is daunting. Extensive in-service professional development is also required for professionals to keep pace with the evolution or, in some cases, the revolution involved in many of these concepts. Each new change in law, regulation, or policy requires that service providers alter practices and develop a new set of skills and accountability measures

(Bartlett, Otis-Wilborn, & Peters, 2017). Although there are many domains and skills that service providers are expected to learn in their preservice training, field experiences, and in-service professional development, there are areas of emphasis required to build a culture that will narrow the research-to-practice gap in the service of people with intellectual disabilities.

If the gap between research and the implementation of research in classrooms and therapy centres is to be narrowed, then the culture of evidence-based practice is something that needs to be a focus of preservice training. There are still significant pockets of resistance to using the products of science in educational settings (Goodley, 2016). Despite the United States having federal laws requiring that specialized interventions have a scientific basis, evidence-based practice is still not the norm (Gambrill, 2006). When teachers are looking for interventions, it is far more likely that they will be looking to Pinterest or other forms of social media than peer-reviewed scientific research (Richmond & Floden, 2018). This is a cultural issue requiring renewed focus in preservice and in-service settings. Of course, some of the onus is to be placed on researchers to develop a mechanism by which research is transparent, credible, useful, and accessible to service providers.

In addition to understanding advances in research and scholarship, the training of educators and other service providers benefits from supporting understanding of disability studies, human rights, advocacy, and other important systemic supports. Sometimes these sociological and cultural domains are considered to be out of the realm or even in opposition to scientific research (Fuchs, Fahsl, & James, 2014). Educational and therapeutic services for people with intellectual disabilities are not simply individually administered interventions that have research-based support; they fit into a system that involves culture, human rights, self-determination, and legal and regulatory compliance. The implementation of evidence-based practices requires the integration of sociological and cultural variables with science-based activities. Preparation of the next generation of teachers and therapists will require integration of these domains for the best possible comprehensive services to all people with intellectual disabilities.

Often the biggest impediment to advances in professions is the reluctance of training programs and professors to evolve by incorporating advances in science and new ways of thinking (Freeman, Simonsen, Briere, & MacSuga-Gage, 2014). Modifying university training programs and the nature of practicum and internship settings is challenging and has significant bureaucratic hurdles. Flexibility and innovation in training is a key variable to ensure that the next generation of teachers and therapists engage in practices that evolve with advances in research and scholarship.

One of the goals of the present volume is to communicate advances in scientific research, which include more than biological, genetics, or medical sciences (Bertelli, Salerno, Rondini, & Salvador-Carulla, 2017). Advances in scientific research also include better understanding of instructional techniques, mental health service delivery, family involvement, and team processes and decision-making. The tools of science have many applications and potential to improve all aspects of service delivery to people with intellectual disabilities. Specialized scientific efforts to improve preservice and in-service training can also result in directly in improved functioning of four people with intellectual disabilities.

Implementation Science

Most of this book reviews advances in research that have appeared in refereed scholarly journals, books, professional conferences, and government reports these advances represent important contributions to the field. However, the often-forgotten challenge is to implement these new ideas by altering treatments, teaching techniques, policy, and service delivery. Translation research, knowledge translation, narrowing the research-to-practice gap, and implementation science have all been developed to address these important issues. Estimates are that for special education, published research literature takes over 14 years before it has a significant national influence on teaching practices (Pearson, 2018). Usually, influences interact as research has a larger effect on laws, regulations, and policies, which in turn influence teaching practices. Converting research into practice has become its own field of study. Implementation science has its own journals and professional societies. There are multiple models and approaches to converting innovations in research into specific practical techniques (Birken et al., 2017). Narrowing the research-to-practice gap is not something that should be taken for granted but requires systematic consideration.

Partnerships

One mechanism by which the gap between research and practice can be narrowed is through university and school partnerships. These are not unusual as a significant amount of research with children with developmental disabilities takes place in school settings. The challenge of conducting school-based research is that there may be advantages in external validity or the relevance of a finding to schools, but it is extremely difficult to maintain internal validity or control of potentially confounding variables. Action research has been a mechanism to evaluate the effectiveness of classroom-based interventions. However, there are limitations and the ability of action research to generalize to other classrooms. Working closely with schools to address their specific needs is an important method for improving the relevance of research. Scientific research is a systematic method of thinking and does not simply involve research that appears in scholarly journals (Feldman, Bosett, Collet, & Burnham-Riosa, 2014). Expanding the definition of research to include practical and functional classroom and therapeutic activities is one method to reduce the research-to-practice gap.

Open Science

Open science is an advancing movement to make scientific research, data and dissemination accessible to all levels of an inquiring society, clinician, policymaker, amateur, or professional (Open Science Collaboration, 2012). Making science accessible and transparent improves the quality of science and the value of science to clinicians and those who wish to use research to guide services for people with intellectual disabilities. Science that is relevant to the needs of professionals and stakeholders has strong research design characteristics, transparent data and analysis, and replicable, also needs to be accessible (van der Zee & Reich, 2018). Problems with the replicability of research in education and psychology have led to strong criticism of scientific psychology and education (Baker, 2016). Addressing these criticisms will not only improve the quality of scientific research but make evidence more compelling and useful in a system of evidence-based practices. In turn, these improvements will increase the quality of interventions to people with intellectual disabilities. Moreover, it is helpful for research data to be completely open, available, and transparent.

Open science is also a response to critiques over questionable research practices that are widely used in medical, psychological, and educational services. Questionable research practices reduce the credibility, utility, and implementation of research (Ioannidis, 2018). Questionable research practices are found in many fields of research such as medical and psychological research (John, Loewenstein, & Prelec, 2012). There are specific questionable research practices affecting the quality of research that serves as the foundation of service delivery to people with intellectual disabilities (D'Intino, Lysenko, & Shaw, 2018; Ioannidis, 2018):

- Publication bias, which is that papers are far more likely to be accepted if they are statistically significant regardless of the quality of the research design and methodology.
- Failure to replicate and reproduce initial findings, which is an essential practice in science.
- HARKing, which means hypothesizing after results are known, which subverts the predictive aspect of the scientific process.
- Low statistical power, which usually stems from small sample sizes. This is a major issue for all work concerning people with developmental disabilities, especially low incidence disabilities.
- Wait-list control groups exaggerate the likelihood of a statistically significant event.
- P-hacking, which is collecting large amounts of data and simply selecting relationships that are statistically significant for further interpretation. This practice usually capitalizes on error and leads to science that is not robust and cannot be implemented.
- Random assignment to condition is often lacking, sometimes because random assignment to treatments may be unethical.

- Blind instructors and assessors, knowing which students receive which forms of intervention, often introduces bias into results.
- Transparency of methodology and analysis is often lacking. If it is not clear exactly what procedures were followed in the study, the implementation or replication is not possible.
- Accessibility of findings for educators is an issue with journals that require subscription and has a paywall. Unless there is an institutional subscription to journals, access to research can be extremely expensive or impossible.
- Conflicts of authors' interests without acknowledgement.

At least one of these questionable research practices has been found in over 98% of research articles in school psychology (D'Intino, Lysenko, & Shaw, 2018). These criticisms of traditional science do not necessarily mean that research is not strong or provide a strong evidence base for practices (Banks, Rogelberg, Woznyj, Landis, & Rupp, 2016). However, there are opportunities to improve. There are three specific suggestions. The first recommendation is increase in the use of Registered Reports, which are a form of empirical journal article in which methods and proposed analyses are preregistered and peer reviewed prior to research being conducted (Chambers, 2017). High-quality protocols are then provisionally accepted for publication before data collection commences. This has the advantage of reducing publication bias, p-hacking, and HARKing and supports publication of the highest quality research methodology (Chambers, 2017). The second recommendation is that journals and researchers would benefit from valuing exact and conceptual replications of research on persons with intellectual disabilities. There needs to be an incentive for replications and reproduction of research, or this basic scientific process will not happen. Third, open science concepts such as increased transparency of procedures and enough detail in the intervention that interventions can be applied in a classroom are necessary for evidence-based interventions to be a relevant concept (Van der Zee & Reich, 2018). All educators must have access to the published literature without a pay wall.

Model for Improvement of the Process

There are opportunities to improve the process of implementing research into classroom and therapeutic settings. One such approach is an analogy to open-source software and a novel framework for implementation of innovation in the classroom (Shaw, Boulanger, & Gomes, 2015). Open-source software is noted for characteristics of free distribution, sharing of the source code, encouraging innovation and changes, and consistently updating operating systems and end-user software. It is often developed in a public, crowd-sourced, and collaborative manner; the source code is made available and allows users the rights to study, change, and distribute the software to anyone and for any purpose. Unlike commercial software that are protected through copyright, patent, trademark, or other proprietary protections, the source code of open-source software can be altered to meet the unique needs of a consumer. Thus, innovation becomes more likely, and the quality of open-source software is hypothesized to be better than commercial software due to the collective wisdom of large groups.

Educational interventions, under the legal and professional pressures to be evidence-based, share many issues with commercial software. Evidence-based interventions must be carefully researched and standardized in terms of target population, domain of intervention, procedures used, and evaluation measures (Alexander et al., 2015). The logic of the proposed open-source analogy model (OSAM), as an enhancement to traditional evidence-based interventions, is that users can adapt the practice to the unique needs of clients, students, resources, training, and systemic needs. From this the model predicts that the majority of altered psychological and educational interventions will result in more effective outcomes than the prototype. However, like open-source software, open-source intervention practices have a structural kernel that cannot be changed. For software, the kernel is known as the structural operating system. For psychological interventions, the kernel is the theory-driven core of the intervention that cannot be changed or the intervention loses all meaning, coherence, and goals.

The open-source analogy model (OSAM) has the following characteristics:

- Materials for all psychological and educational intervention shall be available for free.
- All psychological and educational interventions shall be strongly grounded in theory.
- All psychological and educational interventions have a kernel, or set of procedures linked to theory that cannot be altered by the user.
- A prototype set of implementation strategies shall be described, just as in evidence-based practices.
- Users are free to alter implementation strategies to best meet the needs of the clientele, resources, and systems.

The value of OSAM is to take advantage of the skills and resources currently possessed by those doing the implementation rather than requiring a specific skill set to implement a program with strict treatment integrity. The rationale is that altered interventions are more likely to meet the needs of the immediate environment given the expertise of those implementing the intervention in meeting those needs. Any deviation from the prototypical implementation strategy is to be described in detail (Shaw et al., 2015). In this fashion, the open-source analogy model creates dynamic interventions that are growing, expanding, and improving based on the expertise of the users. In addition, because those conducting the implementation have ownership over the direction and specific resources, they have the benefit of working around obstacles and are invested in seeing the intervention succeed. By tapping into the systemic knowledge, OSAM is far more likely to be implemented and sustained, and the commitment to innovation increases over time.

Outcome data thus far show that OSAM results in improved student outcomes in a variety of academic and mental health measures when compared to the traditional treatment integrity model (Harrison, Falvo, Weiss, & Holland, 2017). Specific programs can easily be implemented at different grade levels, multiple cultural and ethnic backgrounds of students, different schools, and an alternative setting such as hospitals and mental health centres with no need for change in the kernel. Moreover, teachers and those implementing innovation report being more satisfied to have greater ownership and to experience increased feelings of professionalism and being respected when compared to the traditional treatment integrity model.

There multiple models of implementation that are currently being developed to implement and apply research to classroom and therapeutic settings. Rather than serving as a secondary aspect of research, the scientific study of implementation will be a primary contribution to research as a relevant and important contribution to improving the lives of people with intellectual disabilities.

Conclusions

Researchers have made advances in the basic knowledge of the causes and treatment of intellectual disabilities. In addition, there have been significant scholarly advances in-service delivery, education, and management. These advances have potential to improve the functioning and quality of life for people with intellectual disabilities and their families. However, whether the potential is realized will depend on equal advances in educational, social, and medical policies towards preventative activities and service delivery, whether training becomes evidence based and mirrors the advances in research, and whether there is a systematic effort to advance implementation that mirrors advances in research.

Research will continue to advance. However, to improve the functioning and lives of people with intellectual disabilities, research needs to be supported through appropriate levels of funding, effective collaboration, and integration of research among a variety of professions, and involvement of stakeholders and communities. Improving the lives of persons with intellectual disabilities is a communal effort. For the research to continue to advance and to be applied, educational and community systems must be strong to support the complex needs of people with intellectual disabilities.

References

Alexander, J. L., Ayres, K. M., & Smith, K. A. (2015). Training teachers in evidence-based practice for individuals with autism spectrum disorder: A review of the literature. *Teacher Education and Special Education, 38*(1), 13–27. https://doi.org/10.1177/0888406414544551

Altermark, N. (2014). The ideology of neuroscience and intellectual disability: Reconstituting the 'disordered' brain. *Disability & Society, 29*(9), 1460–1472. https://doi.org/10.1080/09687599.2014.953244

Anjum, R. (2016). Evidence-based or person-centered? An ontological debate. *European Journal for Person Centered Healthcare, 4*(2), 421–429. https://doi.org/10.5750/ejpch.v4i2.1152

Bailey, D. B., Raspa, M., Bishop, E., & Holiday, D. (2009). No change in the age of diagnosis for fragile x syndrome: Findings from a national parent survey. *Pediatrics, 124*(2), 527–533. https://doi.org/10.1542/peds.2008-2992

Baker, M. (2016). 1,500 scientists lift the lid on reproducibility. *Nature, 533*(7604), 452–454. https://doi.org/10.1038/533452a

Banks, G. C., Rogelberg, S. G., Woznyj, H. M., Landis, R. S., & Rupp, D. E. (2016). Editorial: Evidence on questionable research practices: The good, the bad, and the ugly. *Journal of Business and Psychology, 31*(3), 323–338. https://doi.org/10.1007/s10869-016-9456-7

Bartlett, M., Otis-Wilborn, A., & Peters, L. (2017). Bending or breaking: Appropriating edTPA policy in special education teacher education. *Teacher Education and Special Education, 40*(4), 287–298. https://doi.org/10.1177/0888406417720188

Bertelli, M. O., Salerno, L., Rondini, E., & Salvador-Carulla, L. (2017). Integrated care for people with intellectual disability. In V. Amelung, V. Stein, N. Goodwin, R. Balicer, E. Nolte, & E. Suter (Eds.), *Handbook integrated care* (pp. 449–468). Cham, Switzerland: Springer. https://doi.org/10.1007/978-3-319-56103-5_28

Birken, S. A., Powell, B. J., Shea, C. M., Haines, E. R., Alexis Kirk, M., Leeman, J., … Presseau, J. (2017). Criteria for selecting implementation science theories and frameworks: Results from an international survey. *Implementation Science, 12*, 124. https://doi.org/10.1186/s13012-017-0656-y

Bitler, M., Hoynes, H., & Kuka, E. (2017). Child poverty, the great recession, and the social safety net in the United States. *Journal of Policy Analysis and Management, 36*(2), 358–389. https://doi.org/10.1002/pam.21963

Bölte, S. (2014). Is autism curable? *Developmental Medicine & Child Neurology, 56*(10), 927–931. https://doi.org/10.1111/dmcn.12495

Bryson, J. M. (2018). *Strategic planning for public and non-profit organizations: A guide to strengthening and sustaining organizational achievement*. Hoboken, NJ: Wiley.

Bushman, G., Victor, B. G., Ryan, J. P., & Perron, B. E. (2018). In utero exposure to opioids: An observational study of mothers involved in the child welfare system. *Substance Use & Misuse, 53*(5), 844–851. https://doi.org/10.1080/10826084.2017.1388406

Chambers, C. (2017). *The seven deadly sins of psychology: A manifesto for reforming the culture of scientific practice*. Princeton, NJ: Princeton University Press.

Clark, C. A. C., Fernandez, F., Sakhon, S., Spanò, G., & Edgin, J. O. (2017). The medial temporal memory system in Down syndrome: Translating animal models of hippocampal compromise. *Hippocampus, 27*(6), 683–691. https://doi.org/10.1002/hipo.22724

Clark, M. M., Stark, Z., Farnaes, L., Tan, T. Y., White, S. M., Dimmock, D., & Kingsmore, S. F. (2018). Meta-analysis of the diagnostic and clinical utility of genome and exome sequencing and chromosomal microarray in children with suspected genetic diseases. *Npj Genomic Medicine, 3*(1), 16. https://doi.org/10.1038/s41525-018-0053-8

Crnic, K. A., Neece, C. L., McIntyre, L. L., Blacher, J., & Baker, B. L. (2017). Intellectual disability and developmental risk: Promoting intervention to improve child and family well-being. *Child Development, 88*(2), 436–445. https://doi.org/10.1111/cdev.12740

D'Intino, J., Lysenko, E., & Shaw, S. R. (2018). Questionable research practices and evidence-based interventions in school psychology. *NASP Communique, 47*(4), 1–3.

Dan, O., Hochner-Celnikier, D., Solnica, A., & Loewenstein, Y. (2017). Association of catastrophic neonatal outcomes with increased rate of subsequent Cesarean deliveries. *Obstetrics & Gynecology, 129*(4), 671. https://doi.org/10.1097/AOG.0000000000001925

dos Santos, J. F., de Melo Bastos Cavalcante, C., Barbosa, F. T., Gitaí, D. L. G., Duzzioni, M., Tilelli, C. Q., … de Castro, O. W. (2018). Maternal, fetal and neonatal consequences associated with the use of crack cocaine during the gestational period: A systematic review and meta-analysis. *Archives of Gynecology and Obstetrics, 298*(3), 487–503. https://doi.org/10.1007/s00404-018-4833-2

Esmonde, I., & Booker, A. N. (2016). *Power and privilege in the learning sciences: Critical and sociocultural theories of learning*. New York, NY: Taylor & Francis.

Feldman, M. A., Bosett, J., Collet, C., & Burnham-Riosa, P. (2014). Where are persons with intellectual disabilities in medical research? A survey of published clinical trials. *Journal of Intellectual Disability Research, 58*(9), 800–809. https://doi.org/10.1111/jir.12091

Freeman, J., Simonsen, B., Briere, D. E., & MacSuga-Gage, A. S. (2014). Pre-service teacher training in classroom management: A review of state accreditation policy and teacher preparation programs. *Teacher Education and Special Education, 37*(2), 106–120. https://doi.org/10.1177/0888406413507002

Fuchs, W. W., Fahsl, A. J., & James, S. M. (2014). Redesigning a special education teacher-preparation program: The rationale, process, and outcomes. *The New Educator, 10*(2), 145–152. https://doi.org/10.1080/1547688X.2014.898493

Gambrill, E. (2006). Evidence-based practice and policy: Choices ahead. *Research on Social Work Practice, 16*(3), 338–357. https://doi.org/10.1177/1049731505284205

Generoso, J. S., Collodel, A., Simões, L. R., Dagostin, C., Dominguini, D., Lodetti, B. F., … Barichello, T. (2018). RAGE inhibitor prevents cognitive dysfunction and reduces inflammatory mediators in experimental pneumococcal meningitis. *The Journal of Immunology, 200*(Suppl. 1), 50.2.

Goodley, D. (2016). *Disability studies: An interdisciplinary introduction*. London, England: SAGE.

Graham, H. (2005). Intellectual disabilities and socioeconomic inequalities in health: An overview of research. *Journal of Applied Research in Intellectual Disabilities, 18*(2), 101–111. https://doi.org/10.1111/j.1468-3148.2005.00239.x

Gupta, K. K., Gupta, V. K., & Shirasaka, T. (2016). An update on fetal alcohol syndrome—Pathogenesis, risks, and treatment. *Alcoholism: Clinical and Experimental Research, 40*(8), 1594–1602. https://doi.org/10.1111/acer.13135

Harrison, C., Falvo, D., Weiss, V., & Holland, B. E. (2017). *Medical and psychosocial aspects of chronic illness and disability*. Burlington, MA: Jones & Bartlett Learning.

Inglis, A., Lohn, Z., Austin, J. C., & Hippman, C. (2014). A 'cure' for down syndrome: What do parents want? *Clinical Genetics, 86*(4), 310–317. https://doi.org/10.1111/cge.12364

Ioannidis, J. P. A. (2018). Meta-research: Why research on research matters. *PLoS Biology, 16*(3), e2005468. https://doi.org/10.1371/journal.pbio.2005468

John, L. K., Loewenstein, G., & Prelec, D. (2012). Measuring the prevalence of questionable research practices with incentives for truth telling measuring the prevalence of questionable research practices with incentives for truth telling. *Psychological Science, 23*(5), 524–532. https://doi.org/10.1177/0956797611430953

Johnson, N. M., Carrillo, G., & Mehta, R. K. (2016). Academic and psychosocial impact of air pollution on children. In C. A. Riccio & J. R. Sullivan (Eds.), *Pediatric neurotoxicology. Specialty topics in pediatric neuropsychology* (pp. 167–180). Cham, Switzerland: Springer.

Lee, H., Park, H., Ha, E., Hong, Y.-C., Ha, M., Park, H., … Kim, Y. (2017). Stability of cognitive development during the first five years of life in relation to heavy metal concentrations in umbilical cord blood: Mothers' and Children's Environmental Health (MOCEH) birth cohort study. *Science of the Total Environment, 609*, 153–159. https://doi.org/10.1016/j.scitotenv.2017.07.074

Matsuda, N., Taki, A., Tsuji, A., Nakajima, K., Takasawa, K., Morioka, C., … Morio, T. (2018). Perinatal factors affecting growth and development at age 3 years in extremely low birth weight infants born small for gestational age. *Clinical Pediatric Endocrinology, 27*(1), 31–38. https://doi.org/10.1297/cpe.27.31

Open Science Collaboration. (2012). An open, large-scale, collaborative effort to estimate the reproducibility of psychological science. *Perspectives on Psychological Science, 7*(6), 657–660. https://doi.org/10.1177/1745691612462588

Pearson, D. (2018). The importance of organisational factors in transferring the principles of effective intervention to offender rehabilitation in the real world. In G. Akerman, A. Needs, & C. Bainbridge (Eds.), *Transforming environments and rehabilitation: A guide for practitioners in forensic settings and criminal justice* (pp. 348–370). New York, NY: Taylor & Francis.

Retrieved from https://researchportal.port.ac.uk/portal/en/publications/the-importance-of-organisational-factors-in-transferring-the-principles-of-effective-intervention-to-offender-rehabilitation-in-the-real-world(d4859cc9-3dc0-48df-91c9-b75bacf71ef8).html

Potier, M.-C., & Reeves, R. H. (2016). Editorial: Intellectual disabilities in Down Syndrome from birth and throughout life: Assessment and treatment. *Frontiers in Behavioral Neuroscience, 10*, 120. https://doi.org/10.3389/fnbeh.2016.00120

Richards, S. B., Brady, M. P., & Taylor, R. L. (2014). *Cognitive and intellectual disabilities: Historical perspectives, current practices, and future directions*. New York, NY: Routledge.

Richmond, G., & Floden, R. E. (2018). Leveraging research for teacher education policy, design, and practice. *Journal of Teacher Education, 69*(1), 4–6. https://doi.org/10.1177/0022487117742131

Shaw, S. R., Boulanger, M. M., & Gomes, P. (2015). Enhancing treatment integrity: A proposed model for improving implementation and supporting teachers. *Communiqué, 44*, 1–18.

Shogren, K. A., Shaw, L. A., Wehmeyer, M. L., Thompson, J. R., Lang, K. M., Tassé, M. J., & Schalock, R. L. (2017). The support needs of children with intellectual disability and autism: Implications for supports planning and subgroup classification. *Journal of Autism and Developmental Disorders, 47*(3), 865–877. https://doi.org/10.1007/s10803-016-2995-y

Singer, L. T., Min, M. O., Lang, A., & Minnes, S. (2016). In utero exposure to nicotine, cocaine, and amphetamines. In C. A. Riccio & J. R. Sullivan (Eds.), *Pediatric neurotoxicology. Specialty topics in pediatric neuropsychology* (pp. 51–76). Cham, Switzerland: Springer.

Singh, N. N., Lancioni, G. E., Myers, R. E., Karazsia, B. T., Courtney, T. M., & Nugent, K. (2017). A mindfulness-based intervention for self-management of verbal and physical aggression by adolescents with Prader–Willi syndrome. *Developmental Neurorehabilitation, 20*(5), 253–260. https://doi.org/10.3109/17518423.2016.1141436

Tomlinson, M., Yasamy, M. T., Emerson, E., Officer, A., Richler, D., & Saxena, S. (2014). Setting global research priorities for developmental disabilities, including intellectual disabilities and autism. *Journal of Intellectual Disability Research, 58*, 1121–1130. https://doi.org/10.1111/jir.12106

Trasande, L. (2017). When enough data are not enough to enact policy: The failure to ban chlorpyrifos. *PLoS Biology, 15*(12), e2003671. https://doi.org/10.1371/journal.pbio.2003671

Van der Zee, T., & Reich, J. (2018). Open education science. *AERA Open, 4*, 1–15. https://doi.org/10.1177/2332858418787466

Wallace, R. A. (2016). Genetic testing of aetiology of intellectual disability in a dedicated physical healthcare outpatient clinic for adults with intellectual disability. *Internal Medicine Journal, 46*(2), 177–185. https://doi.org/10.1111/imj.12946

Wilkinson, D., Skene, L., Crespigny, L. D., & Savulescu, J. (2016). Protecting future children from in-utero harm. *Bioethics, 30*(6), 425–432. https://doi.org/10.1111/bioe.12238

Wojtal, D., Kemaladewi, D. U., Malam, Z., Abdullah, S., Wong, T. W. Y., Hyatt, E., … Cohn, R. D. (2016). Spell checking nature: Versatility of CRISPR/Cas9 for developing treatments for inherited disorders. *The American Journal of Human Genetics, 98*(1), 90–101. https://doi.org/10.1016/j.ajhg.2015.11.012

Index

S. R. Shaw, A. M. Jankowska, *Pediatric Intellectual Disabilities at School*, Pediatric School Psychology, https://doi.org/10.1007/978-3-030-02992-0

The manufacturer's authorised representative in the EU is Springer Nature Customer Service Centre GmbH, Europaplatz 3, 69115 Heidelberg, Germany. If you have any concerns regarding our products, please contact ProductSafety@springernature.com

Printed and bound by CPI Group (UK) Ltd, Croydon, CR0 4YY
30/09/2026
02225444-0011